# Neurotrauma

## Managing Patients with Head Injuries

# Neurotrauma
# Managing Patients with Head Injuries

Edited by

**Nadine Abelson-Mitchell**

Associate Professor (Senior Lecturer)
PhD, BSc (Nursing), RN, RM, Dip Nursing Education, RT, Dip Nursing Administration,
DNA, Dip ICU, ENB148, FHEA
*School of Nursing and Midwifery*
*Faculty of Health, Education and Society*
*Plymouth University*
*Plymouth, UK*

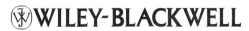

WILEY-BLACKWELL

A John Wiley & Sons, Ltd., Publication

*Library of Congress Cataloging-in-Publication Data*

Neurotrauma : managing patients with head injuries / edited by Nadine Abelson-Mitchell.
       p. ; cm.
   Includes bibliographical references and index.
   ISBN 978-1-4051-8564-6 (pbk. : alk. paper)
   I. Abelson-Mitchell, Nadine.
   [DNLM:  1. Craniocerebral Trauma–therapy.  2. Craniocerebral Trauma–rehabilitation.  3. Evidence-Based Medicine.  WL 354]
   617.5'1044–dc23
                                                                    2012027830

A catalogue record for this book is available from the British Library.

Wiley also publishes its books in a variety of electronic formats. Some content that appears in print may not be available in electronic books.

Cover images courtesy of iStockphoto
Cover design by Steve Thompson

Set in 9.5/12 pt Times by Toppan Best-set Premedia Limited, Hong Kong
Printed in Singapore by Ho Printing Singapore Pte Ltd

1   2013

# Contents

Contents                                                                    ix

*Colour plate section can be found between pages 106 and 107*

# Preface

This book is designed to provide a holistic, evidence-based approach to the primary, secondary and tertiary care of a person with neurotrauma in all settings.

It uses a patient-centred needs approach to enhance the quality of care of head injured patients, their family and carers.

The book content enables the reader to apply the knowledge, skills and attitudes learned to the practice of neurotrauma in all settings.

In addition, as many of the neurosurgical procedures that are undertaken result in trauma to the brain, this neurotrauma book can also be used in wider neuroscience practice by health professionals, families, carers and all personnel committed to the care of a patient with neurotrauma.

Nadine Abelson-Mitchell

# Dedication

This book is dedicated to my inspirational father Harry Abelson (z"l), who taught me to cope with adversity, my wonderful mother, Hilda Abelson, husband, John Mitchell whose help is immeasurable, sister Marissa Rittoff and my aunt Miriam Brener (z"l), a fine nurse.

It is also dedicated to my patients and their families who have strived to achieve their maximum potential.

People who have suffered a head injury *'must have accessible, available, and appropriate health care and wellness promotion services'* to enable the person to lead a *'full life in the community'* (Office of the Surgeon General [US] and Office on Disability [US] 2005: v).

# Acknowledgements

I wish to acknowledge the following for their contribution to the book:

The authors and co-authors who have contributed to the knowledge within the book.

My husband, John Mitchell, for his unstinting support and hours of proof reading.

A special thank you to Claire Butcher for editing the manuscript, Esther Hughes and Hannah Paddon for their continued support and to Fiona Carmichael for the drawings.

The companies who provided me with images for the book:

- SECA Ltd for the ECG images
- Codman Ltd for the ICP monitoring images
- Toshiba Medical Systems for the images of the MRI Scanner and CT Scanner.

The Publishers for agreeing to publish the book.

My patients with whom I have shared many hours of practice.

# Contributor Details

**NADINE ABELSON-MITCHELL**

Nadine is an Associate Professor in the School of Nursing and Midwifery, Faculty of Health, Education and Society at Plymouth University, Devon, UK. She is also an Honorary Nurse Consultant for the Plym Neurorehabilitation Unit, Plymouth Community Healthcare CIC, Plymouth, UK.

Nadine has been actively involved in neurotrauma practice since 1976. In 1987, Nadine completed a PhD entitled the 'Comprehensive care of adults with moderate and severe head injuries'.

Nadine lived in South Africa before moving to the United Kingdom where she was responsible for developing post-registration neurotrauma programmes for Registered Nurses. Her expertise in neurotrauma management has enabled her to be an expert witness and prepare medico-legal reports with regard to medical negligence and road traffic accidents. She opened a very successful nurse-led community-based practice managing neurotrauma patients in the community.

She has written book chapters, has published numerous articles and undertaken national and international conference presentations and workshops. She is a Trustee of Headway, Plymouth, UK.

Having written this book she is preparing a workbook on her experience of community-based rehabilitation for use by all.

**JUDE FEWINGS**

Jude Fewings qualified in 1992 from Caledonia University (formally Queen's College) Glasgow. Following a three year general rotation in Newcastle-upon-Tyne, she moved to a post on the Neuroscience rotation in Sheffield in 1995, working almost exclusively within Neurosurgery and the Neurosurgical ICU. Subsequent promotion culminated in being appointed Team Leader in Neurosciences in 1999.

In this Clinical Specialist role, Jude led the integrated teams of physiotherapists and occupational therapists in the assessment and treatment of all neurological patients and worked closely with Hallam University regularly lecturing on the under- and postgraduate therapy courses, herself gaining a Postgraduate Certificate in Neurological Physiotherapy.

In 2005 Jude was appointed to the post of Consultant Therapist in Neurosurgery at Plymouth. As an experienced clinician she was able to comment on, and therefore influence, the relevant strategic direction of the Trust and its policies whilst remaining involved in the clinical aspects of physiotherapy.

**PENNY FRANKLIN**

Penny Franklin is an independent and supplementary nurse prescriber as well as a community practitioner nurse prescriber and a Fellow of the Institute of Teaching and Learning in Higher Education. She is also an Associate Professor in Health Studies, Medicines Management and Prescribing at Plymouth University.

She is a member of the BMA and British National Formulary Subcommittee for the Community Practitioners Formulary for Prescribing; secretary of the Association for Nurse Prescribing; expert advisor to the National Prescribing Centre (NPC) and NICE for the Updating of Information for Designated Medical Practitioners; practice advisor to the CPHVA for non-medical prescribing/medicines management; academic link for Non-Medical Prescribing for Non-Medical Prescribing Leads in the Southwest Peninsula; external examiner for Prescribing at the University of Reading; education committee member for Community Practitioners and Health Visitors Association and clinical practice as public health nurse.

Penny has co-authored *The Oxford Handbook of Non-medical Prescribing for Nurses and Allied Health Professionals* with S. Beckwith (2011).

## ANTHONY GILBERT

Tony Gilbert is Deputy Head of the School of Social Science and Social Work at Plymouth University, UK. Prior to taking an appointment in higher education, Tony worked for approximately 17 years in health and social care mainly with people with intellectual disability. His research interests are in applied social sciences and social policy where he has been involved in a number of studies in areas such as mental health, safeguarding and the sustainability of community-based organisations.

## HENRY GULY

Henry Guly was a Consultant in emergency medicine at Derriford Hospital, Plymouth, retiring in 2011. He qualified in 1974 and, after initially training in general practice, he started in emergency medicine in 1980 and was appointed a Consultant in Wolverhampton in 1983 and moved to Plymouth in 1986. Before he retired he was a civilian consultant in emergency medicine and civilian advisor in resuscitation to the Royal Navy.

## KATY LEWIS

Katy Lewis was born in Cornwall, where she completed school and sixth form before gaining a BSc in English and Psychology 1997–2000 at Cardiff University, followed by an MSc in Language Pathology at the University of Reading 2001–2003.

Her first post (2003) was as a Research Speech & Language Therapist (SLT) on a research project for the Peninsula Medical School into the intensity of SLT in post-stroke aphasia.

Her second post (2004) comprised a split between the acute hospital setting and a post-acute neurorehab unit, working with clients post ABI, and some MS, GBS and others.

She was then based solely at the Plym Neurorehab Unit in Plymouth where, barring a brief spell working on a Stroke Unit, she has been ever since.

## SUE MOTTRAM

Sue Mottram is Chief Executive of Headway Dorset, a charity for the support and rehabilitation of people with acquired brain injury living in the county of Dorset. At the time of her son's accident, she was managing a mental health rehabilitation unit in Bournemouth. She is a state registered mental nurse, has a 2.1 honours degree in psychology and a postgraduate degree in personnel management.

## ZUHAIR NOORI

Zuhair Noori is a Consultant in Neurorehabilitation in Croydon's Healthcare Trust for in-patient and community neurorehabilitation and has previously been a consultant neurosurgeon in England and overseas. He holds a Specialist Certificate (CCST) in Rehabilitation, London as well as a Certificate of the European Board in Physical Medicine and Rehabilitation. He is trained in neurosurgery, spinal cord injuries and spinal disease rehabilitation. He has had training in amputation medicine. His expertise relates to tone, neurological pain and biomechanics of mobility. He also has experience in the neuropsychological aspects of neurological diseases and more specifically in conversion reactions.

## SIMON PARFORD

Simon Parford is a member of the Law Society's Clinical Negligence Specialist Panel and Action Against Medical Accidents Clinical Negligence Specialist Panel.

He has undertaken claimant clinical negligence litigation since 1986 and has specialised exclusively in this area of work since 1991. Specialist areas of interest are child and adult brain injury claims and spinal injury claims. He investigates Brain Injury Claims involving failures and/or delays in diagnosing and/or treatment. He has investigated dozens of such claims and has achieved many multi-million pound settlements; the largest to date being in excess of £6 500 000. These claims are almost always difficult, complicated claims involving complex medical issues and very substantial quantum.

## MICHELLE SMITH

Michelle Smith is a Consultant Clinical Neuropsychologist, a full member of the British Psychological Society Divisions of Clinical Psychology and Neuropsychology, and registered with the Health Professions Council. Current clinical practice is part-time at the Wessex Neurological Centre, University Hospital Southampton, with the adult specialist epilepsy surgery team, and at Glenside Hospital and Care Homes leading the psychology service and team for the rehabilitation of adults with acquired brain injuries or progressive conditions, complex care and high dependency, and neurobehavioural programmes. Before this she was Head of the Neuropsychology Rehabilitation and Counselling Services for Neurotrauma and Neurological Disease in Southampton for many years, with clinical experience ranging from acute, and in-patient, to long-term community settings. This experience was, and still is, primarily based on multidisciplinary team collaboration. Current professional interests include epilepsy and surgery, impaired consciousness after acquired brain injury, quality of life in people on long-term mechanical ventilation, with previous research regarding rehabilitation of memory problems in Multiple Sclerosis.

## JUDI THOMSON

Judi Thomson qualified as a social worker in 1981 and obtained a Degree in Social Science and a Certificate of Qualification in Social Work. She has worked in a wide range of settings but her core work has been hospital social work. She has worked with adults with disabilities and life threatening illness. She has also worked in local offices in the community and has spent a short time working with children with cancer and their families – a post funded by the Malcolm Sargent Cancer Fund for Children.

Whilst working in hospital she developed an interest in strokes and this led to a post being created dedicated to working with stroke survivors and their carers. It was funded jointly by Health and Social Services and enabled her to carry out a truly multidisciplinary role. She went on to become a Care Coordinator for the Primary Care Trust in the Continuing Health Care team reviewing and assessing eligibility for continuing healthcare and also contributing to multidisciplinary panels.

She then went on to become Carer Support Worker for Headway Dorset where she now remains, supporting carers, families and friends of adults who have an acquired brain injury. She is able to provide support to those with an ABI and help families. Part of her role is to provide education, information and advice but also to assist in navigating the myriad of services which exist and are ever changing. Her background in social work has provided her with extensive knowledge and she feels able to be an effective advocate for anyone who she comes in contact with.

## KEVIN TSANG

Mr Kevin King Tin Tsang was born in Hong Kong and read medicine at Guy's and St Thomas' Hospitals. He is currently working at Frenchay Hospital, Bristol. Previously he worked at Derriford Hospital, Plymouth, as a specialist registrar (ST6) in neurosurgery.

He has also worked in the neurosurgical departments in Queen's Hospital, Romford, and Addenbrooke's Hospital, Cambridge, and also worked with the spine team in Oxford, both at the Nuffield Orthopaedic Centre and at John Radcliffe Hospital.

He has a particular interest in trauma care, both cranial and spinal, and will be looking to further his career in that direction.

## ANDREW WARLOW

Andrew Warlow is a Partner and leads the Head and Spinal Injuries Unit at Wolferstans. He specialises in complex, catastrophic injury claims. He is the contact partner for Wolferstans and has been for a number of years on the Headway – The Brain Injury Association Personal Injuries Solicitors List, as well as the Spinal Injuries Association Directory for Personal Injuries Solicitors. He is also the contact partner for Wolferstans in the Child Brain Injury Trust Legal Directory. Andrew is a Fellow of the Association of Personal Injury Lawyers and a member of The Law Society's Specialist Personal Injury Panel.

Andrew is a member of The Management Committee of Headway Plymouth, a local charity promoting awareness of and helping the victims of acquired brain injury and their carers.

## PETER WHITFIELD

Peter Whitfield is a Consultant and Associate Professor in Neurosurgery at the South West Neurosurgery Centre, Derriford Hospital/Peninsula College of Medicine and Dentistry, Plymouth. His interest in neurosurgery was fuelled by undergraduate training in Southampton. He undertook Basic Surgical Training in Glasgow and Winchester before being appointed a Registrar in Cambridge. He was awarded an MRC Clinical Training Fellowship and undertook a PhD on the molecular mechanisms underpinning cerebral ischaemia. He has a longstanding interest in head injury management and is the lead editor of 'Head Injury: A Multidisciplinary Approach' (Cambridge University Press). He has a keen interest in surgical training and is the Deputy Chair of the Specialists Advisory Committee in Neurosurgery, a member of the National Neurosurgical Selection Panel and an examiner for the Royal College of Surgeons and the European Association of Neurological Surgeons.

## DANIELLE WILLIAMS

Danielle Williams is a senior II occupational therapist at the Royal Hospital for Neuro-disability in Putney, London, specialising in long-term care in disability management of individuals with complex neurological disabilities and is a Bachelor of Science in Occupational Therapy.

Previously she was employed by Headway Dorset for 18 months, following a placement with the organisation during her training and work through the summer as part of the rehabilitation team. The charity is unusual, if not unique in regards to other Headway groups across the UK, in that it has a multidisciplinary team of professionals providing rehabilitation across the county. Working with clients who have survived brain injuries is a challenging and rewarding vocation, and Headway Dorset delivers a fantastic service to its client group. Danielle has found working with the experienced team, including occupational therapists, neurophysiotherapists, neuropsychologists and nurse specialists with decades of experience between them, an excellent learning experience for a newly qualified healthcare professional.

She has a particular interest in the dynamics between the physical, cognitive and psychological challenges experienced by survivors of brain injury, and gets great pleasure from facilitating change and progress in clients' recovery. She also has a keen interest in vocational rehabilitation, and a strong belief in the health benefits of having a productive role in our society, whether it be paid or otherwise.

# Abbreviations

| | | | |
|---|---|---|---|
| ABCDE | Airway, Breathing, Circulation, Disability, Exposure and Environment | DAI/TAI | Diffuse axonal injury/Traumatic axonal injury |
| ABI | Acquired brain injury | DVT | Deep vein thrombosis |
| A&E | Accident and Emergency Department | EBIC | European Brain Injury Consortium |
| ACTH | Adrenocorticotropic hormone | ECF | Extracellular fluid |
| ADH | Antidiuretic hormone | ECG | Electrocardiogram |
| ADL | Activities of living | ED | Accident and Emergency Department/ Casualty |
| AMPLE | Allergies, Medication, Past history, Last ate or drank, Events | EEG | Electroencephalogram |
| ARN | Association of Rehabilitation Nurses | ESP | Early stimulation programme |
| ATLS | Advanced trauma life support | ETT | Endotracheal tube |
| ATMIST | Age, Time, Mechanism of injury, Injuries, Signs, Treatment given | FAST scan | Focused abdominal sonography for trauma scan |
| BBB | Blood brain barrier | FAM | Functional assessment measure |
| BP | Blood pressure | FIM | Functional independence measure |
| BSRM | British Society of Rehabilitation Medicine | FSH | Follicle-stimulating hormone |
| BSDT | Brain stem death testing | GBS | Guillain-Barré syndrome |
| CBF | Cerebral blood flow | GCS | Glasgow Coma Scale |
| CBR | Community-based rehabilitation | GOS | Glasgow Outcome Scale |
| CBV | Cerebral blood volume | HDU | High Dependency Unit |
| CN | Cranial nerve | ICF | Intracellular fluid |
| CNS | Central nervous system | ICP | Intracranial pressure |
| CPAP | Continuous positive airways pressure | ↑ICP | Increased intracranial pressure |
| CPP | Cerebral perfusion pressure | ICSH | Interstitial cell-stimulating hormone |
| CSF | Cerebrospinal fluid | ICU | Intensive Care Unit |
| CT scan | Computerised tomography scan | INR | International normalised ratio |
| CVA | Cerebrovascular accident | IV | Intravenous |
| CVP | Central venous pressure | LH | Luteinizing hormone |
| DH | Department of Health | LOC | Level of consciousness |

| | | | |
|---|---|---|---|
| LMA | Laryngeal mask airway | PTA | Post-traumatic amnesia |
| MAP | Mean arterial pressure | RAS | Reticular activating system |
| MC&S | Microscopy, culture and sensitivity | RNF | Rehabilitation Nursing Foundation |
| MRI scan | Magnetic resonance imaging scan | R/RR | Respiration |
| MS | Multiple sclerosis | RCP | Royal College of Physicians |
| MSH | Melanocyte-stimulating hormone | RTA | Road traffic accident |
| MVA | Motor vehicle accident | RTC | Road traffic collision |
| NANDA-I | NANDA International | RSI | Rapid sequence induction |
| NIC | Nursing Interventions Classification | SAH | Subarachnoid haemorrhage |
| NICE | National Institute for Health and Clinical | SALT | Speech and Language Therapist |
| | Excellence | SNS | Sympathetic nervous system |
| NOC | Nursing Outcomes Classification | T | Temperature |
| NNN | (NANDA, NIC & NOC) | TBI | Traumatic brain injury |
| OPD | Out-patient department | TSH | Thyroid-stimulating hormone |
| P | Pulse | UK | United Kingdom |
| PCWP | Pulmonary capillary wedge pressure | U&E | Urea and electrolytes |
| PCS | Post-concussion syndrome | USA | United States of America |
| PEEP | Positive end-expiratory pressure | WHO | World Health Organization |
| PEG | Percutaneous endoscopic gastrostomy | WTE | Whole time equivalent |
| PNS | Parasympathetic nervous system | | |

# List of Tables and Figures

# Section 1
# FOUNDATIONS FOR PRACTICE

## INTRODUCTION

This book has been designed to empower health and other professionals with applicable knowledge in neurotrauma practice, to support and manage patients, families, carers and communities throughout all stages of a patient's journey to recovery. This is accomplished using a multidisciplinary approach to facilitate recovery and maximise potential, whatever this level may turn out to be.

The management of patients with neurotrauma has improved over the last decade. This has resulted in patients, who previously would not have survived, surviving their head injuries and requiring extensive rehabilitation (House of Commons 2001). This has had a major effect on the use of available resources (Christensen *et al.* 2008). Services, including rehabilitation, are neither equitable nor accessible to all neurotrauma patients (Aronow 1987; Beecham *et al.* 2009; British Society of Rehabilitation Medicine [BSRM] 2008a; Bulger *et al.* 2002; RCP 2010; United Kingdom Acquired Brain Injury Forum (UKABIF) 2004; Zampolini *et al.* 2012). Not all patients with moderate or severe head injuries are able to access neurosurgical centres (Treacy *et al.* 2005). The majority go home, some with a follow-up appointment or a GP referral, others without any follow-up, yet patients requiring rehabilitation should be able to access this at any stage within their journey (RCP 2010).

It is said that the costs for a person injured in a road traffic accident can vary between £35 000 and £60 000 per incident (Beecham *et al.* 2009) and costs for an injured pedestrian are estimated at £57 400 per incident (Crandall *et al.* 2002). The estimated cost per patient experience is presented in Table 1.

People with neurotrauma may achieve a good recovery. However, a lack of recovery, or partial recovery, may be devastating for them, their families and communities.

This book examines the journey related to health, illness and recovery, in particular for neurotrauma. In order to maximise outcome, cost-effectiveness, efficiency and quality of care, it is necessary to accompany the patient along the journey in the primary, secondary and tertiary settings.

---

### Key objectives

On completion of this section you should be able to achieve the following:

- Define neurotrauma.
- Define the patient's journey.
- Describe factors that affect the patient's journey.
- Determine how to ensure the patient has a seamless journey regarding neurotrauma.
- Evaluate the various care pathways for neurotrauma patients.
- Describe various models of wellness.
- Apply these models to neuroscience practice.
- Apply the Needs Approach Model in practice.
- Determine how using the Needs Approach Model will assist in providing holistic, patient-centred care in a multidisciplinary milieu.
- Describe effective multidisciplinary management.
- Describe the role of the neuropsychologist.
- Describe the techniques one can use to provide a therapeutic milieu.
- Manage difficult patients.
- Describe behaviour modification.
- Describe how to communicate with patients, families and carers.

**Ethical/legal considerations**

Debate the ethical issues related to this section.

Consider and apply the legal and ethical issues highlighted in these chapters to neurotrauma practice:

- Patient Charter.
- Human Rights.
- Accountability and responsibility.

- Consent.
- Confidentiality.
- Record-keeping.

**Table 1** Estimated costs for 18–25 year olds experiencing head injury.

| Severity of injury | Admission location | Discharge location | Sequelae | Use of health and social services | Costs | |
|---|---|---|---|---|---|---|
| | | | | | Per annum | Per person |
| Mild head injury | A&E | Return home<br><br>1:5 have follow-up appointment | Up to 6 months | Low | £23.8 million | £240 |
| Moderate–severe head injury | Neurosurgical unit<br><br>Rehabilitation centre | Return home <1 year<br><br>Need some personal support<br><br>Require frequent OPD visits | | Low–moderate | £6 million | £17 160 |
| Moderate–severe head injury | | Live in supported accommodation<br><br>Paid carers<br><br>Community housing | Limited independence – independence | Moderate–high | £30.9 million | £32 900 |
| Severe head injury | | Home/<br><br>residential facility/<br><br>nursing home | Severely disabled | | £10.4 million | £33 900 |

Beecham *et al.* (2009).

# Chapter 1
# The Patient's Journey

*Nadine Abelson-Mitchell*

School of Nursing and Midwifery, Faculty of Health, Education and Society, Plymouth University, Devon, UK

## INTRODUCTION

A person is on a journey through life which runs from the ante-natal period to the time of death. It is to be anticipated that, through experience, a person can manage obstacles in their pathway and continue on their journey in a productive and positive manner. This life journey contains a number of pathways. These pathways, such as financial circumstances, interpersonal relationships and health, do not always run smoothly and may lead to various deviations. The health pathway is a continuum of wellness, illness, recovery or death and includes all occasions of ill-health.

Primary prevention is an important aspect of the patient's journey. Preventing disease or ill-health through early education will decrease morbidity and mortality. A particular pathway along the patient's journey commences once the patient has been diagnosed with a particular health condition/problem. Unfortunately, due to the nature of neurotrauma, there is seldom a pre-arranged plan in place as there is for elective surgery. This part of the health journey usually comes as a shock and 'emergency resources' may need to be called upon to be able to continue the journey. It is important to provide a smooth route throughout the patient's journey in order to ensure that quality care is provided, decrease stress, increase compliance and decrease deviant or destructive behaviour. The patient's journey takes place within a particular environment and involves the patient, family and the wider community. It is a journey that needs to be patient-centred and focused on the patient's perspective, expectations, motivation and

behaviour. When considering the journey the patient's life experience, their strengths, abilities, capabilities and any fears or weaknesses must be considered. The patient's health journey, interrupted by the neurotrauma, is influenced by a number of existing factors:

*The patient:*

- Age.
- Gender.
- Pre-existing conditions.
- Social practices.
- Health status.

*The factors:*

- Peri-natal care.
- Environment.
- Education.
- Family support.
- Community support.

Planning the patient's journey may be referred to as 'process mapping' whereby the team and the patient work out the pathway a patient is expected to follow. This requires taking into account all aspects of holisitic, person-centred care that the patient may require, as well as the resources needed to achieve the proposed plan. The team is then able to examine the patient's situation in terms of patient outcome and consider and identify potential challenges that may occur along the pathway that may hinder achievement of the patient's goals.

*Neurotrauma: Managing Patients with Head Injuries*, First Edition. Edited by Nadine Abelson-Mitchell.
© 2013 Blackwell Publishing Ltd. Published 2013 by Blackwell Publishing Ltd.

## CARE PATHWAYS: POLICIES AND GUIDELINES

Numerous care pathways have been developed to ensure cost-effective, efficient patient care to help create a seamless journey through this episode of altered health. Internationally, specific policies and standards have been developed that focus on neurotrauma throughout the patient's journey (Espinosa-Aguilar *et al.* 2008; Seeley *et al.* 2006; Sesperez *et al.* 2001; Zampolini *et al.* 2012). The National Institute for Health and Clinical Excellence (NICE) (NICE 2007) has developed guidelines for the management of head-injured patients. The National Service Framework for Long-term Conditions (DH 2005a) has a particular focus on the needs of people with neurological disease and considers some of the generic issues, including rehabilitation, that are of relevance to people with long-term conditions and disabilities. The introduction of these policies addresses some of the inequities for patients requiring rehabilitation (Pickard *et al.* 2004).

Guidelines have been produced by a number of sources, nationally and internationally, to assist in clinical decision making, prevention, diagnosis and management, including rehabilitation, of patients with neurotrauma. Guidelines make specific practical recommendations based upon rigorous and available scientific data (RCP 2010).

The health professional is responsible and accountable for the quality of care a patient receives. Basic care in today's climate is often protocol driven, particularly as many basic tasks are undertaken by non-professional personnel under the direct or indirect supervision of registered personnel.

## INTEGRATED CARE PATHWAYS

Internationally (Espinosa-Aguilar *et al.* 2008; Seeley *et al.* 2006; Sesperez *et al.* 2001) and nationally (BSRM 2002; BSRM 2008a; 2009; NICE 2007; Royal College of Physicians [RCP] and BSRM 2003) interprofessional, integrated care pathways have been developed to improve the management of patients with neurotrauma and are useful in managing specific issues such as depression (Turner-Stokes *et al.* 2002).

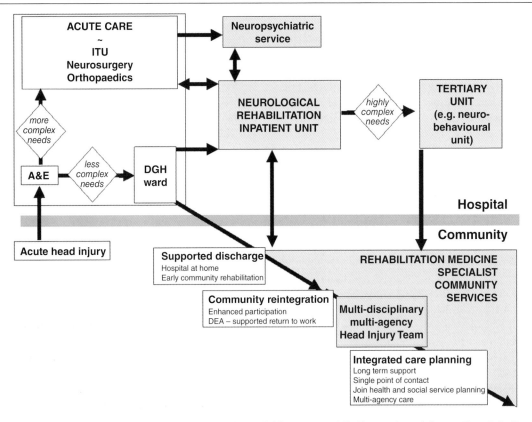

**Figure 1.1** Care pathway for traumatic brain injury (RCP 2010: p. 28). Reproduced from: Royal College of Physicians. Medical rehabilitation in 2011 and beyond. Report of a working party. London, RCP, 2010. Copyright © 2010 Royal College of Physicians. Reproduced by permission.

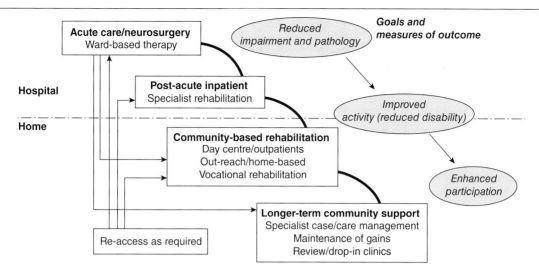

**Figure 1.2** The 'Slinky' model of phased rehabilitation (RCP and BSRM 2003: p.10). Reproduced from: Royal College of Physicians and British Society of Rehabilitation Medicine. Rehabilitation following acquired brain injury: National clinical guidelines (Turner-Stokes, L. ed). London, RCP, BSRM, 2003. Copyright © 2003 Royal College of Physicians. Reproduced by permission.

The National Service Frameworks stress the importance of integrated care pathways in the development of quality healthcare. These pathways, if developed and implemented effectively, will increase interprofessional co-ordination, efficiency of healthcare, reduce sequelae of head injury and reduce healthcare costs (Coetzer 2009; Singh *et al.* 2012; Vitaz *et al.* 2001; Zampolini *et al.* 2012).

Patients able to access these recommended pathways should experience a seamless transition from incident to home or final destination.

**Activity 1.1**

**Scenario**

An 18 year old boy was admitted with a GCS of 14/15 with a scalp injury that required suturing after a skate boarding accident in the park.

**Exercise**

1. Interview the patient and his mother to gain a picture of the patient's life journey thus far.
2. Plan a session with the mother and son to decrease the risk of further head injuries.

**Activity 1.2**

1 Select a patient in the unit who has had neurotrauma (GCS 5/15) and plot the patient's journey.
2 Are there any aspects related to professional practice that you need to consider in the patient's journey?
3 Develop a communication plan for patient.
4 Develop a communication plan for family and carers.

**Activity 1.3**

1 Do you use an integrated care pathway in the unit?
2 If yes, see Chapter 16, Activity 16.1 and describe a possible pathway for Trevor.
3 If no, why does your organisation not use an integrated care pathway?
4 Would you consider developing such a pathway with a team of colleagues?

# Chapter 2
# Philosophy

*Nadine Abelson-Mitchell*

School of Nursing and Midwifery, Faculty of Health, Education and Society, Plymouth University, Devon, UK

## INTRODUCTION

Beliefs and values determine the philosophy that underpins the quality of service provided to neurotrauma patients. Neurotrauma practice is an approach, an attitude and a process. The philosophy behind neurotrauma practice is one of ensuring comprehensive quality holistic care that spans all ages and applies to all settings, individuals, families and communities. It is a philosophy that believes in the worth and value of each human being as an individual, family member and member of a community.

A model of care, or a particular approach to care, underpins this philosophy. There are numerous models of care that can be applied to neurotrauma practice. There are models that provide a framework, a logical systematic approach to quality care. The most commonly used are the 'medical model' (Mountain and Shah 2008), with a focus on functional ability, and the social model (Sharpf 2002) that encompasses the whole person. In their pure form, most models do not include all that is required in nursing. In order to achieve the goals of nursing an adapted, integrated model (Joubert *et al.* 2006) of care is appropriate. This integrated model takes into consideration the World Health Organization (WHO) International Classification of Functioning (ICF), Disability and Health components (WHO 2001). The integrated model is a patient-centred model that enables a comprehensive holistic approach to

the patient incorporating a multidisciplinary team rather than an illness/disease orientated model.

The focus of the model changes as the patient progresses throughout their journey. Within secondary health services acute and sub-acute management is the priority. As the patient progresses along their journey to tertiary services, the focus changes to a wellness model of care (Hattie *et al.* 2004; Hettler 1984; Myers and Sweeney 2004; Myers *et al.* 2000).

The wellness model focuses on health and lifestyle and includes aspects such as:

- Holistic health that encompasses the integration of body, mind and spirit.
- Making informed choices.
- Approaches to wellness.
- Facing challenges.
- Changing lifestyles.

The WHO (1958: p. 1) defines health as 'a state of complete physical, mental and social well-being, not merely the absence of disease or infirmity'. This definition enables a holistic approach to healthcare and engenders the concept of wellness. It may require a culture change to embrace a wellness model rather than a disease-based, medical model. The concept of wellness implies that the individual will be proactive, aware of the advantages of a healthy lifestyle and

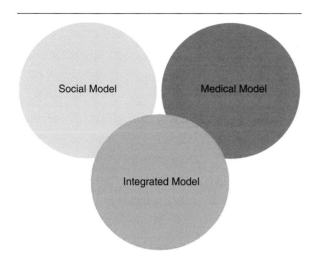

**Figure 2.1** Model of neurotrauma management. For a colour version of this figure, please refer to the plate section.

the appropriate health promotion and lifestyle choices to maintain wellness. The wellness model empowers and enables people to progress towards wellness, health and independence; to accept challenges, to encompass integration and creativity, in order to lead a fulfilling life. When all the patient's needs are in balance the person is in a state of homeostasis and harmony (Figure 2.1). In this respect, primary prevention and health promotion are very important. Should disease or injury occur, the patient's equanimity of life is disrupted. Once this adverse event has been managed the patient can expect to return to optimal wellness.

Wellness, for all patients who have experienced neurotrauma, is the objective of health management. The philosophy behind the wellness model is the patient's right to wellness and recovery, to enjoy life and to strive for health, safety and wellbeing.

The challenge is how to achieve this state in patients who may have an altered level of consciousness and physical, emotional, psychological and cognitive deficits. The wellness model involves a whole person approach. It implies that it is a holistic approach that includes the physical, psychological, social, spiritual, intellectual, emotional, environmental, educational and leisure needs of the patient (Avery 1996; Kiefer 2008; Wade 2011). It emphasises the holistic view of health. The individual is considered as a unified whole progressing towards high level wellness (Hattie *et al.* 2004; Hettler 1980; Travis and Ryan 2004). It is about life choices and living a meaningful existence. It enables integrated functioning that maximises an individual's potential within a particular environment.

A person determines the level of wellness they wish to achieve for the lifestyle choices they make. It is an active choice to pursue optimal health and wellbeing. As this may not be possible in the patient with neurotrauma, intervention is planned to empower the patient to achieve and maintain their maximum level of wellness. With today's technology individuals who survive neurotrauma are faced with the need to significantly adjust their attitudes and approaches to life, to become a leader of the team, control their own destinies and adjust to the real world.

Alternatively, low-level wellness is the inability of the individual to meet their needs in a way that allows for adequate functioning. People with neurotrauma may fall into the 'sick role' as opposed to a wellness role. Being sick becomes the focal point of their lives, they function poorly, readily deplete their energy reserves and may slip into a life of submission and dependency.

The Needs Approach Model (NAM) developed by Abelson (Abelson-Mitchell 2006) is based within the framework of a wellness model and incorporates core components of wellness such as physical, psychological, emotional, environmental, lifestyle, social, leisure and independence (Kiefer 2008) (see Chapter 3). The Needs Approach Model is appropriate for use in all care settings as the patient's needs are determined by the patient, or caregivers in the event that the patient is unable to determine his own needs. The Needs Approach Model can be applied in a primary, secondary or tertiary setting as the needs are relevant to health and wellbeing in primary prevention, acute illness and throughout the process of rehabilitation and recovery.

There are numerous authors who have developed theories of wellness; namely Travis and Ryan (2004), Witmer *et al.* (1998) and Hettler (1980). These can be related to the wellness model and Needs Approach Model that has been developed (Abelson-Mitchell 2006). Spirituality, psychological and physical dimensions are key to all theorists (Hettler 1984; Kiefer 2008; Myers *et al.* 2000; Travis and Ryan 2004).

Witmer *et al.* (1998) developed the ecological Wheel of Wellness (Figure 2.2). Albeit that the theoretical Wheel of Wellness was initially developed for counselling, it can certainly be applied to health. The Wheel of Wellness represents the whole person, body, mind and spirit (Myers *et al.* 2000). Any change in one aspect of the wheel may lead to change in some or all of the other aspects. Spirituality is at the centre of the wheel and from there the various individual life tasks radiate to the other circles at the edge of the wheel. The Wheel of Wellness includes 'five life tasks' namely spirituality, self-direction, work and leisure,

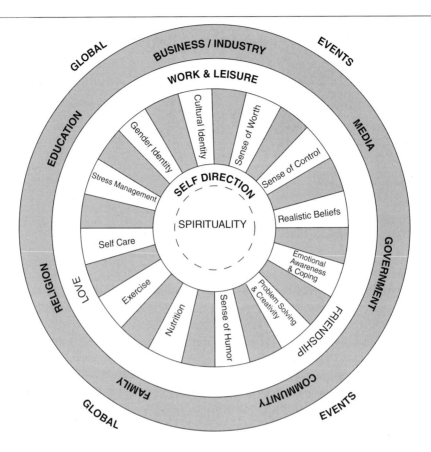

**Figure 2.2**   The wheel of wellness. Witmer, Sweeney and Myers. Copyright © 1998 J.M. Witmer, T.J. Sweeney, & J.E. Myers.

friendship and love. Self-direction is further divided into 12 life tasks, namely sense of worth, sense of control, realistic beliefs, emotional awareness and coping, problem solving and creativity, sense of humour, nutrition, exercise, self-care, stress management, gender identity and cultural identity. These 12 life tasks determine the person's response to the contents of the next wheel which relate to work and leisure, love and friendship. The outer wheel relates to government, media, business, industry, education, community, family and religion (Myers and Sweeney 2008: p. 483). For further details regarding the Wheel of Wellness see www.uncg.edu/ced/jemyers/wellness/docs. In addition, Myers and Sweeney (2004) have developed the Indivisible Self, which underscores the holistic nature of wellness.

Travis developed a wellness model for health as a continuum from ill-health to wellness (http//:thewellspring.com/flex/the-wellness-paradigm/1951/) (Figure 2.3).

The continuum has two sections either side of a neutral point. To the left of the neutral point, where disability and illness are represented, treatment is used to manage these issues. To the right of the neutral point, the person is well and attains high-level wellness through awareness, education and growth. The person is perpetually trying to achieve wellness. Achieving high-level wellness requires lifestyle choices, determination and active participation. It is important for a person to establish their position on the continuum. More importantly, when establishing their position they need to consider the direction they wish to follow. The direction should be towards high-level wellness rather than premature death (Travis and Ryan 2004).

With regard to wellness, Travis and Ryan (2004) advocate the Iceberg Model (Figure 2.4) to understand wellness and health.

What is visible above the surface is the tip of the iceberg. One needs to look at the rest of the iceberg to discover what is happening below the surface. Travis and Ryan (2004) suggest that there are three levels below the iceberg that need to be considered:

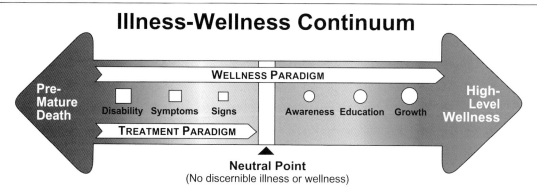

**Figure 2.3** Illness–wellness continuum. www.thewellspring.com. Travis, Copyright © 2004, 1988, 1972 JW Travis. Reproduced with permission. For a colour version of this figure, please refer to the plate section.

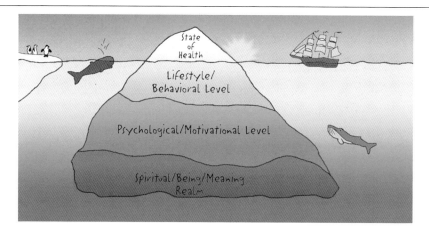

**Figure 2.4** The Iceberg Model. www.mywellnesstest.com/IcebergModel.asp. Travis © 1978, 1988, 2004 JW Travis. Reproduced with permission. For a colour version of this figure, please refer to the plate section.

Level I   The lifestyle and behavioural level relates to a person's physical being, eating, exercise, safety and stress management.

Level II  The psychological and motivational level helps a person understand their chosen lifestyle and the influence of cultural norms.

Level III The spiritual, being and meaning realm relates to reality, a place within reality, spirituality, philosophy in the unconscious mind and the real meaning of life.

According to Travis and Ryan (2004) it is these three levels that underpin wellness or ill-health.

Hettler (1980) developed a hexagonal six-dimensional model of wellness (Figure 2.5) that includes social, occupational, intellectual, spiritual, physical and emotional aspects of life, wherein he stresses that it is necessary to have balance in all dimensions of life. It is each dimension,

as well as all dimensions together, that will determine one's wellness status and it is important to strive for high-level wellness (Box 2.1).

**CONCLUSION**

The Needs Approach Model incorporates many of the aspects of the Wheel of Wellness (Myers and Sweeney 2008), the Health–Illness Continuum (Travis and Ryan 2004) and Hettler's Hexagon Model (Hettler 1980) in a different format. Wellness theories and the Needs Approach Model are concerned with the integration of mind, body and spirit. Wellness is the focus and health and wellness are the first priorities. Belief in the wellbeing and wholeness of an individual is a priority to help them function at maximum capacity and achieve full potential, irrespective of what that level will be; determining and meeting a patient's needs are the main concerns. Lifestyle and life choices affect happiness and potential for achieving goals.

**Box 2.1** Strategies that can be used to enable high-level wellness

1. Maximise assets. Build on the patient's positive attributes or assets. Patients' feelings of normality can be increased by building on their physical and psychosocial assets. Patients should be encouraged to use their creative talents to engage in activities which match, enhance or exceed their capabilities.
2. Work to reduce limitations and negative factors. Help compensate for negative factors by identifying them and developing strategies to cope with them e.g. using a memory log or an electric wheelchair. Explore ways in which the environment can produce more growth and become less restricting for these patients.
3. Help to use available energy efficiently and conserve energy whilst striving to achieve maximum wellness. Activities must be balanced and paced allowing adequate rest.
4. Assist the patient to become progressively aware of the ramifications of, and the limitations imposed by, challenges and to come to terms with 'this is the way it is going to be' and 'making the best of it'.
5. Resolve external or internal conflicts.
6. Maintain integrity of the patient's ego. Feelings of ego integrity involve a positive self-concept and self-worth. Enable the patient to gain and use their own personal power. Feelings of empowerment may enable individuals to experience a sense of control and mastery over their lives. Allow patients to accept responsibility for their life, programme, role in society, etc. Avoid intrusions by caregivers and protectors.
7. Achieve maximum level of self-integration. Inspire hope by focusing on and maximising the moment, by living in the present, by appreciating the aesthetics in the environment, by maximising experiences and sustaining relationships and interconnecting with others.
8. Having a positive attitude spreads outwards to others.

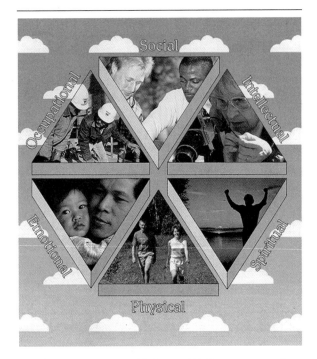

**Figure 2.5** Model of Wellness. Wellness promotion on a university campus, B. Hettler, *Family & Community Health* 3 (1). Copyright © 1980 B. Hettler. Reproduced with permission.

Activity 2.1

1. Is the care in the Unit based on a medical model, social model or integrated model?
2. Analyse the advantages/disadvantages of the model in current use.
3. Describe how the model in use could be improved.
4. Apply the Witmer, Sweeney and Myers Wheel of Wellness to your practice with neurotrauma patients.
5. How can you use the Wheel of Wellness in practice to improve patients' lifestyles and choices?
6. Using Travis's Health–Illness continuum, consider the state of your health.
7. Using Travis's Health–Illness continuum, consider the state of a patient's health.
8. Using Travis's Iceberg Model, consider the state of your health.
9. Use Hettler's Hexagonal Model to facilitate patient or family understanding of their condition.
10. Include information from the Iceberg Model when considering planning for the patient.
11. Relate Hettler's concept, Travis's concept and Witmer, Sweeney and Myers' concept to the Needs Approach Model.

# Chapter 3
# The Needs Approach Model

*Nadine Abelson-Mitchell*

School of Nursing and Midwifery, Faculty of Health, Education and Society, Plymouth University, Devon, UK

## INTRODUCTION

Based on the integrated model of health, and the wellness model, a new model of care called the Needs Approach Model (Figure 3.1) has been developed (Abelson-Mitchell 2006). The model is a patient-focused, needs-led, integrated model of care. The model incorporates aspects of Roper, Logan and Tierney's model of Activities of Living (Roper *et al.* 2000), Orem's model of self-care (Orem 1983) and Maslow's hierarchy of needs (Maslow 1968).

---

### Reflection

Whilst working in the neurosurgical unit as the 'clinical teacher' I overheard a conversation about a patient. The patient had been admitted with an acoustic neuroma. The patient stayed for three days and then discharged himself. The staff were not pleased with the situation but refrained from making further enquiries. On the third occasion when this happened I asked the staff if I could talk to the patient. Whilst talking to the patient I discovered the reason for his leaving the hospital after three days. He had a farm and his wife had had a stroke and he could not leave her for more than three days at a time. He had been assessed by members of the interdisciplinary team yet this had been missed by everyone. How could this important aspect of his life be missed? This incident was the basis for the development of the Needs Approach Model.

---

## WHAT IS A NEED?

Human beings have needs. A need can be defined as an element that is required for the body to maintain physical, psychological and social wellbeing. Needs are what individuals must gratify for normal functions to happen. Humans have certain needs, one of which is the basic requirement to maintain health and wholeness.

## STRUCTURE OF THE NEEDS APPROACH MODEL

The Needs Approach Model is comprised of a circle, or wheel, of needs which are represented individually, as well as collectively, in the circle. If one need is affected this may affect other needs within the circle. The Needs Approach Model enables a holistic approach to patient care.

In the circle there are 22 needs relating to the physical, psychological, social, cognitive, spiritual, vocational and educational needs of patients in all settings, including home-based care. Some of the needs have been subdivided to enable appropriate assessment and planning within the overall need, e.g. hygiene. Within the model there is a sector called 'other', should an additional need be identified. Within the continuum of health and wellness, needs may be partially or fully achieved. An Extended Needs Approach Model has also been developed for use in community-based rehabilitation (see Chapter 27).

In the model the bio-psycho-social individual is viewed as a self-care agent, the key participant in the attainment

*Neurotrauma: Managing Patients with Head Injuries*, First Edition. Edited by Nadine Abelson-Mitchell.
© 2013 Blackwell Publishing Ltd. Published 2013 by Blackwell Publishing Ltd.

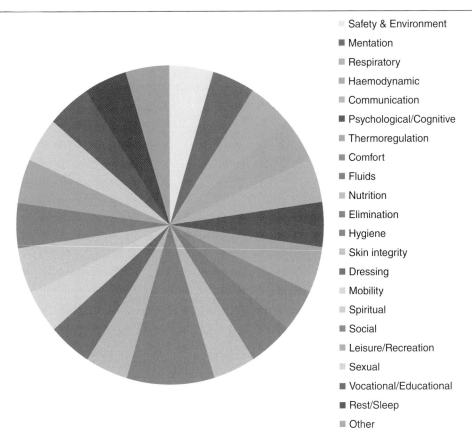

- Safety & Environment
- Mentation
- Respiratory
- Haemodynamic
- Communication
- Psychological/Cognitive
- Thermoregulation
- Comfort
- Fluids
- Nutrition
- Elimination
- Hygiene
- Skin integrity
- Dressing
- Mobility
- Spiritual
- Social
- Leisure/Recreation
- Sexual
- Vocational/Educational
- Rest/Sleep
- Other

**Figure 3.1**   Needs Approach Model. For a colour version of this figure, please refer to the plate section.

of health/wellness and responsible for their own care, where possible. This model views neurotrauma practice and rehabilitation as a process through which an individual's movement towards health is facilitated. A dynamic process of planned and adaptive change in lifestyle, as a response to an unplanned change imposed on the individual by disease or traumatic incident. The focus may not be on a cure, but on living with as much freedom as possible, at every stage, and in whichever direction the condition progresses.

It is anticipated that patients will be able to meet their needs independently. Where patients are unable to meet their needs independently, the health team will facilitate the attainment of their needs in a conducive environment.

**USE OF THE MODEL**

The model is simple to use, and is particularly user-friendly enabling nurses, the interprofessional team, patients, families and carers to continue with care along the patient's

journey (Abelson-Mitchell and Watkins 2006). The Needs Approach Model ensures that neuroscience guidelines and standards are incorporated in practice (National Health Service Institute of Innovation and Improvement 2011a, 2011b; DH 2001a, 2005a, 2010c).

The Needs Approach Model utilises a problem-solving approach to assess, plan, implement and evaluate appropriate needs of the patient. The basic structure for the model is shown in Figure 3.2.

**ASSESSING THE PATIENT'S NEEDS**

Assessment of the patient takes place at various stages along the journey, according to the patient's needs and health status. A detailed assessment will enable the multidisciplinary team to plan appropriate care, including rehabilitation for the patient. This assessment may include a full central nervous system (CNS) assessment depending on the patient's needs (Chapter 18).

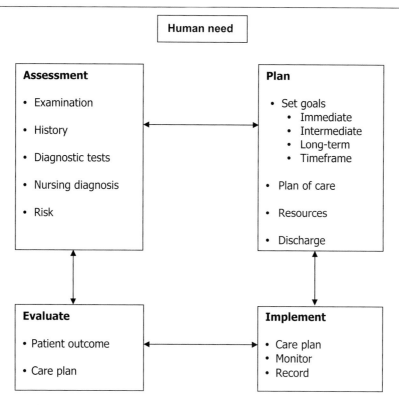

**Figure 3.2**   Human needs.

Whilst it is necessary to initially undertake a comprehensive assessment in order to establish the patient's needs, it may not be necessary to assess all needs on all occasions. The assessor, together with the team, can decide which needs are relevant to the individual. In order to complete the assessment, depending on the circumstances, it may be necessary to meet family and carers. It is important to maintain confidentiality and respect at all times.

A comprehensive assessment involves history taking, physical examination, evaluating the results of investigations prior to establishing nursing diagnoses, and establishing any real or potential risks that are present.

A comprehensive assessment includes the needs listed in Table 3.1.

Details and comments of the specific needs are given in Figures 3.3, 3.4, 3.5, 3.6, 3.7, 3.8, 3.9, 3.10, 3.11, 3.12, 3.13, 3.14, 3.15, 3.16, 3.17, 3.18, 3.19, 3.20, 3.21, 3.22 and 3.23.

**PLANNING**

Once the assessment of the patient's needs has been completed and the nursing diagnoses established, the next step in the process is to plan management in relation to those particular needs.

It can be seen that the process is continuous; assessment, planning, implementation and evaluation based on the nursing diagnoses.

It is extremely important that the plan be reviewed regularly to establish changes in the patient's status. Depending on the patient's condition the plan may be reviewed hourly, daily, weekly or at regular specified periods of time. The plan and any adjustments must be documented in the patient's notes and reported at team meetings.

The plan of care must be practical and pragmatic and the resources required to implement the plan must be considered. These resources may include accommodation, equipment and staffing levels.

**Table 3.1** Comprehensive needs of an individual.

| Need | Page |
|------|------|
| Safety and environmental | 15 |
| Mentation | 16 |
| Respiratory | 16 |
| Haemodynamic | 17 |
| Communication | 17 |
| Psychological/Cognitive | 18 |
| Thermoregulation | 18 |
| Comfort | 19 |
| Fluids | 19 |
| Nutrition | 20 |
| Elimination | 20 |
| Hygiene | 21 |
| Skin integrity | 21 |
| Dressing | 22 |
| Mobility | 22 |
| Spiritual | 23 |
| Social | 24 |
| Leisure/Recreation | 24 |
| Sexual | 25 |
| Vocational/Educational | 25 |
| Rest/Sleep | 26 |
| Other | |

**Tips for effective goal setting**

- Appoint key worker to co-ordinate care.
- Patient-centred goal setting.
- Focus on patient's needs.
- Set goals with patient, family and carer.
- Set team goals.
- Set therapy specific goals.
- Decide on timeframe in which goals to be achieved.
- Set goals in terms of accepted outcome measures.

## IMPLEMENTATION

Once the care plan has been formulated it must be implemented by the relevant team member. It is important to ensure that there is adequate communication between the named key worker, the patient, family and the team. Document the care that the patient receives. In the event that the planned care, or any part of the planned care, is not undertaken, this must be documented and the reason the patient did not receive the care must especially be included.

## EVALUATION

Evaluation is undertaken on a regular basis. Evaluation is undertaken both in terms of patient outcome and care outcome.

**Tips for planning care**

- Assess patient using Needs Approach Model.
- Establish nursing diagnoses.
- Involve the patient, family and carer in decision-making.
- Enable patient to undertake as much activity as possible.
- Ensure patient feels safe whilst undertaking activity.
- Encourage independence.
- Praise achievements.

**Implications for practice**

It is important to regularly ask the question:

Has the intervention achieved what it was expected to achieve in the set timeframe?

## GOAL SETTING

When planning the care programme it is necessary to set immediate, intermediate, short, medium and long-term goals. Short-term, medium-term and long-term goals must be realistic, measurable and achievable in a set timeframe. Where possible, the patient, family and carer should be involved in the goal setting process.

Any variance needs to be discussed and the programme redesigned to achieve the set goals.

## RISK

Risk assessment is extremely important when assessing a patient prior to admission, on admission and throughout their stay in the unit.

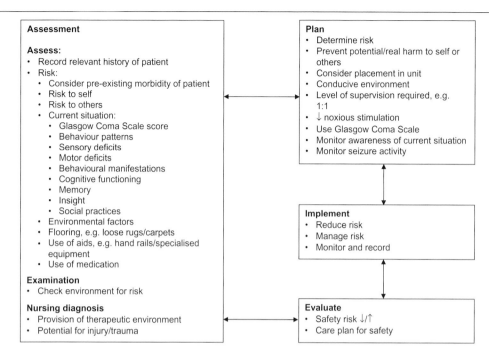

**Figure 3.3** Safety and environmental needs.
Definition: Safety and environmental needs refers to safety and ergonomics (e.g. light, heating, space) of the therapeutic environment to enable minimal disruption to patient.

Risk assessment includes:

- A pre-admission assessment.
- Staff preparation.
- The use of patient dependency rating scores to decide whether the necesssary resources, such as staff and equipment, are available for the particular patient. An example of a dependency rating score is the Northwick Park Dependency score (Turner-Stokes *et al.* 1998, 1999a).

- Establish the risk to self and others.
- Establish whether the patient is to be admitted to the unit.

Self-care is defined as the individual's ability to attend to self-care needs independently. Numerous activities are included in self-care, e.g. nutrition, elimination, mobility, hygiene, dressing and feeding.

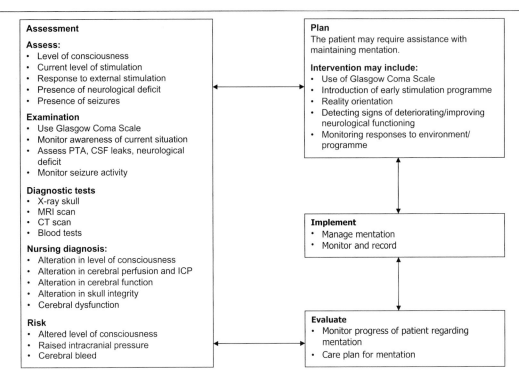

**Figure 3.4**  Mentation needs.
Definition: Mentation needs refers to state of awareness of patient.

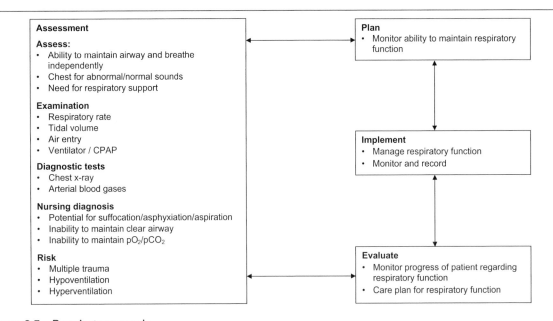

**Figure 3.5**  Respiratory needs.
Definition: Respiratory needs refers to patient's ability to maintain normal respiratory status in environmental air.

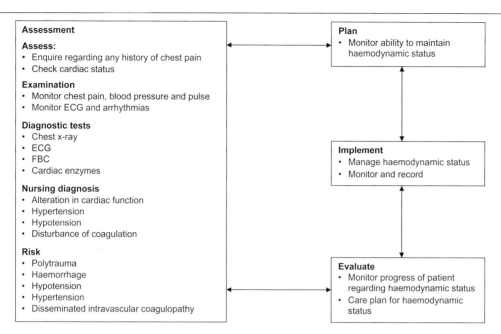

**Figure 3.6** Haemodynamic needs.
Definition: Haemodynamic needs refers to patient's ability to maintain blood pressure and circulation within normal limits.

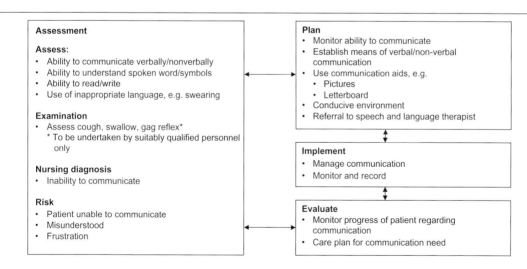

**Figure 3.7** Communication needs.
Definition: Communication needs refers to patient's ability to understand, be understood and communicate with others in various settings.

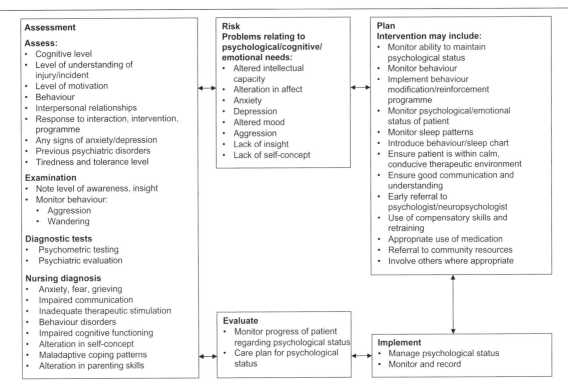

**Figure 3.8**  Psychological/Cognitive needs.
Definition: Psychological/Cognitive needs refers to patient's ability to maintain effective cognitive, psychological and emotional status.

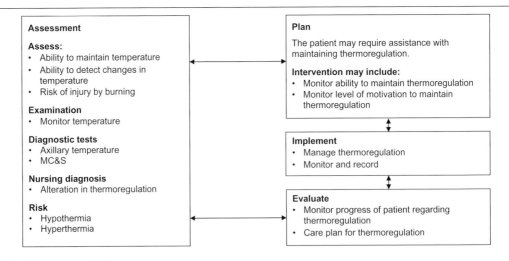

**Figure 3.9**  Thermoregulation needs.
Definition: Thermoregulation needs refers to ability to maintain normal body temperature: 37°C.

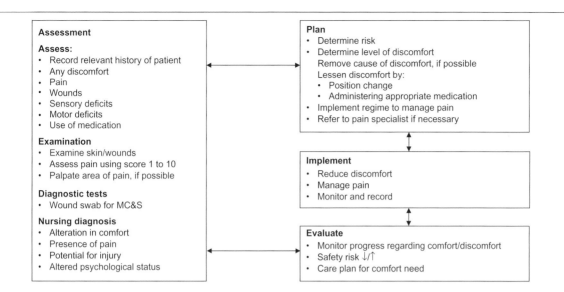

**Figure 3.10** Comfort needs.
Definition: Comfort needs refers to ability of patient to maintain comfort, minimize pain and discomfort.

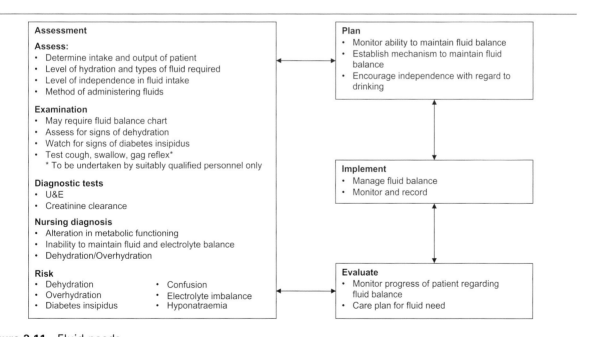

**Figure 3.11** Fluid needs.
Definition: Fluid needs refers to patient's ability to maintain homeostasis with regard to fluid and electrolyte balance.

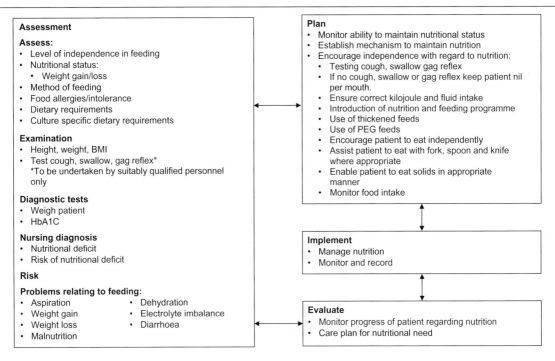

**Figure 3.12** Nutritional needs.
Definition: Nutritional needs refers to patient's ability to maintain nutritional status, BMI and body mass.

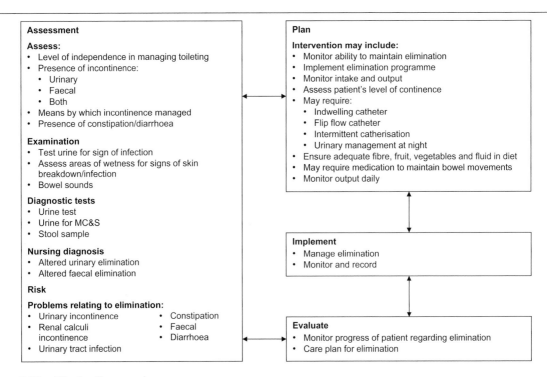

**Figure 3.13** Elimination needs.
Definition: Elimination needs refers to patient's ability to maintain bowel motility, normal elimination of urine and faeces.

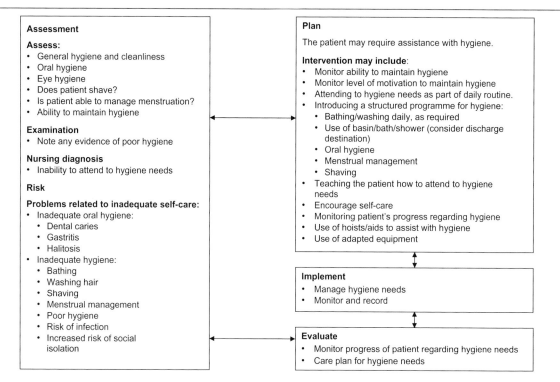

**Figure 3.14** Hygiene needs.
Definition: Hygiene needs refers to patient's ability to maintain personal hygiene.

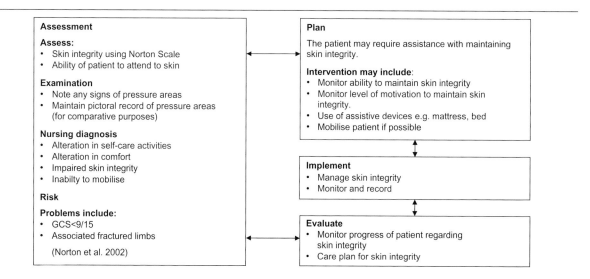

**Figure 3.15** Skin integrity needs.
Definition: Skin integrity needs refers to patient's ability to maintain skin integrity independently at all times.

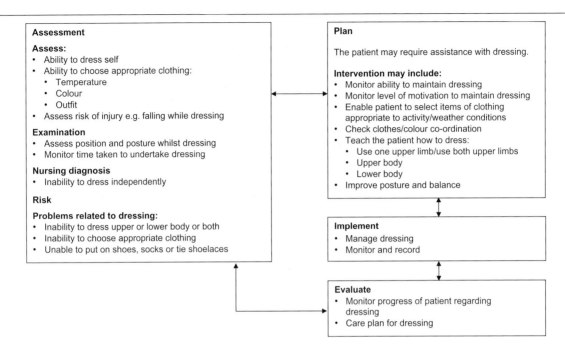

**Figure 3.16** Dressing needs.
Definition: Dressing needs refers to patient's ability to dress independently.

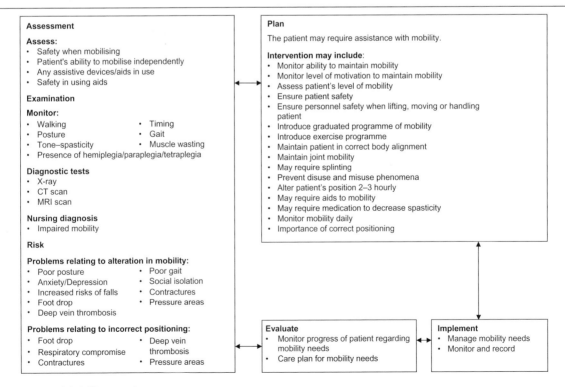

**Figure 3.17** Mobility needs.
Definition: Mobility needs refers to patient's ability to maintain normal posture, position and mobility.

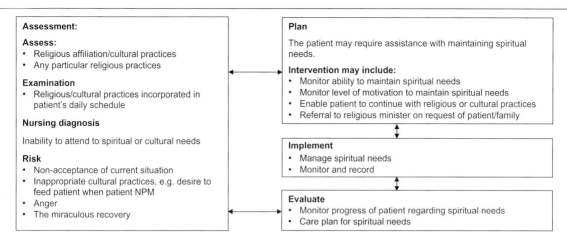

**Figure 3.18** Spiritual needs.
Definition: Spiritual needs refers to ability to maintain religious and cultural practices in all settings.

## THE MIRACULOUS RECOVERY

In the immediate aftermath of being told that their family member has had a head injury families may find it difficult to face up to the situation. Within the first six weeks post-injury, it is so traumatic that it is difficult for families to accept what has happened. At this stage it is important to remember the five stages of grieving as described by Kubler-Ross and Kessler (2005) i.e. denial, anger, bargaining, depression and acceptance. Families often believe that a miracle will occur, that their loved one will somehow return to normal. They believe that their family member will be fine. They pray for a miracle irrespective of their religious affiliation. Families may wish for the miracle to occur, say special prayers, arrange for other to say prayers, anoint the person with oil that has been blessed and other similar practices. What is the position of the health professional in such circumstances? The safety and wellbeing of the patient is the first priority. Provided that what the family wants to introduce cannot harm the patient, does not interfere with the medical and health regimen, nor causes any distress to the patient, there is no reason to deter them.

Families need to be realistic. They pray for a miracle but when it does not occur the families may need appropriate support. The realisation that a miracle has not occurred is one of the stages of grieving (Kubler-Ross and Kessler 2005). If a miracle does occur it will be a reason for joy and celebration.

---

### Reflection

A 16-year-old boy suffered a severe head injury, GCS 3/15. Based on the CT scan the medical team did not expect him to pull through. It was recommended that he be placed in a long-term residential facility but his family, who were deeply religious, chose to take him home and they implemented a home-based rehabilitation programme. Daily prayers were undertaken asking for his recovery. Today he is a happily married, employed person contributing to his family, community and society.

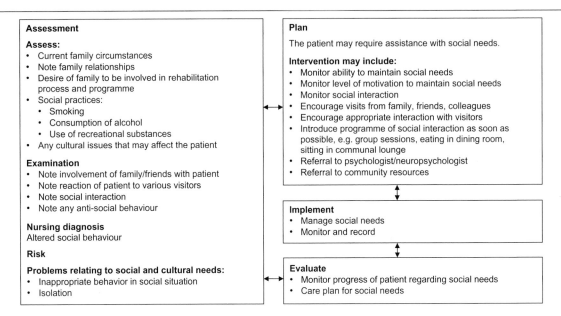

**Figure 3.19**　Social needs.
Definition: Social needs refers to patient's ability to develop and engage in social interaction and maintain healthy social practices and social behaviour.

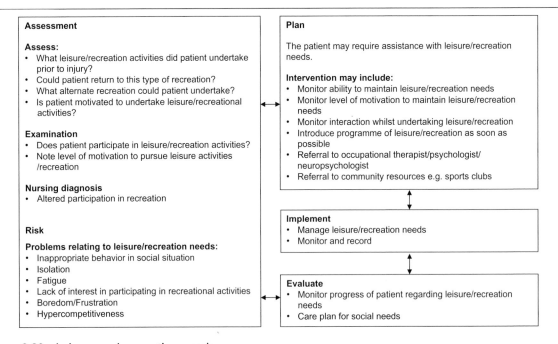

**Figure 3.20**　Leisure and recreation needs.
Definition: Leisure and recreation needs refers to patient's ability to actively participate in previous leisure and recreational activities or develop new leisure and recreational interests.

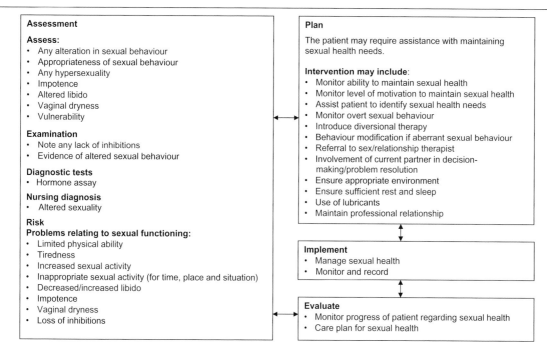

**Figure 3.21** Sexual health needs.
Definition: Sexual health needs refers to patient's ability to maintain feelings of love, belonging and sexual health, not merely the act of sexual intercourse.

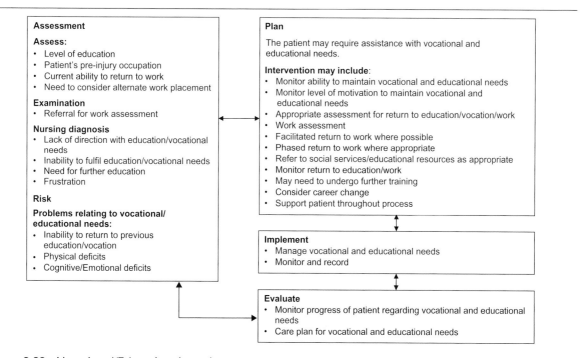

**Figure 3.22** Vocational/Educational needs.
Definition: Vocational/Educational needs refers to patient's ability to maintain interest and ability to return to previous vocational/educational abilities or learn new abilities.

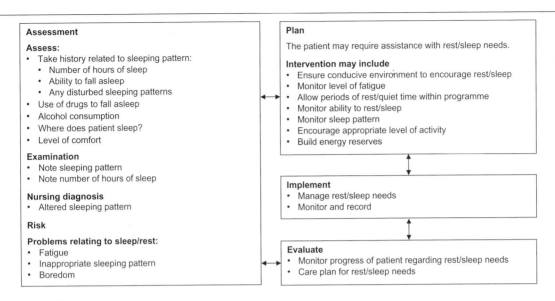

**Figure 3.23**  Rest and sleep needs.
Definition: Rest and sleep needs refers to patient's ability to rest and sleep in appropriate manner.

## NURSING DIAGNOSIS

Advancing nursing education and roles provide the nurse with the opportunity to utilise knowledge, expertise and skills to improve the quality of care of patients. Nursing diagnoses are used to plan, deliver and measure the outcomes of nursing (ARN and RNF 2006, Hoeman 2008). The use of nursing diagnoses improve cost-efficiency and cost-effectiveness with regard to nursing and health management (Müller-Staub *et al*. 2007, 2008). Utilising a nursing diagnosis framework within the Needs Approach Model enables nurses to provide care that is scientifically based and measurable in terms of the goals that are set (NANDA-I 2012). Nursing professionals, based on a sound foundation of unique knowledge as well as interprofessional and interagency knowledge, within the remit and scope of practice of the registered nurse, make nursing diagnoses on which appropriate decisions may be based. When considering a nursing diagnosis, the nurse takes into account knowledge of anatomy, physiology, pharmacology, pathology, microbiology, sociology, psychology, research, ethics as well as nursing knowledge.

Once the information from the history, examination and investigations, e.g. blood gases or chest x-ray, is available

it is necessary to compile appropriate nursing diagnoses that reflect the intervention required and the timeframe in which the outcome should be achieved.

It may be possible to utilise the Nursing Intervention Classification (NIC) to decide on appropriate intervention/s (NANDA-I 2012). The nursing intervention needs to be undertaken within a specific timeframe, i.e. the predicted timeframe to achieve the specific goal. It may also be possible to utilise the Nursing Outcome Classification (NOC) to decide on appropriate outcome/s (NANDA-I 2012).

### What is a nursing diagnosis?

A nursing diagnosis is a 'clinical judgment about individual, family or community experiences/responses to actual or potential health problems/life processes. A nursing diagnosis provides the basis for selection of nursing interventions to achieve outcomes for which the nurse has accountability' (NANDA-I 2012, back cover).

For a detailed nursing care plan incorporating nursing diagnoses see Chapter 23.

### Establishing relevant nursing diagnoses

Different organisations/institutions utilise varying nursing diagnoses (ARN and RNF 2006; Hoeman 2008). In practice, diagnoses are made depending on the patient's needs therefore not all nursing diagnoses are relevant to all patients. Nursing diagnoses from NANDA International (NANDA-I 2012) are used as well as other nursing diag-noses more specific to patients with neurotrauma (Abelson 1987). Additional nursing diagnoses may need to be estab-lished if the patient is suffering from polytrauma and co-morbidities.

**Table 3.2** Nursing diagnoses relevant to neurotrauma.

| Nursing diagnoses related to physical needs (Abelson 1987) | Nursing diagnoses related to physical needs (NANDA-I 2012) |
| --- | --- |
| Provision of therapeutic environment | Excess fluid volume |
| Potential for injury/trauma | Deficit fluid volume |
| Potential for infection | Impaired skin integrity |
| Alteration in level of consciousness | |
| Alteration in cerebral perfusion | |
| Alteration in ICP | |
| Alteration in cerebral function | |
| Alteration in skull integrity | |
| Cerebral dysfunction | |
| Alteration in respiratory function | |
| Respiratory dysfunction | |
| Potential for suffocation | |
| Alteration in cardiac function | |
| Alteration in cardiac output | |
| Maintenance of body fluids | |
| Impairment of kidney function | |
| Alteration in bowel elimination | |
| Nutritional deficit: | |
|    Risk of nutritional deficit | |
|    Alteration in metabolic functioning | |
| Alteration in thermoregulation | |
| Alteration in self-care activities | |
| Altered ability to attend to personal hygiene | |
| Altered ability to attend to dressing | |
| Alteration in comfort | |
| Impaired mobility | |
| Alteration in rest/sleep pattern | |
| Other nursing diagnoses may also need to be established | |
| **Nursing diagnoses related to family needs (Abelson 1987)** | **Nursing diagnoses related to family needs (NANDA-I 2012)** |
| Alteration in parenting | Anxiety |
| Role alteration | Fear |
| Adequacy of family coping | Grieving |
| Other nursing diagnoses may also need to be established | |

*(Continued)*

**Table 3.2** *(Continued)*

| Nursing diagnoses related to cognitive/emotional/psychological needs (Abelson 1987) | Nursing diagnoses related to cognitive/emotional/psychological needs (NANDA 2012) |
|---|---|
| Impaired communication | Anxiety |
| Inadequate therapeutic stimulation | Fear |
| Behaviour disorders | Grieving |
| Impaired cognitive functioning | Social isolation |
| Alteration in self-concept | |
| Alteration in socialisation patterns | |
| Altered spirituality | |
| Altered sexuality | |
| Maladaptive coping patterns | |
| Other nursing diagnoses may also need to be established | |

Nursing Diagnoses – Definitions and Classification 2012–2014. Copyright © 2012, 1994–2012 by NANDA International. Used by arrangement with Blackwell Publishing Limited, a company of John Wiley & Sons, Inc. (Abelson 1987; NANDA-I 2012)

## CONCLUSION

Using the Needs Approach Model, including nursing diagnoses, will enable health professionals to provide evidence-based holistic health care to meet the ever-changing needs of the patient and promote maximum recovery throughout the patient's journey.

---

## Activity 3.1

### Scenario

Mr Jones, 21 years old, was involved in a road traffic accident. He presented in Accident and Emergency with the following:

- GCS score 10/15.
- Restlessness.
- Fractured left ankle.
- ? abdominal injuries.

He is unaccompanied.

### Exercises

1. Using a needs approach, assess Mr Jones' needs.
2. Prepare a care plan for Mr Jones whilst in the A&E department (6 hours only).
3. Consider any aspects that are of significance to patient rehabilitation and recovery.

Utilise the following format:

| Nursing diagnosis | Potential problems | Possible causes | Intervention | Outcome/Evaluation |
|---|---|---|---|---|
| | | | | |
| | | | | |

## Activity 3.2

### Scenario

Mr Davidson, 28 years old, was involved in a road traffic accident. He has been in Accident and Emergency for the past 6 hours and has been transferred to the unit where you are working. He presents with the following:

- GCS score 9/15.
- Restlessness.
- Fractured ankle in plaster of paris.
- No blood in abdomen.
- Intravenous therapy in place in right forearm.
- Nil per mouth.

He is accompanied by his wife, Joanna, who is extremely distressed at the 'state of her husband'.

### Exercises

1. Using a needs approach assess Mr Davidson's needs.
2. Prepare a care plan for Mr Davidson whilst in the ward (24 hours only).
3. Consider any aspects that are of significance to patient rehabilitation and recovery.

| Nursing diagnosis | Potential problems | Possible causes | Intervention | Outcome/Evaluation |
|---|---|---|---|---|
|  |  |  |  |  |
|  |  |  |  |  |

## Activity 3.3

### Scenario

Mrs Priscilla Hopkins, 46 years old, has been admitted to A&E after suffering a 'blackout' after falling and hitting her head. She was brought to hospital by ambulance. She presents in A&E with the following:

- GCS score 14/15.
- Very tired.
- No neurological loss.
- She is very concerned as this has not happened previously.
- She has a fractured right wrist.
- Her scalp wound has bled profusely.

- She reports to you that she is on anticoagulant therapy as she has Atrial Fibrillation.

She is unaccompanied and is admitted to the 24 hour observation unit for monitoring.

### Exercises

1. Using a needs approach, assess Mrs Hopkins's needs.
2. Prepare a care plan for Mrs Hopkins whilst in the A&E department (6 hours only).
3. Consider any aspects that are of significance to patient rehabilitation and recovery.

| Nursing diagnosis | Potential problems | Possible causes | Intervention | Outcome/Evaluation |
|---|---|---|---|---|
|  |  |  |  |  |
|  |  |  |  |  |

## Activity 3.4

### Scenario

Mr van Vuuren, 65 years old, has suffered a left-sided hemiplegia after a head injury.

He presents in the ward with the following:

- GCS score 11/15.
- Restlessness.
- Dense left hemiplegia.
- He is unable to talk and is very frustrated.

He is accompanied by his wife, Martha, who is extremely distressed that her husband will be permanently disabled.

### Exercises

1. Using a needs approach assess Mr van Vuuren's needs.
2. Prepare a care plan for Mr van Vuuren whilst in the ward (24 hours only).
3. Consider any aspects that are of significance to patient rehabilitation and recovery.

Utilise the following format:

| Nursing diagnosis | Potential problems | Possible causes | Intervention | Outcome/Evaluation |
|---|---|---|---|---|
|  |  |  |  |  |
|  |  |  |  |  |

## Activity 3.5

### Scenario

A month ago Mr Wilson, 34 years old, was in a motor vehicle accident. He suffered from polytrauma.

His injuries included:

- Head injury with a GCS of 5/15.
- Fractured ribs 3, 4 and 5 on the right-hand side for which he has been on a ventilator.
- Fractured pelvis.
- Fractured left femur which is pinned.

His current functional ability is reported as:

- Current GCS 9/15. Disorientated.
- Left sided hemiparesis.
- Difficulty with speech and eating.

### Exercises

1. Prepare a cognitive rehabilitation programme that can commence in the unit as it will be some while before Mr Wilson can be transferred to the Rehabilitation Unit.
2. In the accident Mr Wilson's girlfriend, Samantha, was killed. Mr Wilson keeps on asking you why Samantha has not been to see him. Describe how you will manage this situation.
3. Mr Wilson's family are most distressed at the lack of information that has been provided to them regarding head injuries. Describe how you will manage the situation and develop a resource for the family.

# Chapter 4
# The Patient Matters

*Nadine Abelson-Mitchell[1], an anonymous carer and Sue Mottram[2]*

[1]School of Nursing and Midwifery, Faculty of Health, Education and Society, Plymouth University, Devon, UK
[2]Headway, Dorset, UK

## THE PATIENT

Neurotrauma care is a patient-centred process. Involving the patient and family within the team from the outset is essential for effective care planning. Throughout the patient journey it is essential for the multidisciplinary team to encourage the patient to take an active role, to develop a sense of belonging, to be valued as an individual, to participate in decision making, when appropriate, and to be an integral part of the system.

## FAMILY AND CARERS

It is important to obtain the family's co-operation for they retain the major responsibility for the patient. The role of carers within rehabilitation is ever increasing and for effective family relationships and rehabilitation, communication with the patient and family is essential.

The role of the multidisciplinary team with regard to the family includes:

1. Recognising the needs of the family in order to promote recovery.
2. Initiating family therapy, individual and group therapy, an essential element of neurotrauma care. Counselling and emotional support must occur as early as possible, in order to prepare the family for changes in the patient's behaviour and to avert inappropriate reactions that complicate the rehabilitation process.
3. Arranging regular meetings to keep the family fully informed, giving complete, honest answers and sensible advice to the family. Severe anxiety, denial, information overload, intimidation by the complexity of the injury, contradictory information provided by health professionals, timing of content and relevance of content all inhibit learning, retention and absorption of information. Aids to learning include web-based learning, group sessions and the use of helplines as well as access to community organisations.
4. Allowing and encouraging the family to work in, and with the programme, where appropriate. Use the family as a resource, as a support tool in the preventive rehabilitation programme and for reality orientation.
5. Referring the family to social services and a support group if this is available. Encouraging the patient and carer to contact voluntary organisations such as Headway (UKABIF 2004).
6. Assisting the family through the grieving process.
7. Preparing the relatives regarding the patient's recovery, interim and long-term goals. The attitude of the family towards the patient, the rehabilitation programme and recovery will affect the patient's rehabilitation outcome.

*Neurotrauma: Managing Patients with Head Injuries*, First Edition. Edited by Nadine Abelson-Mitchell.
© 2013 Blackwell Publishing Ltd. Published 2013 by Blackwell Publishing Ltd.

A positive, realistic attitude to the patient and recovery will aid the rehabilitation process. It is important to explain the emphasis on independence and self-care in the programme so that the family does not regard it as neglect, nor spoil the patient. A barrier to the patient's progress towards independence can be caused by others who utilise the patient's dependence as a prop for their own existence.

8. Allowing the family to express fears, anxieties and feelings, as they may be devastated. Stress is highest in the months following the accident and often the anxiety level of the family is related to the degree of eventual recovery.

The trauma disturbs the family's routine and affects both the injured patient and the family. The injured patient, because he is concerned about coping with additional financial costs and his future role in the family, and the family because of their reaction to seeing their loved family member in this state and their difficulty in coping with the uncertainty of the patient's outcome. Patients with residual psychological and cognitive impairment present a stressful situation for both themselves and the family. Issues that arise may relate to dependence, economic difficulty, dealing with support agencies regarding financial or other benefits and the change in role of the head injured patient, e.g. a competent housewife or a breadwinner in the house becoming dependent on financial support from other members of the family, the state or society (McCabe *et al.* 2007).

Family members and carers who accept responsibility for the care of the neurotrauma patient need physical, psychological and emotional strength. When the carer is a family member, it is important to assess their needs to ensure they are physically and psychologically able to care for the person. The carer may suffer from depression, anxiety and distress. It is therefore vital for carers to be provided with appropriate information and support to lessen their burden (McCabe *et al.* 2007).

The important effects of traumatic brain injury (TBI) include:
• The stress caused by the actual demand of caring for an individual with disability and the ensuing dependence on family members (McCabe *et al.* 2007).

• The difference between the burden of the patient with TBI on the family, compared to that of a patient with a spinal cord injury or debilitating illnesses, is that the patient with TBI exhibits greater dependency on the family.
• When the injured person is a sibling, the stress of caring for a sibling affects the behaviour and well-being of other siblings.
• The feeling that all the responsibility is falling on one person. The perception that 'no one will be there to care in the future' or 'nobody appreciates my efforts' is often found in carers. This personal concern is sometimes associated with the preference for institutional care.
• The stresses associated with the cost implications to the family, resentment and lost opportunities.
• Often carers report that prior to traumatic brain injury there was unhealthy family functioning or emotional stress (Sander *et al.* 2003). This finding makes carers more vulnerable to the stress associated with the injury and results in greater difficulties with coping.

9. Encouraging normal family relationships. An adverse effect on the relationship between spouses is mainly due to the behavioural problems of the injured person, especially if there is a young family at the time of injury. This is due to the lack of an established social support network and the dependency of the injured person on the spouse and any other children for social interaction, like friendship and confidence. In an established family where the patient is an injured adult, there is the risk that previous social contacts will disappear due to a change in interests, age and other factors. When the severely injured is a child, the opportunity to develop societal norms and a network of close friends is also reduced.

It has been found that marital relations are affected significantly, causing general loss of self-esteem and ultimately loss of marital cohesion. Domestic abuse as a cause of neurotrauma, or as a result of neurotrauma, must be considered and managed appropriately. The most common characteristic of brain-injured people is the loss of ability to empathise with others and this is an important source of marital difficulty. The divorce/separation rate five to eight years after injury is 49% (Wood and Yurdakul 1997).

## Case Study 1: From a carer's point of view

**Anonymous carer:**

One moment everything is 'normal', perhaps some excitement going on holiday the next day, all the preparation going well, we were looking forward to a nice easy few weeks. And then it happened. BANG. Everything changes in an instant; my husband was rushed to hospital in a coma.

I went from excitement to despair, fear of the unknown, and frightened. I was in an alien place; people rushing, machines beeping and the person I love motionless. There was no one to talk to, everyone doing something but me. I felt useless, out of control and all I did was try not to cry and keep a brave face.

What's going to happen to him? What's going to happen to me? 'Survival or the Unthinkable'. What will I do? What if? And silly things popping into my head; did I lock the door? I started to panic, trying to breath slowly, but all that was going through my head was what if . . . ? How am I going to manage . . . ? What are they doing to my husband? Why can't I see him? Why won't they tell me? Where is everyone? I can't sit still. I feel as if I'm going mad.

And then finally someone tells you what's happened. You only accept what is said at that time, but I was not able to take it in. I felt I was really on my own. At last I was able to see my husband, he looked the same, but I was not prepared for all the equipment and this was very frightening, but I thought 'Everything will be alright. He will be back to normal soon.'

I felt angry, 'How dare he cause such problems and now be peacefully asleep.' I still thought he would be OK and that life would resume as before (how wrong I was).

Trying to carry on a normal life was very difficult, because family and friends were concerned and asking questions that I could not answer. I wanted answers but there was never anyone to talk to. He was being cared for, but what about me? Visiting the hospital after a period of time, I found tiredness and resentment crept in because there was no response from him.

Time's going on and there are no clear signs of him getting back to normal, and then he's discharged home. I had no help, no discharge package, no social worker, no information on any changes there would be to him, or even how much damage he had suffered. He looked OK, he walked OK, but there was something not right!!!!!

BACK HOME, at last I thought life was back on track and it would only be a matter of time before he would be going back to work. Once again how wrong I was. My husband felt there was nothing wrong with him. As far as he was concerned he had not changed, nothing wrong with his memory, balance, behaviour. Ha! Ha!

For me it was frustration. I wanted to scream. I did not understand what had happened and my whole world was upside down in a split second. I lost my patience with him and myself, who can help me? Things were going downhill fast. Why, when he has been discharged from the hospital, is he not back to normal?

Financial difficulties were now setting in. I found I was overloaded with paperwork, telephone calls, finding the money to pay bills, coping with my husband's anger and frustration and I found that I was running on adrenaline. How much more can I take? It was time to visit my GP again. My husband was the priority, now it's more medication to face.

Thankfully it was my brother-in-law that told me that we may be entitled to some benefits; more paperwork to complete and what a mine field. I really could have done with some help.

By chance, in a local shop, I was able to make contact with an off-duty social worker who advised me to make an official contact for an appointment. Things started to improve for me, from having equipment, financial review, and most importantly Headway, which has changed both our lives completely. They have become OUR life-line. I value counselling as it has helped me to understand the enormity of the loss we have had, and that I am important. I am now able to make appropriate changes to my life after brain injury.

Life is still difficult and has numerous challenges, but I no longer feel alone or isolated. There are no answers, nothing prepares you for the future or the outcomes to living with someone with a brain injury. Everyone's experience is different and unique, however, there are some common factors when 'caring' for someone.

## Case Study 2: Consequences of head injury – a précis of a personal experience

On September 9th 1985, my 16 year old son gave me a broad grin as he rode past me in a bicycle race. The next time we saw him was two hours later in the resuscitation unit at hospital, convulsing and arching his back as a tube was being inserted to help him breathe. He had received severe head injuries as a result of hitting unmarked road works. He was transferred to intensive care, ventilated and put into a drug-induced coma to help relieve secondary swelling of his brain. We were told that he would likely die. We were given conflicting advice at the hospital. On the second day the neurologist said he would wake up and there would be no damage! Another doctor said that he would not recover but 'people like that are happy'. He remained in ITU for nine days, by which time he was breathing on his own. Once the sedation was removed he opened his eyes but remained a thin, jerky, vacant looking individual. He became very active and kept pulling at his tubes incessantly and even managed to dislodge his endotracheal tube.

On Monday, 16th September he slept all night without the ventilator and his respirations were good.

The nurses and doctors were extremely kind and worked hard to save him. One of us was always at the hospital and we did our best to stimulate and reassure him, whilst the other explored all avenues of possible help. We would have loved to have spoken to someone who had been through the same experience but were told that this was not possible. I read up about acquired brain injury in the post-graduate library but any information there was extremely depressing. I found a book by Joan Collins in a '10p bin' outside a newsagents 'Katy: A Fight for Life', which catalogued her daughter's recovery from a similar accident. It was a great help and comfort to us. We chased up specialists and facilities that they had found helpful. It also gave us an idea of what we should expect and how to deal with it. A day later, on Tuesday, he was moved into the ward as his bed was needed in ICU; he was still gravely ill. Basic care was very poor; no-one was assigned to him and we felt extremely vulnerable. It became apparent that there was very little knowledge of, and often no interest in, brain injury and rehabilitation. His first memory is of falling out of bed because no-one put his cot-sides up. I took him to all his therapy sessions and continued to carry out the exercises on his return to the ward. We spent many hours trying to

stimulate him – reading to him, playing games with him (when he was able to concentrate), and for many weeks trying to keep him in bed when he threw himself around whilst semi-conscious.

After repeatedly asking for a room of our own in the daytime, after many weeks, we were given the use of a side-room and were able to play and talk to our son in privacy each afternoon, rather than suffer the embarrassment of many curious eyes on us and many sniggers as he threw the bed clothes off (he was nursed naked) and made strange noises.

We felt that we could organise his rehabilitation more effectively at home and about two months later, on November 11th, he returned home after spending a weekend and many afternoons there. He could not walk unaided. He was now able to speak, although this was soft and slurred. He continually asked what had happened to him and whether he would walk again. He was now continent, although I had had a battle to stop them re-catheterising him after he pulled his catheter out. He needed continuous care and encouragement. His weight on discharge was just over 6.5 stone and his height was 5′ 10″, so both his physical and mental dependence was great.

Therapy sessions took place off the ward and there was no sharing of information between the various disciplines or to us. We were not made aware of any plans for the future and when I asked for a referral to a rehabilitation centre was told by the neurologist that he would recover just as well in a darkened room.

One day an occupational therapist brought flash cards for him but when my husband gave him a pen he wrote that he had a dreadful headache. Although he perseverated, we were able to communicate with him and we found our son again. He was able to joke with his sister. We also found out that case conferences had been held without our knowledge. After being dropped on his head three times, he was transferred to the neurogym and adult physiotherapy services. Although he had never sworn whilst regaining consciousness, when he was put into a standing-frame and stood up, he asked me whether, if the physiotherapist broke his legs, I would kill her. On hearing this she refused to treat him! We were then transferred to two brilliant physiotherapists, who we are extremely grateful to.

He returned to the hospital five days a week for physiotherapy and occupational therapy as well as medical appointments. Often occupational therapy sessions were cancelled but we were not informed until we got there. Due to his disinhibited and inappropriate behaviour he was given many 'holidays' from occupational therapy. No-one, apart from us, attempted to tackle this behaviour, thus he was rewarded for it.

Speech therapy was also patchy and became a battle of wills. The therapist said she could not continue to treat him until he accepted his difficulties. He had at that point tried to kill himself and was very distressed at his disabilities but would not admit this to her. He was given yet another 'holiday'.

We took him for singing lessons and to an elocution teacher. Both were invaluable. The elocution teacher tolerated no nonsense and he responded well to this. He also had private physiotherapy at the weekends. The physiotherapists were excellent and had a 'can do' philosophy. On their recommendation, as the hydrotherapy pool in the hospital was always unavailable, we hired a pool at a local school for children with disabilities. He found he could walk in water, which gave him so much pleasure and encouragement. We attended the Bobath Centre and they helped us continue with the therapy and exercises.

Over the next few months he continued to improve but became very depressed when the true state of his life hit him. He would try to hang himself from the stairs and threaten to kill himself. Many nights I slept with the door keys under my pillow in case he ran out. By early December he would walk (a few steps) unaided. Once he could stagger across the neuro-gym there was pressure to discharge him. The physiotherapists fought to keep him. I was doing a post-graduate degree in personnel management and they let me leave him with them for the day as a physiotherapy aide. By early spring (after much trying) he could ride his bike. He became very frustrated by the lack of freedom and on many occasions ran away on his bike (usually leaving a note). He was in no way safe to ride as lack of balance and control, together with his poor eyesight, made it most dangerous for him to be on the road. We had to notify the police on a number of occasions.

He was very sorry when he returned, or was returned, but still repeated this very worrying way of behaving. He kept repeating the same questions ad nauseum all day long and it was extremely wearing for his family for example, will I ever get better? Will I be able to ride my bike as I used to? What happened to me? We took him

skiing against medical advice and this was very successful for us all.

We persisted and he received an appointment at a rehabilitation centre after he had been at college for a year. In April 1986 it was decided to send him back to school part-time. I had previously contacted educational psychology for advice but was told that if he had an average IQ then it was nothing to do with them. He attended school 2.5 days per week and continued with his various therapies the other 2.5 days, as well as the private physiotherapy at the weekends. I returned to work. In retrospect this was premature, as he was extremely disinhibited in word and deed and caused much pain and embarrassment to his sister by his behaviour. He was also immature and could not settle in work. We had to take him to and from school and to and from the Hospital for his various therapies. These were often cancelled with short or no notice and I eventually gave up work. He still ran away from home on occasions. He lost his school friends due to his behaviour. He suffered five blackouts in the first week at school and epilepsy was diagnosed. It was felt that he needed individual tuition and a college in Southampton was found where he could re-sit his O-levels part-time.

I first had to take him and assess how he should travel. The railway station was too far away and the pavement very uneven, so there was a risk of him falling. The coach station was nearby so he was shown how to get to it – over and over again. The bus times and numbers had to be rehearsed and written down because of his poor memory. For two weeks I travelled with him to begin with until I felt satisfied that he was able to cope on his own. Almost all his activities involved such planning before he was able to manage. I had to organise a programme whereby steps were followed so that he would become competent, in safety. Simple tasks like going into a shop to buy a newspaper had to be rehearsed prior to him carrying it out.

During this very trying time I repeatedly asked for help from psychology as well as mental health. He was deemed inappropriate for mental health services and by the time psychology was available we were on to another problem. I asked for help with his social skills but he was put on a course devised for people with learning disabilities – nothing was tailored to his needs. He hit two people and started to steal from us but we dealt with this as best we could. At this time a clinical psychologist kindly allowed me to attend one of her courses for trainee clinical psychologists, which was invaluable. After his year at college where his grades improved I approached a Disability Employment Adviser. Careers advice was not helpful and he left them bemused with his contradictory answers. He has been assessed and deemed unemployable on two occasions based on working on electronic circuit boards and shelf-stacking.

This is a person with sight problems and a left hemiplegia!

He has attended college courses, worked in my husband's architectural practice, worked in retail, in a hotel belonging to friends of ours and for a while ran his own delivery business. Nothing has been successful for long. We all feel that we have failed in that he can now only do voluntary work. He now drives; I went with him to Banstead to be assessed prior to his taking driving lessons. He has been married and divorced, been to America, China and Europe with various girlfriends.

Even now I see him every day and we are there to sort out any problems he may have. These have included suicide attempts, assaults (on him), gambling and speeding convictions amongst many others. Headway is crucial in that he has a support system and a role (he fetches and carries; does the banking for the charity).

The trauma of our son's injury and the limited knowledge and help available to effect a significant rehabilitation for him, leaves us with feelings of guilt and helplessness, even when knowing that we have tried every avenue, professional and non-professional (e.g. faith healer, dance therapy, yoga, etc.) in our efforts to assist him.

I think both parents, the fathers more so; feel trapped and very isolated by the dependent child situation that now exists. Our daughter has had difficulty in coping with the changes in him. As a teenager she was in a position to go out with him to aid his social rehabilitation.

This she has found difficult and embarrassing due to his uninhibited behaviour (e.g. producing condoms whilst she and a friend were having coffee with him in Bournemouth) and slurred speech in front of her friends. His inability to settle also caused problems, for soon after arriving he always wanted to leave; he either pesters one incessantly or just walks off. Another consequence is the loss of an older brother. He is very much the immature member of the family who has to be looked after and this has both long and short-term consequences for our daughter; longer-term consequences should his parents reach a position where they are unable to look after him.

There have been, and will continue to be, significant financial consequences for the family as a result of his disabilities. We went through a successful compensation claim.

Finally we all have to try and plan a longer term way of life which will enable us to function in a continuing support situation for him. The consequences, which we will continue to deal with for our son, are a total change in our family, work and social lives, which has imposed huge strains on all members of the family.

As a consequence of his injury the family has gone through a number of stages in terms of the impact of the injury on them:

- Grief and despair when it was not certain that he would survive.
- Anxiety and bewilderment as the changes in him became apparent.
- A pre-occupation with helping him (mother gave up her career, both parents gave up virtually all leisure time after the accident, searching out rehabilitation services, visiting them, and initiating rehabilitation activities). This pre-occupation with helping our son in all available time led to a neglect of the needs of the remaining members of the family.
- Feelings of helplessness, despair and mourning, as the realisation that a much loved son and brother has changed, that the changes were long-term and permanent and that expert help that existed was insufficient to effect a recovery.
- Emotional turbulence between members of the family as they sought to come to terms with the long-term/permanent changes in him.
- Attempts (continuing) to re-organise our lives and adapt to the fact that he is faced with permanent disability, which threatens the resumption of the family, work and social life and has altered the lifestyle of the family totally.
- One of the hardest things for us to bear is seeing his frustration and unhappiness at what his life has become. He already feels that such normal desires as a job and a family of his own are unlikely to be fulfilled for him. This is a real tragedy for us all.

As a result of our journey I question whether acquired brain injury (ABI), after acute stage, is relevant in an acute hospital where the medical model is practiced. Rehabilitation should be placed under the social care model. Over the years it has become apparent that there is still no organised care pathway, no joined up working. Apart from Headway it is not needs-led (people sent back to work too soon), no designated housing, benefits, etc.

In 1993 Headway Dorset was founded as it was still apparent that services for ABI were inadequate. We aim to provide a client-centred, needs-led service. Referrals for clients with ABI come from many and varied sources. These referrals may come from any one of a number of agencies and organisations dealing with different services provided to these clients, and the same client may be referred to several agencies at the same time. This situation leads to duplication of effort for some clients and for others it may mean that they get missed altogether. In order to simplify and streamline this situation, it is suggested that a Single Point of Access (SPA) be considered. The proposal for the SPA approach is drawn from the Gold Standard Pathway for ABI Services drawn up by Sussex Acquired Brain Injury Forum (SABIF) and West Sussex Acquired Brain Injury Network.

One point I want to stress is although the professionals were not providing what was needed, when it was needed, they kept approaching me saying that they were there if I needed to talk. I felt that this was inappropriate and when setting up Headway ensured that carer support was separate from rehabilitation. What we find now is that the therapists all want to counsel the relatives but most of the relatives' anguish could be alleviated if their cared for person received proper rehabilitation.

## CONCLUSION

The carers' stories are a poignant reflection of the issues raised when a person has a TBI. On reflection, it appears that concerns raised by the families are not being addressed. Families retain the major burden of care for the patients. Services are neither accessible nor equitable and more needs to be done for patients with TBI to enable them to return to a positive role within the family and community.

# Chapter 5
# Multidisciplinary Management

*Nadine Abelson-Mitchell[1] and Katie Searle[2]*

[1]School of Nursing and Midwifery, Faculty of Health, Education and Society, Plymouth University, Devon, UK
[2]Plymouth Community Healthcare CIC, Devon, UK

## INTRODUCTION

The most effective means of achieving high quality care for the head-injured patient is through a multidisciplinary team approach from the outset until ultimate recovery (BSRM 2009, 2008a; RCP 2010). In order to meet the needs of the head-injured patient adequately, co-ordination of patient management by a multidisciplinary team will lead to one co-ordinator directing, but not necessarily supervising, many disciplines. Each team member, within the scope of practice of his or her profession, has independent, dependent and interdependent functions and is responsible and accountable for the prescribed therapeutic intervention. The professionals are consultants, teachers and resource persons who function as peers in decision-making. Rehabilitation is interprofessional collaborative patient care carried out as a continuing programme with general medical care (RCP 2010). Continually changing government agendas, initiatives, technology, the pressure of finances and demographics, and conflicting demands of professional interests, will inevitably lead to changes in the make-up and responsibilities of the rehabilitation team providing rehabilitation services (DH 1998, 2000a, 2000b, 2000c, 2001a, 2001b, 2004a, 2004b, 2005a, 2006a, 2007a, 2007b, 2007c, 2008a; RCP 2010).

> **Reflection**
>
> 'Imagine, if you can, that you are permanently confined to a wheelchair or a bed. You have to wait to be fed, wait to be put on a bedpan, then be stripped and bathed with the door wide open and people coming in and out. You have to wait for someone to bring you your drink of water, turn on the TV for you, comb your hair, clean your filthy glasses. You have to wait for someone to come sit down and talk with you or give you a hug.
>
> You wait for a letter from anyone, a visit, a friendly nod, some sign that you still exist as a person – not just a body to be moved around several times a day, bathed, fed, changed and put to bed. . . .
>
> You have a past history. You used to matter to somebody, and you want to matter today. Imagine all this, if you can, and then you might begin to have just an inkling of what it must be like to be helpless and dependent, to lose your dignity and your pride, to be trapped and know that you have years of this ahead of you. Imagine all of this and maybe you could try just a little bit harder for that human touch. Remember, these people raised us. They were young people with hopes and dreams just like us, and we will be old just like them. These people are our future.'
> (Anonymous)

The patient passes through various specialities during their journey, from care at the scene, the Emergency Department, neuro ICU, HDU, a ward and rehabilitation services. There are also many other stops along this journey. This can be a prolonged and frightening experience as the patient is exposed to numerous professionals and unknown situations along the way. An empathetic and gentle orientation and training for the patient and family about the system, as well as how to navigate through it, is important and necessary as it builds a healthy alliance. An atmosphere of trust and mutual understanding aids the process of rehabilitation. The central focus of the team is the patient. Every endeavour must be made to involve the patient where possible in the rehabilitation process. The patient and the family need to be given an opportunity to be part of the team because it is the family that knows the patient best.

---

In order to achieve an effective team, personnel require certain characteristics:

- A caring attitude.
- Confidence.
- The ability to do activities with, rather than for, patients.
- The ability to laugh with, not at, patients.
- A good sense of humour.
- Patience: the ability to repeat the same activity or statement many times.
- Tolerance.
- Forgiveness: sometimes patients and families can be very demanding.
- Good interpersonal skills.
- Good communication skills.
  - To listen and hear.
  - To observe and see.

---

## STAFFING

Within the various care settings, it is difficult to give the precise number of personnel required without knowing: the type of unit, acuity of patients, resources available, availability of specialised rehabilitation personnel, accessibility of support systems, and community resources. The members of the health team that may be involved in the

care and rehabilitation of the head injured patient include those shown in Figure 5.1.

### The physician

The rehabilitation medicine consultant is regarded as the rehabilitation team leader who is legally responsible for the patient's overall management (RCP 2010). The rehabilitation team may be headed by a physiatrist (medical practitioner trained in rehabilitation medicine) who is responsible for supervising the patient's rehabilitation programme.

The question of which medical practitioner should have final accountability for the patient's management remains debatable. The head-injured person is primarily the responsibility of the neurosurgeon, but if all head-injured patients were admitted under the neurosurgeon's direct surveillance an increased number of neurosurgical beds would be necessary. In the acute phase, most head-injured patients are cared for by doctors whose speciality is not the brain (RCP 2010).

The role of the rehabilitation medicine consultant includes, but is not limited, to that shown in Table 5.1.

### The nurse

The role of the nurse in the pre-hospital, emergency unit, ward situation, physical and psychological rehabilitation from the outset, must not be underestimated (American Association of Rehabilitation Nurses (ARN), www.rehabnurse.org/advocacy/content/roleofnurse.html). The ARN stresses the need for rehabilitation nurses to be employed 'where ever rehabilitation is provided' (www.rehabnurse.org). Quality nursing care is supported when the nursing department functions on an equal and integrated basis with all other departments and is strengthened when effective collaborative relationships exist between nurses, physicians and allied health professionals. The nurse is a full member of the team with responsibility for comprehensive care of patients. It is essential that nurses, within their scope of practice, support the work of the team. Rehabilitation commences as soon as the patient is admitted and includes nursing input from acute treatment until the patient has resumed a positive role in society.

The nurse's attitude and approach may affect the entire therapeutic milieu. In the acute phase, the nurse is the one member of the health team who is with the patient constantly, has the most contact with the patient, medical and allied health personnel and families. The personnel involved in the care of the head-injured patient rely on the nurse's assessment of the patient via verbal or written feedback in order to make management decisions. This raises a number of issues within the multidisciplinary team. Nurses cannot do 'follow-on therapy' for a physiotherapist or occupational therapist. When nurses accept to undertake an activity with the patient, it must be within their scope of practice, and they must be trained and competent to perform the delegated activity.

## SPEECH AND LANGUAGE THERAPY SERVICES

The speech and language therapist (SALT) provides detailed and individualised assessment/diagnosis, treatment and management of patients with varied and complex needs and backgrounds within the multidisciplinary team (MDT). A 'Care Aims' Model is used to prioritise the case load and aims to treat high priority patients at least daily.

Aspects of patient recovery included in SALT responsibilities are:

- **Aphasia/dysphasia**: acquired language impairment.
- **Dysarthria**: disturbance in muscular control of the speech mechanisms.
- **Apraxia of speech**: impaired motor programming and co-ordination of speech muscles.
- **Dysphagia**: swallowing difficulties, including tracheostomy.
- **Cognitive communication impairment**: impaired communication resulting from combination of linguistic and cognitive deficits.

The role of the SALT is to optimise the patient's communication potential, support and educate family/carers, the MDT, and liaise with outside agencies regarding the impact of the person's communication impairment.

Intervention is tailored to the person and takes place in one-to-one sessions, group/joint sessions, and in combination with other team members/therapists where appropriate. SALT intervention can be directed at the level of impairment, disability, participation and psycho-social adjustment – often simultaneously. Treatment is strictly goal-led, with a strong focus placed on enabling the person to set their own goals, wherever possible. Intervention aims to remediate the person's communication difficulties, whilst working to educate the person and significant others about the nature of the difficulty and how to compensate for lost skills.

In people with aphasia, comprehension of written and spoken information is often affected, meaning the SALT often works with the person to re-inforce key information regarding their rehabilitation (goals, discharge planning, etc.).

Communication impairments present as very subtle changes in patients with TBI, but have a profound impact on maintaining and forming relationships. A high level of experience and knowledge is therefore required in order to diagnose and manage these cases sensitively and effectively.

SALTs play an important role in the MDT in establishing the capacity of a patient to make fundamental decisions around their care and future needs. This is often a complex issue, with significant implications for the person, their family and the focus of intervention.

The SALT is responsible for identifying the need for alternative means of communication (communication aids) and referring to the appropriate centres for assessment and purchase of appropriate equipment.

SALTs are responsible for the management of dysphagic patients, which includes liaison with the dietician, nursing and housekeeping staff. Intervention with these patients often takes place at mealtimes, in a setting best suited to the individual. This frequently takes place with occupational therapists to establish safety and independence when feeding.

SALTs make referrals for videofluoroscopy assessments and to other departments where necessary, for example to the Ear, Nose and Throat Department.

SALTs play a key role in the management of patients with tracheostomies. Alongside physiotherapists, nursing and medical staff, SALTs work to establish safe oral intake and effective verbal communication, where possible.

SALTs work closely with occupational therapists and neuropsychologists to assess the presence of language and cognitive deficits, and the impact of these on the person's communication and capacity to make informed decisions.

Due to the nature of TBI patients, a large part of the SALT role is, by necessity, to establish sufficient insight into their difficulties in order to have effective intervention, whilst enabling the person to communicate their needs and feelings effectively. This involves close working with the neuropsychologist, using video recording, education and work with families.

SALTs facilitate communication with outside agencies regarding the wishes of the person, by explaining the options and their implications for the person in an accessible way. These agencies may include social services, residential/nursing homes, the police and solicitors, amongst others. SALTs are able to facilitate more community work to implement therapeutic advice in functional settings, in readiness for a timely and successful discharge.

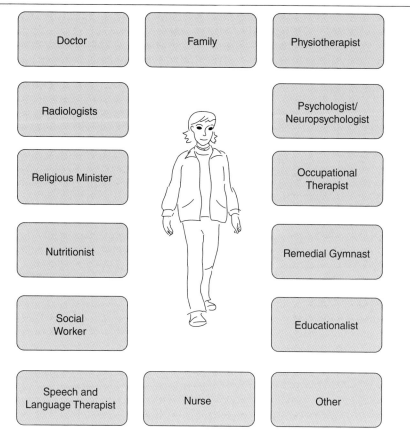

**Figure 5.1** The multidisciplinary team.

**Table 5.1** Role of rehabilitation medicine consultant.

| In-patient | Out-patient | Community |
|---|---|---|
| Ward rounds | Unidisciplinary medical out-patient clinics | Multidisciplinary team meetings |
| In-patient multidisciplinary team meetings | Special clinics, e.g. spasticity clinics Young adult clinics | Outreach clinics |
| Referral work | | Home visits |
| Interdisciplinary liaison | | Scheduled visits to specialist nursing homes |
| Case conferences | | |
| Clinically related administration | | Home-based interagency review meetings |
| Specialist on call | | Outreach or network-based activity |

(RCP 2010)

SALTs, as members of the multidisciplinary team, play a role in:

- Being a Key Worker.
- Training and participation in the use of goal setting, outcome measures (FIM+FAM), and the role of Key Worker.

- Providing in-service training on communication and swallowing difficulties in ABI.
- Arranging and chairing progress meetings.

---

## Activity 5.1

1  In your practice is there a multidisciplinary team?
2  Design a programme to improve multidisciplinary function and communication.
3  Prepare a multidisciplinary, holistic discharge plan for a 22 year old patient who is to be discharged in three weeks, including available resources.

Current status:

- GCS 10/15.
- Continent.
- Able to eat with assistance.
- Mobilising with frame.
- Loss of memory.
- Difficulty speaking but can use some words and gestures to communicate.

Discharge destination: staying with parents in house with 14 stairs to bedrooms.

# Chapter 6
# Physiotherapy

*Jude Fewings*

South West Regional Neurosurgical Centre, Plymouth, Devon, UK

## INTRODUCTION

Early intervention aims to maintain optimal respiratory function – thereby limiting secondary brain damage, avoiding weaning delays, preserving the integrity of the musculoskeletal system and starting the process of regaining motor control. In order for multidisciplinary teams, particularly nursing and therapy staff, to manage patients with TBI they must have an understanding of neural and muscle physiology, pathophysiology of the brain injury and a working knowledge of all rehabilitation concepts and clinical experience. An accurate assessment needs to be made. A problem list and individual treatment plan is then constructed; no two head injured patients will have the same deficits/medical problems (Campbell 2000; Clini and Ambrosini 2005).

Recent research advocating the need for early rehabilitation has been supported by government initiatives identifying the importance of timely rehabilitation (Audit Commission 1999; DH 2004a, 2005c; RCP 2010). Prolonged ICU stays have been associated with reduced function and greater mortality, as well as increased costs (Chang *et al.* 2004).

Advances in medical technology allow patients with extensive neural injuries (who in the past would most certainly have died) to live and be maintained for indefinite periods of time, irrespective of the ultimate outcome. The severity of the primary injury directly relates to the period of unconsciousness, during which time they are more susceptible to secondary adaptations of the musculoskeletal system compared with their conscious counterparts, and thus have poorer functional outcomes (Stucki *et al.* 2005).

## RESPIRATORY CARE

Early physiotherapeutic, nursing and medical interventions in the acute ICU stages are initially to facilitate and maintain the parameters of optimal cerebral oxygenation in the presence of raised intracranial pressure (ICP), which is said to occur in about 70% of severe head injuries (Bullock and Teasdale 1990). Potential problems can arise from the impact of the damage to vital centres within the brain, causing respiratory depression, abnormal breathing patterns and risk of infection from aspiration, local injury or merely immobility.

## POSITIONING

The optimum position, initially with respect to maintaining cerebral perfusion, is one of the head up at 15–30° with the neck in a neutral position, whereby venous drainage is facilitated without compromise to the systolic blood pressure thereby maximising the cerebral perfusion pressure (Chudley 1994).

*Neurotrauma: Managing Patients with Head Injuries*, First Edition. Edited by Nadine Abelson-Mitchell.
© 2013 Blackwell Publishing Ltd. Published 2013 by Blackwell Publishing Ltd.

As the patient's clinical condition develops so too does the positioning regime. If a chest infection becomes an issue then postural drainage and side-lying positions can be used (strictly no head down due to potential ICP rises), bone flap deficits need careful consideration when side lying a patient. Additionally when used in conjunction with sedation and paralysation agents assisting medical management of the patient, the use of positioning has benefits in preventing or slowing the changes in skeletal muscle structure which have been said to occur within hours (Williams 1990). These changes occur more rapidly in the neurologically-impaired patient (Grossman 1982).

## MUSCULOSKELETAL INTEGRITY AND NEUROMUSCULAR STATUS

Spasticity results from any lesion in the upper motor neurone pathway, causing absence (or disruption) of extrapyramidal inhibitory influence on alpha and gamma motor neurones. Reflex arcs are disinhibited giving rise to hyperreflexia and increased tone, typically in the antigravity muscles – the upper limb flexors and lower limb extensors. A velocity dependant increase in the tonic stretch is seen, i.e. greater resistance to faster stretch.

Spasticity can occur early following TBI and may result in limb deformities, compromising patient care and delaying early rehabilitation (Mortenson and Eng 2003; Pohl *et al.* 2003; Pope 2002; Verplanke *et al.* 2005).

Muscle stretch/lengthening is resisted by hypertonia. As a consequence muscles remain in a shortened position for prolonged periods of time which results in changes to the physical properties of muscle and associated soft tissues. Sarcomeres in series, responsible for determining the distance and force of contraction, are reduced thus decreasing length and extensibility (Verplanke *et al.* 2005).

The muscle and soft tissue changes result in loss of joint range and movement (Campbell 2000; Edwards and Charlton 2002). Muscle function can also be compounded by pain associated with heterotopic ossification and the presence of skeletal fractures in the patient with multiple injuries (Hurvitz *et al.* 1992) (see Chapter 26 on sequelae).

Stretch, either active or passive, is recommended to prevent contracture formation. The optimum degree and frequency is unknown, however prolonged stretch has been shown to reduce spasticity (Mortenson and Eng 2003; Schmit *et al.* 2000). This is achieved by casting, which is now an established means of controlling contractures and spasticity in both adults and children (Edwards and Charlton 2002). Proactive casting is frequently employed early

in the course of TBI. This provides the prolonged stretch required to maintain joint range during the initial unconscious period and is commonly applied prior to weaning from ventilation (Campbell 2000; Edwards and Charlton 2002; Singer *et al.* 2003). The optimum method of casting (removable and non-removable) remains debatable. Removable casts are custom made to allow a passive range of movement exercises to maintain tissue and joint extensibility. Potential drawbacks of non-removable serial casting include muscle atrophy, pain, increased DVT risk and pressure ulceration. The most suitable method of casting depends on the patient's diagnosis, cognition and conscious level (Mortenson and Eng 2003; Pohl *et al.* 2003; Singer *et al.* 2003).

From the management point of view, spasticity has two components amenable to treatment – the biomechanical and neural (Barnes 2001; Pope 2002; Verplanke *et al.* 2005). The biomechanical aspect is managed by physiotherapy – passive movements, positioning, splinting and casting are all commonplace (Barnes 2001). Alleviation of the neural component is achieved by antispasmodic drugs: Baclofen and Tizanidine are commonly used, others include Sodium Dantrolene and Clonidine. All these drugs have potential side effects (Barnes 2001) and some have been implicated in possibly delaying cognitive recovery following brain injury (Dobkin 2000; Jackson-Friedman *et al.* 1997).

In cases of focal spasticity or severe spasticity – Botulinum Toxin A (BTX-A) can be used. BTX-A is a powerful neurotoxin which inhibits pre-synaptic acetylcholine release at the neurotransmitter junction producing a localised temporary muscle weakness (Barnes 2001). Its effects can be seen within 24–72 hours and last on average three to four months. Used in conjunction with passive movements and casting, it has been shown to significantly reduce tone, allow toleration of the cast and improve functional recovery (Kay *et al.* 2004).

## SUMMARY

The multidisciplinary team's care of the patient, while they are on bed rest and potentially unwell, has been outlined so far. The 24-hour management of these patients, their chest care and musculoskeletal integrity is of paramount importance.

The physiotherapy team will assess, treat, advise and instigate treatment plans, which will then be discussed with and implemented by the nursing team.

It is essential that the nursing team are able to understand and provide this tandem approach to care in order to ensure that the patient's recovery is optimised. This essentially is the beginning of the rehabilitation process for the patient.

Nursing staff should have an awareness of the splints being used, know why they are being used and be able to passively move the patient's limbs in order to:

- Maintain muscle length.
- Accurately place limbs in splints.
- Provide comfortable therapeutic positioning for the patient.

## REHABILITATION AND MOTOR CONTROL THEORIES

The wide variety of treatment approaches in rehabilitation have their foundations in an array of motor control theories (Horak *et al.* 1997; Mathiowetz and Haugen 1994). The challenge for the physiotherapist is to develop their own model of practice, where the treatment methods they select have a scientific, physiotherapeutic and practical knowledge base.

Plant (1998) states that physiotherapy practice in neurology falls into three broad categories:

1. Neurodevelopmental or neurophysiological, i.e. Bobath (1969, 1990).
2. Motor learning and relearning, i.e. Carr *et al.* (1995).
3. Eclectic.

The eclectic approach is a mix of the real world of physiotherapy practice (Plant 1998).

Movement between different positions (postural sets) aims to stimulate proprioceptive input and thereby enhance efferent activity (Allum *et al.* 1998). Excitation of the vestibulospinal tract involves recruitment of lower limb extensors, proximal musculature and head movement (Kandel *et al.* 1995). This is closely linked with reticulospinal tract activity, influencing extensor tone and involving the cerebellum in maintaining equilibrium. Since the feet afford afferent input into the vestibulospinal tract, standing can be used as a therapeutic means of activation.

The tilt-table is a useful adjunct to facilitate early, safe standing. It is particularly useful for patients who are unconscious and require total support (Edwards 1996). Additionally, the use of weight-bearing helps maintain length in the plantarflexors (Richardson 1991). Brain injured recumbent patients have impaired autonomic orthostatic responses, initially only small angles of tilt should be used with continued monitoring of BP, $SaO_2$, HR, RR and pallor. Malalignment should be avoided as this impairs normal proprioceptive input (Chang *et al.* 2004).

Trunk control is equally as important as respiratory care and spasticity management in the rehabilitation of the head injured. The role of the trunk is fundamental to head control and limb function via the shoulder and pelvic girdles (Davies 1994).

Physiotherapy treatment of the trunk therefore needs to be incorporated; for this reason treatment plans frequently involve alternating sessions of standing (tilt-table initially, therapist facilitated later) and working in sitting position.

Positioning attained by the tilt-table and sitting enables normal head–neck alignment, stimulates visual and vestibular facilitated pathways and promotes dynamic stability of anterior neck muscles. The anterior neck muscles are important for tongue movements and swallowing as they help stabilise the hyoid bone (Mohr 1990). Early active and passive oro-facial movements are encouraged as this helps with respiratory care, nutrition and communication recovery (Davies 1994).

Movement modulation mediated by the cerebellum can be targeted to assist motor learning by means of task(s) repetition (Frank and Earl 1990; Horak *et al.* 1997). Movement and control of movement against gravity encourages balance control, i.e. facilitation of the vestibular system; weight bearing and recruitment of postural tone can be assisted by using a smaller base of support and movement between postural sets. As improvements in proximal trunk control, head control and selective lower limb movements occur, treatments gradually incorporate facilitation of gait. The therapist should continually strive to rehabilitate patients beyond their present functional ability in order to attain their maximal future functional status.

## POSTURE AND SEATING

Posture and seating are important to normalise proprioceptive feedback as postural stability is necessary for functional activity. Seating systems are frequently used for patients with severe neurologic impairment and are used as adjuncts to the previously mentioned treatments. The range of ankle movement and tone management are fundamental to wheelchair dependant patients, the ability to achieve plantar grade contributes to ease and safety of transfer into the chair, and also reduces the risk of pressure areas associated with poor alignment (Singer *et al.* 2003).

By applying external supports to the patient in the most functional and least restrictive positions, a stable posture can be attained (Pope 2002). It is important to consider appropriate orientation of the trunk in space. Rearward tilting is used in many seating systems (Green *et al.* 1992). The use of gravity to assist stability is considered vital in the severely posturally incompetent patient but must be used with caution to limit any further detrimental effects of social, visual and environmental isolation (Andersson *et al.* 1974). Additionally a wedge cushion, bilateral thoracic supports and head support along with the inclusion of a table (to assist in supporting the upper limbs and encourage midline orientation), can be used to build a stable posture (Pope 2002). Stability in the sitting position confers better oro-facial control, swallowing and speech; social interaction and communication are enhanced thus re-inforcing recovery of function and improving the patients' quality of life (Pope 2002). Nurses are equally responsible for mobilising patients. The type of seating system used has important rehabilitation considerations and the act of sitting out of bed can be used as a rehabilitation technique since significant levels of endurance, muscle strength and muscle tone will be required. An ability to understand and use seating systems is necessary for nurses to be instrumental in the rehabilitation process. If done incorrectly, this everyday task causes significant lifetime complications and poor functional outcome for patients.

## CONCLUSION

For a multidisciplinary team providing 24-hour care to a head-injured patient, it is imperative that, as the patient's condition stabilises, the early phases of rehabilitation commence. For nurses working within the MDT in an acute setting, the demands on their time are multifold. Nurses are with the patient for the longest part of any day. It is important, therefore, that once the therapy team has assessed the patient's functional abilities these are handed over to the nursing team with the appropriate recording of those abilities.

In the early stages following TBI, patients have a limited ability to tolerate even the most simple of interventions. Maintaining optimal conditions for brain recovery and avoiding secondary brain damage are the principle treatment maxims. An accurate functional and respiratory assessment and multidisciplinary treatment approach are vital. The demands and priorities of the brain injured patient frequently change and therefore treatment regimes should consistently be reviewed and updated. Close observation and assessment must continue even when medical stability is achieved. There is a need to stimulate the body via proprioceptive input and enhance movement and the control of movement, as well as providing other aspects of coma stimulation to those remaining in PTA. The emphasis is on sitting patients both upright in bed and out of bed, ensuring that the environment around them attempts to increase their level of awareness (see Chapter 28).

Early and timely rehabilitation is vital to limit and promote recovery from any neurologic deficit. Improving and shortening ITU stays ultimately reduces mortality, improves functional outcome and reduces cost (Audit Commission 1999; DH 2004a, 2005a).

# Chapter 7
# Neuropsychology

*Michelle Smith*

Wessex Neurological Centre, University Hospital Southampton, UK

## INTRODUCTION

The aim of this section is to introduce neuropsychology in traumatic brain injury (TBI) rehabilitation for the nurse who is perhaps relatively new to this clinical field and to encourage further interest in those with more experience, but it cannot hope to cover all aspects in depth. The content has been inspired by the queries from the various nursing colleagues I have worked with over many years in neurorehabilitation settings.

## WHAT IS CLINICAL NEUROPSYCHOLOGY?

Clinical neuropsychology is a specialist area of applied clinical psychology that derives a theoretical knowledge base from several sources, but especially the neurosciences and cognitive psychology. This helps to provide an understanding of brain functions (cognition, behaviour, emotion) against a background of neuroanatomy, neurophysiology and neuropathology.

## WHO IS A CLINICAL NEUROPSYCHOLOGIST?

In the UK, a clinical neuropsychologist is usually a clinical psychologist who has post-qualification training in the field. Some neuropsychologists may come from other backgrounds, including education and academic settings.

## WHAT IS THE ROLE OF THE CLINICAL NEUROPSYCHOLOGIST IN THE MANAGEMENT OF TBI?

Roles vary but include:

- Helping to define and describe the neuropsychological changes following TBI and monitoring the progress of these over time.
- Using theoretical knowledge, evidence-based practice, and clinical experience to assess neuropsychological functioning.
- Helping other people to understand profiles of residual and changed abilities, and the impact and implications of these.
- Working with multidisciplinary colleagues to create appropriate rehabilitation and therapy programmes.

Some areas of knowledge and expertise overlap with those of other professional colleagues, such as speech and language therapists and occupational therapists.

## NEUROPSYCHOLOGICAL FUNCTIONS

The neuropsychological consequences of TBI can involve cognitive, behavioural and emotional systems. The

*Neurotrauma: Managing Patients with Head Injuries*, First Edition. Edited by Nadine Abelson-Mitchell.
© 2013 Blackwell Publishing Ltd. Published 2013 by Blackwell Publishing Ltd.

following briefly outlines some of the neuropsychological impairments that can occur after TBI.

## Attention and information processing

These abilities enable maintaining focus on tasks, dealing with distractions and taking in different kinds of information.

These skills include:

- Sustained attention – concentration over time.
- Focused attention – ignoring distractions.
- Selective attention – choosing the appropriate stimuli.
- Divided attention – multi-tasking.

TBI can affect the efficiency of these functions and reduce someone's capability of dealing with the speed, quantity and complexity of information (Mathias and Wheaton 2007).

## Memory and learning

Learning means the ability to acquire new information and skills, and this ability is particularly vulnerable after TBI. Memory processes include being able to register, encode, retain and retrieve information (see Chapter 12).

There are different kinds of memory:

- Short-term or working memory – information held on a temporary basis for short period of time, such as looking up and then dialling a telephone number.
- Long-term memory – information retained for much longer periods, even permanently. This includes recent memories and remote memory of information and events from many years ago.
- Prospective memory – remembering to do something in the future.

Other terms refer to the sort of information held in memory.

- Semantic memory – general knowledge about the world.
- Episodic memory – personal experiences and events.
- Procedural memory and learning – particularly for behavioural skills.

Impairments of memory and ability to learn new things are very common consequences of TBI (Barker-Collo and Feigin 2008; Vakil 2005).

## Language

Very simply, language skills enable processing and understanding of spoken and written information and enable one to speak and write.

- Receptive dysphasia – problems understanding spoken communication.
- Expressive dysphasia – difficulties with spoken language, such as problems finding words and names.
- Dyslexia – deficits affecting reading and spelling.

When these are changed by TBI, changes can range from very mild and subtle to very severe. Mild deficits may not easily be identified without the professional skills of a speech and language therapist or clinical neuropsychologist.

## Verbal skills

Other verbal intellectual abilities include calculation skills and logical reasoning.

## Perceptual and constructional skills

Perceptual abilities are those that help us recognise and make sense of the information received by the brain. This information may be received via visual, auditory or tactile routes.

- Agnosia – impaired ability to recognise visual, auditory or tactile stimuli.
- Sensory inattention or neglect – inability to consciously register information presented to the opposite side of the particular area of the brain damage. This most frequently occurs for stimuli presented on the left. The patient is often unaware of the problem.
- Apraxia or dyspraxia – difficulties with producing organised sequences of behaviour to perform a task. This is sometimes more of a problem when the person is asked to deliberately follow an instruction. Because the task can sometimes be carried out successfully when the person does it almost accidentally or incidentally, this may be mistaken for lack of co-operation or compliance.

Occupational therapists as well as clinical neuropsychologists are skilled at identifying these kinds of problems.

## Executive functions

Executive functions comprise a number of high-level cognitive abilities that enable a person to plan, organise and implement actions to achieve purposeful goals. These abilities are mostly associated with the frontal lobes of the brain. It is rather like the board of directors of a cognitive company, and other cognitive systems are the specialised departments. A particular department may not be seriously impaired following TBI, but if the board of directors is damaged, then that department does not operate effectively without direction. In contrast, if the executive board retains good function, then compensatory strategies can be developed to support a damaged cognitive department. Again, unfortunately, the executive systems are also very vulnerable to TBI and, when impaired, can contribute to long-term reduced independence (Rassovsky *et al.* 2006) and occupational functioning (Strucken *et al.* 2008).

### Neurobehavioural changes

Changes in behaviour and character are frequently associated with frontal damage and are not easily assessed with formal tests of cognitive abilities. It is important to discuss this with the family or others who are familiar with the patient prior to the TBI to clarify what has changed, and to help them understand why it has. It may also be helpful to make systematic observations of particular behaviours and environmental influences on those behaviours (Vetruba *et al.* 2008). This can help the clinical neuropsychologist and other professional team members to offer guidance for managing behaviour if necessary. Some behavioural changes persist in the long term and may be a prominent limitation on independent functioning and community integration (Cattelani *et al.* 2008; Reid-Arndt *et al.* 2007).

### Emotional changes

Emotional changes may be a direct result of the TBI, but also a result of the patient's reactions to the consequences, such as impaired abilities and personal loss. These will vary with the stage of recovery and progress. Depression should be recognised and treated, and the patient should be able to discuss fears and anxieties as they arise (Bay and Donders 2008; Bornhofen and McDonald 2008; Draper *et al.* 2007; Pagulayan *et al.* 2008).

### THE PATIENT'S NEUROPSYCHOLOGICAL JOURNEY

### Post-traumatic amnesia (PTA)

After emergence from coma or other states of impaired consciousness, the patient may still be very confused. The duration of PTA for any one individual may vary from a few seconds or minutes, to hours, days, weeks or months for those with more severe TBI. It has been defined as a failure of everyday memory, but is usually characterised by a range of other disrupted cognitive functions and behaviours, which can easily be misunderstood if not recognised.

Some features of PTA include:

• Confusion and disorientation.
• Fatigue.
• Irritability and agitation.
• Impaired everyday memory.
• Confabulation.
• Other cognitive impairments.

### Case study 1

A young man with a severe TBI, but minor physical injuries, was in PTA for several weeks. At one point it was thought he could be experiencing hallucinations as he complained of bombs going off during the night. Careful exploration revealed subtle expressive language difficulties and he was actually referring to someone having dropped a metal tray in the middle of the night.

### Case study 2

A woman sustained severe head injuries during an assault. Although very disorientated for time and place, she confidently and repeatedly described details of the assault and her assailant. She was socially and vocally very plausible but unfortunately all the information was entirely confabulatory.

During the period of PTA, the person is unlikely to be able to focus and maintain attention, will fatigue easily and become overwhelmed by too much stimulation. They can be supported by simplifying the environment, engaging in simple short activities, planning rest times and particularly encouraging visitors to attend in small numbers for short periods. Orientation information may be provided, but directly confronting confabulatory information may result in re-inforcing incorrect beliefs and can provoke agitation. Clinical experience suggests distraction and diversion can be more productive tactics.

### After PTA

At this stage, more formal and detailed assessments of cognitive functions can be informative to determine on-going cognitive changes and residual cognitive strengths. This profile contributes to understanding the consequences of traumatic TBI for that person, family members and friends. Physical injuries and difficulties are often more obvious and tend to capture attention. Cognitive, behavioural and emotional changes can be extremely subtle and difficult for both the patient and layperson to understand, but do impact on rehabilitation programmes and frequently contribute to distress.

### Case study 3

An elderly lady suffered a right cerebral hemisphere stroke. She was orientated and able to hold good conversations with the clinical staff, but became very distressed and agitated when the orthodontist 'stole' her false teeth, despite reassurances that they were in a glass on top of the locker on the left side of her bed. She was found to have a left visual inattention which meant she was unaware of the locker and her teeth!

### Case study 4

A middle-aged man suffered a diffuse TBI with widespread damage to both frontal lobes. Many of his cognitive abilities appeared to be relatively preserved on formal testing, but some of the most difficult aspects for his family revolved around changes in behaviour and character associated with the frontal damage. He showed poor judgement, safety awareness and ability to initiate action. This passivity had initially made home visits relatively simple for his family until an incident occurred where his wife choked on some food. She eventually managed to help herself, but was very upset that her husband just sat and watched apparently unable to initiate help.

### Long-term neuropsychological changes

There may be noticeable changes and improvements for many people in the months following TBI. These are slow and appear to plateau. Further improvements over many years can still be achieved through compensation and adaptation. Ecologically valid activities, such as getting up in the morning, preparing food, etc. can have therapeutic benefits on cognitive functioning and behaviour, and provide motivation to engage in rehabilitation. Patients are more likely to engage in neuropsychological and other rehabilitation activities if they have a functional reason and need to do so. It is important that these needs continue to be recognised in planning for further support and input

after discharge. The highly structured in-patient environment can often cushion the impact of neuropsychological changes, which only become more apparent when this level of support is reduced. For instance, there are many cues in a ward or rehabilitation unit to support someone remembering what to do at the right time. But, once in the community, any cognitive problems such as memory and executive difficulties become more exposed.

### Case study 5

After several months in a rehabilitation unit following a severe TBI, a young woman was discharged home to live with her parents, who were out at work during the day. At first, she would get confused about day, date and time, and how and when to carry out her daily activities. With the support of carers and her family, a structured set of compensatory memory and planning strategies, such as a diary and goal-setting, were developed and implemented in order for her to become more independent. After several months, she was able to spontaneously use the memory and planning aids to manage many of her every day needs.

## ADDITIONAL FACTORS INFLUENCING NEUROPSYCHOLOGICAL FUNCTIONING

### Medication

Side effects of some medication, such as anticonvulsants and antispasticity drugs, may reduce cognitive efficiency. It is helpful to be aware of any potential side effects of medication a patient is taking routinely.

### Seizures

TBI increases the possibility of developing seizures which, if they do occur, can also be disruptive to cognitive systems, especially memory (Lowenstein, 2009).

### Insomnia

Disturbances of sleep are common following TBI and can interact adversely with other aspects, such as cognition, emotions and health (Ouellet *et al.* 2004).

### Emotional states

Clinical depression and anxiety can reduce the efficiency of cognitive performance and therefore will also have an impact on damaged cognitive systems.

## OTHER ISSUES AND CONSIDERATIONS

### Cognition and mental capacity

Information regarding neuropsychological changes and current status can be helpful when queries regarding capacity arise (DH 2007e, Mental Capacity Act 2007). Not only in defining impairments that may have a bearing on capacity decisions, but also in assisting the capacity assessment process by recommendations on how the patient may best be supported in the light of cognitive impairments such as memory problems. The presence of neuropsychological deficits does not necessarily mean someone does not have capacity to make specific decisions.

### Multidisciplinary team working

The strengths of a multidisciplinary team lie in individual and shared professional expertise about TBI and the potential consequences and subsequent management and rehabilitation. An agreed formulation is important for consistency of the rehabilitation programmes and goals as the many facets of human systems and functions, from physical to psychological and social, are intrinsically integrated. This will impact on management and rehabilitation, for instance, memory or language impairments can interfere with a physical therapy programme and the physiotherapist may find input from other professional colleagues helpful to maximise therapeutic gains. Those in the nursing role are in a unique position to be aware of the patient over 24 hours, providing a very particular perspective about the person and his or her needs. Nurses are also often the first port of call for family and friends of the person with a TBI (Hudson *et al.* 2008).

### The family

If TBI professionals sometimes struggle to understand the subtlety of neuropsychological changes following a TBI, it is only going to be very much more difficult for families and others in the patient's life and they will need time to develop understanding and time for adjustments.

---

### Implications for practice

Always remember that the person you are working with has a brain injury which changes how they can interact with the world.

#### Guidelines

- Review the environment and how it might be adapted to help them.
- Consider how personal interactions, yours and others, can facilitate or hinder a specific situation.
- Take into account any known cognitive difficulties.
- Implement recommendations from the MDT.
- Be aware and identify other factors, such as mood, medication, etc. that may be important.

---

### Activity 7.1

#### Scenario

A 43 year old lady was involved in a car accident two weeks ago. She was unconscious for a week, and is now talking and partially mobile, but is still in PTA.

#### Exercise

1. What aspects of current cognitive functioning would the nurses need to be particularly aware of?
2. How might these be managed and helped?

# Chapter 8
# Social Considerations

*Judi Thomson[1] and Anthony Gilbert[2]*

[1]Headway, Dorset, UK
[2]School of Social Science and Social Work, Plymouth University, Devon, UK

## THE ROLE OF THE SOCIAL WORKER

Traumatic brain injury (TBI) changes life for the individual in an instant. The effect can be long-term and far-reaching, impacting on relationships, work, finance, education, self-esteem, image and aspirations for the future. The social worker plays a significant and important role in providing support, information and care, which can substantially influence how these experiences are managed. The ideal scenario in which the social worker, patient and his or her family can best work together is outlined in this chapter.

Many hospitals have a social worker attached who can get to know a person's situation from the outset and support them through the minefield of the early days and weeks ahead.

When the initial crisis occurs, and throughout the patient's journey, the social worker provides literature and information relating to brain injury and imparts this in a timely fashion when people are ready, finds information appropriate for children and assists parents in how they might communicate.

The social worker assists with financial and practical difficulties. They may be able to advise about grants to help with travel or other sudden expenses, e.g. Headway has an emergency fund whereby amounts up to £500 can be obtained to help with accommodation and other expenses incurred when a family member has a TBI. Finances may be of great concern and advice can be given about appropriate welfare benefits and referrals made to benefits specialists. Practical advice about services for people with a disability, advice about services and opportunities for the disabled, e.g. Blue Badge scheme, other services such as meal provision, assistance with managing medication and advice about housing issues, all may be needed. Citizens Advice Bureau are particularly useful. Social workers can also apply for any grants that may provide financial assistance and there are often many local resources. Often advice is needed about how relatives can access money, particularly if their loved one is in a coma or unable to deal with their own affairs. The social worker will be trained in how to assess mental capacity and will be able to work with colleagues to manage the situation best, as time for recovery will be crucial and decisions often cannot be made immediately. Even if the patient has cognitive difficulties this will not necessarily mean that they are unable to manage their affairs. The social worker can also act as an advocate in these situations or refer to appropriate advo-

*Neurotrauma: Managing Patients with Head Injuries*, First Edition. Edited by Nadine Abelson-Mitchell.
© 2013 Blackwell Publishing Ltd. Published 2013 by Blackwell Publishing Ltd.

cacy services. They can give advice about enduring power of attorney and the Court of Protection. The social worker can put the patient and their family in touch with other appropriate services and ensure they have support from solicitors, police and other organisations. Solicitors can then appoint case managers who will then represent the patient, ensure they have all services available to them and are provided with interim finance whilst any compensation claims are undertaken.

The social worker provides emotional support and helps to interpret feelings of initial shock and devastation. Patients and their relatives all experience huge changes and, most importantly, are coping with the loss of the person they once knew. Their grief moves through shock, hope, depression and hopefully final adjustment, but all need great support from a range of individuals to enable them to complete this journey in a way that is right for them.

The social worker promotes interagency and multi-disciplinary working, refers patients to other professionals if additional help is needed and also links with general practitioners. They can also create links with medical and nursing colleagues to try to ensure that all questions are answered in order to try to reduce the enormous anxiety.

When discharge from hospital is being planned, the social worker will then have a role in organising any care that may be needed. It is important to remember that the hospital has a duty to undertake a safe and timely discharge and any worries should be discussed before going home. Under s47 of the NHS and Community Care Act 1990, councils are required to assess the need for community care services for the people in their area who appear to be in need of such services, and decide, in the light of this assessment, whether services should be provided for that person. Although they have a duty to assess everyone who is eligible, they are not automatically able to offer services to everyone who contacts them. Nowadays, with greatly stretched resources, services inevitably have been very squeezed.

An assessment includes talking to the patient about their situation and their care needs and, with their consent, discussing these with any professionals who may be involved.

Family, friends and neighbours can also be involved, if appropriate. A process called the 'Single Assessment' means that all involved can contribute to a single document, which cuts the need for repeated questioning. The patient can also take part in self-assessment, which means they can emphasise what is important to them and can

determine their own outcomes and goals with the help of the social worker.

Social services use guidelines, which they call eligibility criteria, to find out if people's level of need qualifies for a service. The criteria divide into Critical, Substantial, Moderate and Low. They also complete a financial assessment as their services are means-tested, and each social worker can provide more specific details and information.

Patients also have the option of individual budgets, which allow much greater flexibility when purchasing care. Patients can have a direct payment and use this to pay directly for a service, and they can combine this with other monies that may be available such as the Independent Living Fund. All social services departments have organisations that they commission to help with the employment of carers and personal assistants; many people prefer this to having social services commission the care on their behalf.

When being assessed for social services care patients can also be assessed for their eligibility for continuing healthcare if they are deemed to have a primary healthcare need. The social worker can advise and link in with local health services to make assessments. Health funding and screening should be completed prior to discharge but they can be looked at again at any time. The social worker can remain involved, although care may be transferred to the patient's locality. Any care packages are subject to regular review.

Councils also have a duty to inform carers of their right to an assessment of their needs under the Carers (Equal Opportunities) Act 2004, which is independent of the assessment of the patient. When undertaking a carer's assessment the Local Authority must consider whether the carer works, undertakes any form of education, training or leisure activity, or wishes to do any of these things.

Carers often have enormous feelings of guilt and betrayal and need an opportunity to express these feelings in a safe, trusting environment on their own. Carers may need to be seen separately because there may be potential conflicts of need. GPs also keep registers of carers and provide services via their practices. There are also separate services that exist to support young carers, who are often very isolated and need an opportunity to meet with others. In many circumstances, particularly with older head-injured patients, there may be people who are cared for at home who require carers. These carers can link in with the local services.

Throughout the patients' and families' journey the social worker is instrumental in helping ensure best practice to make sure the patient's needs are met.

## SOCIAL ISSUES

### Personalisation and safeguarding: twin pillars of contemporary social support

Personalisation has arisen as a part of the consumerist agenda embedded in Western social policy (Powell 2009; Powell and Gilbert 2011). It is partly a response to the expectations of individuals and populations that the State should tailor support to meet health and social care needs in a flexible and individualised way (Dittrich 2009; Samuel 2008). Since the 1980s in the United Kingdom there has been growing interest among policy makers and service users alike in developing ways that enable adults who need support and help with day-to-day activities to exercise choice and control over that help (Powell 2005). Growing dissatisfaction has been articulated, particularly by working disabled people, about the inflexibility and unreliability of directly-provided social care services. These have been argued to create dependency rather than promoting independence, and impede disabled people from enjoying full citizenship rights (Dowson and Greig 2009). Instead, disabled people have argued for the right to exercise choice and control over their lives by having control over the support they need to live independently. This, they have argued, can be achieved by giving them the resources with which to purchase and organise their own support in place of services provided in-kind (Samuel 2008). These increased expectations are strongly felt in public services and challenge the traditional relationship between the State and vulnerable groups such as patients with neurotrauma, older people, the physically, mentally, intellectually and emotionally challenged and people who are frail and sick. Significantly, the personalisation agenda dissolved all these traditional user groups and their corresponding specialist provider groupings in local authorities into a single entity of 'adult social care'.

In policy terms the foundations of personalisation in the 1993 community care reforms (NHS and Community Care Act 1990) made front-line care managers responsible for purchasing individualised 'packages' of services from a range of different providers, tailored to meet individual needs and preferences (Powell 2005). At that time, the position of monopolistic authority service providers was challenged by the active encouragement of a 'mixed economy' of social care services, funded by local authorities but provided by a range of charitable and for-profit organisations (Gilbert and Powell 2010; Powell 2009). The potential of the 'mixed economy' shifted radically when the Community Care (Direct Payments) Act (1996) was incorporated by the Green Paper *Independence Wellbeing and Choice* (DH 2005b) which set out the basis for personalised care and support. Policy commentators argued for the active involvement of users in the co-production of services, as this is seen as a means to introduce new incentives for social and health care providers to respond to individual demands. The new incentives for service users will optimise how the resources under their control are used in order to increase cost-effectiveness. This has been repeatedly stated in key policy documents including *Improving the Life Chances of Disabled People* (published by the Prime Minister's Strategy Unit in 2005), and the 2006 Community Services White Paper, *Our Health, Our Care, Our Say* (DH 2006a), which announced the piloting of individual budgets, a development of direct payments. Later *Putting People First* (DH 2007d) promoted a system-wide revision of adult care and support, coining the slogan 'the personalisation agenda' as the centrepiece of a general strategy that included the extension of personalisation to the NHS as envisaged by Lord Darzi's review (DH 2007c). The current administration extended this commitment with *Capable Communities and Active Citizens* (DH 2010b) supported by the cross-sector statement *Think Local, Act Personal* (DH 2011a); firmly linking personalisation to the notion of the 'Big Society'.

The move away from state-directed resource allocation to user-controlled support mirrors developments in North American such as the consumer led Cash and Counseling schemes (Doty *et al.* 2007; Glendinning *et al.* 2008; Simon-Rusinowitz *et al.* 2000, 2002) and northern European examples such as those in the Netherlands, France, Austria and Germany (Boxall *et al.* 2009; Da Roit and Le Bihan 2008; Kreimer 2006; Ungerson and Yeandle 2006; Wiener *et al.* 2003). Such developments, generally referred to as 'cash for care schemes' brought with them a new language of responsibility (Dittrich 2009) involving debates about how social welfare might best achieve the balance between civil liberties and self-constraint. Put simply, personalisation, in Lundsgaard's (2005) language of sustainability, argues for the effective use of resources, empowerment, participation, control, choice and human rights. In the process, this effectively re-casts the focus for health and social support away from the State and onto the individual. Users of welfare services are now responsible for meeting their own needs from a 'personalised' individual budget while parallel processes of risk management and safeguarding protect the state from unnecessary exposure (Manthorpe *et al.* 2009).

Personalisation is underpinned by the notion that every person who receives support, whether this is provided by statutory services or self-funded, will have choice and control over the shape of that support in all care settings (DH 2008c; Glendinning *et al.* 2008). Carr (2008) suggests the overall aim is for social care service users to have control over how money allocated to their care is spent. Personalisation includes within its remit direct payments, individual budgets, personal budgets, user-led services and self-directed support (Glendinning *et al.* 2008). Self-assessment is the cornerstone of personalisation. It gives service users the opportunity to assess their own care and support needs and decide how their individual budgets are spent, while at the same time providing the dynamic for transforming social care (Carr 2008). In circumstances where the service user has limited capacity to either engage in self-assessment or direct their support, a range of possibilities arise such as family and friends, community-based organisations, community-based advocacy groups, brokers and agency staff (Social Care Institute for Excellence [SCIE] 2011), which may be supported by the provisions of the Mental Capacity Act (DH 2007e) such as powers of attorney.

The introduction of personalisation is not without challenges and the extent to which the objectives will be realised is far from certain, as currently the evidence base in relation to the critical success factors is small (Glendinning *et al.* 2008; Moran 2006; Rabiee and Moran 2006). However, both the previous and the current administrations have shown great enthusiasm for the wholesale extension of individual budgets in some form, such that implementation and investment has run ahead of evaluation. Nevertheless, it is easy to see the attractions of personalisation in policy terms as governments look to distance themselves from decisions over the shape of welfare, how it should be delivered, who delivers and at what quality. New Labour under Gordon Brown (2007–2010) identified personalisation as a mechanism to promote individual rights and transform the shape of adult health and social care services. Following the principle that the relationship between the service user and the State is one where citizens are encouraged and enabled to take full control of their needs, the service user has a budget through which they can purchase goods and services to meet a range of self-assessed needs in ways they choose (Leadbeater 2008). Consequentially, social care is transformed from a system where people have to accept professionally-driven definitions of need and corresponding services to one where people have greater control, not only over the type of support offered, but also how and when it is offered, how it is paid for and how it helps them achieve the outcomes that are important to them (Dowson and Greig 2009).

According to Carr (2008), personalisation has the potential to re-organise the way we create public goods and deliver public services. Leadbeater (2004) suggests that to understand personalisation we must locate it in its broad political context of 'participation', as service users become actively involved in selecting and shaping the services they receive. By engaging the tradition of participation, personalisation makes the connection between the individual and the collective, linking the public and the private spheres of life by enabling users to have a more direct, informed and creative say in 'rewriting the script' by which the services they use is designed, planned, delivered and evaluated. Furthermore, service users should be supported and enabled by professionals rather than be dependent on their judgements, with the opportunity to question, challenge and deliberate while also making suggestions about and making demands for more appropriate forms of support. Consequentially, personalisation changes the degree to which the state impinges on individual autonomy.

Critically, invoking the tradition of participation ensures that service users are not merely consumers, choosing between different packages offered to them. Rather, service users should be intimately involved in shaping and 'co-producing' the service they want. This has five key implications: (i) finding new collaborative ways of working and developing local partnerships, which (co) produce a range of services for people to choose from and opportunities for social inclusion; (ii) tailoring support to people's individual needs; (iii) recognising and supporting carers in their role, while enabling them to maintain a life beyond their caring responsibilities (DH 2008b); (iv) access to universal community services and resources – a 'total system' response; and (v) early intervention and prevention so that people are supported early on and in a way that's right for them. Implementing self-directed support is therefore as much about changing cultures as it is about changing systems (Gilbert and Powell 2010).

There are concerns that service users engaging in self-assessment may under-assess their needs. In order to counteract this, many service users, are turning to the voluntary sector to act as advocates and help them to complete the self-assessment forms and to imagine a desirable lifestyle. In some areas a dual system of care manager or social worker assessment alongside self-assessment has emerged. The ease with which individuals adapt to self-assessment differs across patient groups, with people with physical or sensory impairments adapting the easiest to individual budgets (Moran 2006). The inclusion of older people in individual budgets proved more difficult. There was also some reluctance from health service staff to offer individual budgets to mental health service users (Moran 2006). Nevertheless, people receiving an individual budget were significantly more likely to report feeling in control of their daily lives, welcoming the support obtained and how it was delivered, compared to those receiving conventional social care services (Glendinning *et al.* 2008).

Other personalisation concerns relate to the increased opportunity for abuse with the increasing deregulation of the workforce, particularly the employment of personal assistants (Breda *et al.* 2006), and financial abuse including fraud and theft. Before moving on it is important to recognise the importance of risk and risk-taking to personhood and adulthood (Mitchell and Glendinning 2008). Nevertheless, many individuals using care and support are vulnerable when exposed to particular situations. The 'personalisation agenda' sets out the way risk management enables flexibility, while safeguarding provides the mechanism through which concerns, omissions and violations are managed. In this sense, personalisation and safeguarding provide the twin pillars of adult social care policy and practice. All health and social care agencies, both statutory and non-statutory, within a specific local authority administrative area are covered by the multi-agency safeguarding procedures based on the policy guidance included in *No Secrets* (DH 2000d), which defined abuse in the context of an abuse of human rights. These set out the appropriate actions when a case of abuse is suspected. With respect to the governance arrangements covering individual budgets, these are set out in the Chartered Institute of Public Finance and Accounting (CIPFA 2007) guidance, which provides an enabling framework for managing individual budgets within a risk assessment framework. However, issues around safeguarding have already arisen, with financial abuse becoming the second most common form of abuse

reported (Boxall *et al.* 2009; Manthorpe *et al.* 2009; Stanley *et al.* 2011).

## CONCLUSION

This chapter has covered the conceptual and policy underpinnings of personalisation and its relation to substantive issues in self-directed care in communities across the UK. The personalisation agenda has brought significant changes to the way adult care and support is envisaged. The move to various forms of individual budgets means a major shift in the way social care and individual support providers approach providing services. Central to the process is the notion of self-assessment enabling service users to frame their needs in their own terms. This brings with it a greater focus on individual choice and responsibility while, at the same time, drawing in family, friends and community-based organisations. Professionals, particularly those in social service agencies, are seen as having an enabling rather than a directing role. This shift acknowledges the desire of many disabled people for autonomy and citizenship at the same time as it effectively distances the State from individuals. In addition, personalisation produces debates and moral dilemmas about what are appropriate choices and legitimate goods to meet needs.

Personalisation is intended to liberate the creativity of individuals in meeting their own needs, which brings with it an element of risk. It is important to see risk and risk-taking as crucial aspects of adult life. Risk is managed in part by supported and individualised planning and in part by the multi-agency safeguarding policies and procedures developed by all local authorities to prevent abuse (DH 2000d). However, it is acknowledged that personalisation brings with it new opportunities while the deregulation of many of the people working as personal assistants increases risk. Opportunities for financial abuse have also increased making this one of the most prevalent forms, if not the most prevalent form, of abuse. Nevertheless, personalisation does provide a strategy for support that acknowledges the status of adults receiving care and support as citizens with rights to participate in the definition and provision of that support.

# Chapter 9
# Occupational Therapy

*Danielle Williams*

Royal Hospital for Neuro-disability, London, UK

The aim of the occupational therapist, throughout the patient journey, is to assist in the development of their patient's potential towards their maximum competence and minimal dependence wherever possible. Occupational therapy is diverse and often complex, especially when working within a community-based, multidisciplinary rehabilitation team with people who have had a TBI.

This chapter will focus on issues related to working with patients who have suffered TBIs, although the process of assessment and intervention, the cognitive, physical and psychological effects, and the nature of the patients' journey can also relate to patients who have had a CVA, brain damage due to infections or haemorrhage.

Occupational therapists, as with all healthcare professionals when referred a new patient, spend time information-gathering. The amount of background information received with a referral can vary; an initial assessment with the patient can give a wealth of information, and health professionals, carers and family can all add further details to the picture of the patient as they are now, and who they were prior to their injury. It is important to gain a picture of a patient from all these sources, with the consent of the patient, wherever possible.

Whilst many patients may have been comprehensively assessed and may have been in-patients in hospitals and rehabilitation units, having been seen by a multidisciplinary team, there are many patients for whom this may not be the case. Some patients may have been seen briefly in A&E, with some follow-up from their GP, but their ongoing difficulties may not have been immediately obvious. Others, who have been seen in an acute setting, may have had obvious and urgent medical needs that have been addressed, and have made extensive physical recovery. However, cognitive and psychological difficulties may not have revealed themselves during a hospital stay due to the supportive and structured environment. Once a person is discharged home, different problems may come to the fore. A thorough process of information-gathering ensures that what has gone before is not simply relied upon, which can lead to patients 'falling through the gaps'. It is essential to have an open dialogue with the patient, and not to rely on discharge summaries and previous assessments, or on the account given by well-meaning family or friends. It is the individual who is living the experience and who has a unique perspective and is, after all, the person who should be at the heart of any rehabilitation plan.

*Neurotrauma: Managing Patients with Head Injuries*, First Edition. Edited by Nadine Abelson-Mitchell.
© 2013 Blackwell Publishing Ltd. Published 2013 by Blackwell Publishing Ltd.

However, it is also very important to be mindful of the impact of two important concepts within any long-term condition: insight and acceptance. Insight, or an individual's understanding and awareness of the effects of their injury, can be reduced as a consequence of a brain injury. Specifically, damage to the frontal lobe can affect an individual's metacognition, and therefore their ability to self-monitor. This can often lead to a patient being unaware of difficulties that they may have, even when there may be evidence to strongly suggest otherwise to an observer. For example, the patient who misses or forgets to attend several appointments but when questioned about cognitive deficits, states they don't feel they have any significant memory problems.

Acceptance is to do with the psychological journey a patient goes through following a TBI. At early stages post-injury, it is often a protective psychological coping strategy for the patient to deny difficulties, and believe that they are fine and that everything is 'back to normal' rather than accepting that their situation is the result of direct damage to their cognitive functions. Once again, this can lead to the patient not recognising their difficulties and therefore they may not always be a reliable source of information. This is not a reason for not interviewing the patient. It is essential to ask them about their experience and their perception of their levels of function and it also highlights the importance of triangulation.

At this stage, just talking with and observing a patient can give a wealth of information outside of what they are actually saying. A picture of the patient's physical and social environment will be built up. Levels of performance in functional activities will be discussed, including activities of daily living (ADLs), self-care, medication management, food preparation, leisure and vocational activities, etc. The patient will be asked about changes experienced in their physical, sensory, cognitive and psychological condition since the injury. Any communication difficulties will likely be revealed, whether this is dysarthria, expressive or receptive dysphasia. Psychological concerns, possible post-traumatic stress disorder symptoms or signs of anxiety or low mood, may be revealed. When it comes to cognitive changes, this is often the hardest area for patients to describe or understand. Terms like memory, attention, information processing, visual processing and executive functioning are not commonly understood, in the clinical sense, by the general public. Often, a patient will report memory difficulties, but to a professional involved in cognitive rehabilitation, listening to how these problems manifest can sound more like an attentional deficit. Therefore, when asking a patient about their cognitive difficulties, leading them into a conversation around functional activities may demonstrate the cognitive deficits they are experiencing. As examples, asking the patient to recount their experience of shopping in the supermarket will often give an excellent insight into many of these difficulties. Asking a patient if they find it difficult to locate the thing they are looking for on a crowded shelf can indicate visual processing or visual attention difficulties. If a patient says they don't go to the supermarket as they cannot deal with all the noise, this might indicate selective attention or information processing deficits. Reports of getting to the shop and then realising that they have left their list at home might indicate memory or attention deficits.

Using the knowledge from the initial information-gathering, it is often useful to carry out standardised assessments to clarify the deficits that are evident. Further assessment of additional cognitional needs can be attained using the Test of Everyday Attention (TEA), Rivermead Memory Test, Behavioural Assessment of Dysexecutive Syndrome (BADS) and the Chessington Occupational Therapy Neurological Assessment Battery (COTNAB) (Wilson *et al.* 2009). Whilst standardised assessments give a useful insight, observational assessments of patients engaging in functional activities are also important. Road safety assessments, kitchen assessments, observing patients in groups, or visiting the supermarket together are all important ways to establish levels of function.

Once a clear picture of a patient's presenting problems has been formulated, in terms of their physical, cognitive and psycho-social skills, the start of an intervention plan can be put together. This will involve finding out the patient's goals and then identifying the specific skill deficits that are barriers to achieving those goals. This is when activity analysis becomes important. For example, if the patient's goal is to be able to use their telephone, all the stages involved in making or receiving a call need to be considered. This includes recognising the phone is ringing, being able to operate the phone, being able to process verbal information, and to respond verbally with no visual cues, retaining information, remembering or reading numbers, having confidence, etc. A patient may have a range of deficits that make this difficult, so each one will need to be targeted in order to build up skills before the patient can practise using the telephone and learn to do so with confidence. A start may be made with work on identifying numbers, learning strategies to use when speed of information processing is impaired; exercises to improve fine motor skills could be implemented and role-play can give the patient a chance to practise. The type of intervention will be dictated by the individual, their skills, knowledge and motivation and may include activities which to healthy people are relatively simple tasks, such as: cooking independently, mobilising with a stick instead of a frame, gaining paid or voluntary work or accessing public transport.

Occupational therapy is the professional speciality that enables the development of the traumatic brain-injured person towards achieving their maximum physical and psychological potential.

# Section 2
# PRE-REQUISITE KNOWLEDGE

**INTRODUCTION**

This section enables the reader to understand the background to neurotrauma. Information included in this chapter relates to epidemiology and primary prevention of head injuries in adults, applied anatomy and physiology, investigations, microbiology and pharmacology. This information is necessary to enable health professionals to manage patients effectively.

---

**Key objectives**

On completion of this section you should be able to achieve the following:

- Understand the epidemiology of head injuries.
- Debate the key aspects of primary prevention.
- Relate neuroanatomy and neurophysiology to the pathophysiology of neurotrauma.
- List the investigations that may be undertaken.
- Discuss the dangers of investigations mentioned.
- Describe the pre-investigation and post-investigation care required.
- Apply knowledge of microbiology to practice.
- Apply knowledge of neuropharmacology to practice.

---

**Ethical/legal considerations**

Debate the ethical/legal issues related to this section.

Consider and apply the legal and ethical issues highlighted in these chapters to neurotrauma practice:

- Substance abuse.
- Social practices.
- Relevant acts, e.g.
  - Human Tissue Act 2004.
  - Road Safety Act 2006.

# Chapter 10
# Epidemiology

*Nadine Abelson-Mitchell*

School of Nursing and Midwifery, Faculty of Health, Education and Society, Plymouth University, Devon, UK

## INTRODUCTION

As neurotrauma is a major public health problem worldwide it is necessary for health professionals to be aware of epidemiological findings in order to develop effective preventive measures and plan health services (Abelson-Mitchell 2008; Faul *et al.* 2010; Greenwald *et al.* 2003; Kay and Teasdale 2001; Langlois *et al.* 2006; Mauritz *et al.* 2008; Seeley 2007; Tennant 2005) (see Chapter 11). International and national epidemiological data are described to enable personnel to develop strategies for prevention and the delivery of appropriate services.

Epidemiology is defined as 'the study of the distribution and the determinants of disease and problems of health, disease or injuries in human populations' (Barker 1982: p. 1).

There is no universal means of recording and classifying epidemiological data (Seeley 2007) or defining neurotrauma (Cassidy *et al.* 2004; Dawodu 2003, 2008; Servadei *et al.* 2002). The comparison of epidemiological studies may result in divergent estimates of numbers and may lead to false impressions and/or incorrect data interpretation (Andersson *et al.* 2003; Baldo *et al.* 2003; Cassidy *et al.* 2004; Chaudhry *et al.* 2003; Greenwald *et al.* 2003; Kleiven *et al.* 2003; Steudel *et al.* 2005; Tagliaferri *et al.* 2006). However, when inclusion and exclusion criteria are considered, the relative incidences and trends are congruent (Basso *et al.* 2001; Bruns and Hauser 2003).

## SEVERITY OF INJURY

'Mild head injury' is described as a brief period of unconsciousness with GCS 13–15/15. Many patients with mild injuries either seek no medical attention or attend A&E and are sent home. Reasons identified for people with mild head injuries not attending hospital include: the stigma of having a head injury, the effect that a head injury may have on job/sport/driving, not recognising they have suffered a head injury and distance from a medical centre (Jennett 1996).

> '"Moderate head injury" is defined as loss of consciousness for between 15 minutes and 6 hours with GCS 9-12/15 and a period of post-traumatic amnesia (PTA) of up to 24 hours' (Headway 2011).

'Severe head injury' occurs where GCS is <8/15 and a patient has been in a coma for 6 hours or longer, or there is PTA > 24 hours.

See Chapter 16 for further discussion of severity of injury.

*Neurotrauma: Managing Patients with Head Injuries*, First Edition. Edited by Nadine Abelson-Mitchell.
© 2013 Blackwell Publishing Ltd. Published 2013 by Blackwell Publishing Ltd.

**Table 10.1**  Number of A&E attendances for England (July–September 2011).

| Attendance | Totals |
|---|---|
| First attendances | 5 213 363 |
| Follow-up attendances | 175 902 |
| Total | 5 389 265 |

## HOSPITAL ATTENDANCE

The number of A&E attendees for England according to the Department of Health (2011b) are shown in Table 10.1.

With regard to hospital attendance in the UK:

- About 3.4% of the population, per annum, attend A&E after head injury, 80–90% are not admitted (Greenwood 2002).
- 1.4 million people attend hospitals in England and Wales with head injuries (NICE 2007).
- The British Society of Rehabilitation Medicine (BSRM 1998) reports an incidence of 300/100 000 of the population per year attending hospital after sustaining a head injury: 90% are mild injuries, 5% moderate and 5% severe (Kay and Teasdale 2001) and 60–70% are discharged within 48 hours (Jennett 1996).
- The true A&E attendance rate may be 700 000 per annum (NICE 2007).
- In Scotland attendance at Emergency Departments was 1967/100 000 population.
- In North Thames this equates to 118 000 attendances per year (Palmer 1998).

In the USA:

- Annual head injury incidence (not necessarily TBI) ranges from 600 to 900/100 000 USA population. Of these, 200 to 500/100 000 are treated in A&E or other out-patient settings (Bruns and Hauser 2003).
- Per annum, 1.4 million head injuries occur, of these 1.1 million attend hospital (Langlois *et al.* 2006).
- The incidence of TBI related A&E visits for non-admitted patients is 392/100 000 population per annum or 1 027 000 visits to A&E per annum (Guerrero *et al.* 2000). This figure is comparable to that quoted for the UK.

## INCIDENCE

The incidence of head injury in developed countries has decreased; this is mainly for injuries related to motor

vehicle accidents, whereas head injuries in the elderly are increasing (Susman *et al.* 2002). Langlois *et al.* (2006) and Cassidy *et al.* (2004) report that the incidence of head injury is underestimated.

The general incidence of TBI in developed countries is frequently stated to be 200/100 000 population at risk per year (Bruns and Hauser 2003). This estimate, typically, includes only TBI patients admitted to hospitals.

The BSRM (1998) reports the incidence of head injury of all ages per year in the UK as 300/100 000 of the population.

In the USA:

- In 2003 there were 1 565 000 TBIs, that is 538.2/100 000 population (Brown *et al.* 2008).
- Incidence of mild TBI is ± 130/100 000 of the population.
- Incidence of moderate TBI is ± 15/100 000 of the population.
- Incidence of severe TBI is ± 14/100 000 of the population. If one includes pre-hospital deaths in this category the incidence rate is 21/100 000 (Dawodu 2003).

International findings reveal:

- In North Sweden the incidence rate for mild TBI for 16–60 year olds is 220/100 000 (Johansson *et al.* 1991 cited in Andersson *et al.* 2003), whereas the Andersson *et al.* (2003) figure is 204/100 000 population.
- In Norway the incidence rate of head injury is 207/100 000 population for patients visiting a hospital and 157/100 000 for patients admitted to hospital. The overall reduction in head injury incidence rates is related to the introduction of preventive measures (Heskestad *et al.* 2009).
- In Germany the overall incidence rate for head injury is 337/100 000 of the population. For severe head injuries the incidence rate is 33.5/100 000 population (Steudel *et al.* 2005).
- In Denmark there has been a decrease of 41% in the incidence rate from 265 to 157/100 000 population as a result of the introduction of preventive campaigns (Engberg and Teasdale 2001).

## PREVALENCE OF HEAD INJURY

The prevalence of head injury within the UK is 228 per 100 000 with long term problems (The Neurological Alliance 2003). In Glasgow the prevalence was estimated at 3 000–4 500/100 000 population (Greenwood 2002: p. i8). Prevalence of head injury for the USA is 439/100 000 and for Canada 54/100 000 (Jennett 1996). Currently an estimated 5.3 million Americans live with the long-term effects of TBI (Greenwald *et al.* 2003; Langlois *et al.* 2006).

## AGE DISTRIBUTION

Age is an important variable in relation to the recovery of the head injured patient. Although TBI incidence varies with population and locale, with high rates in late adolescence/early adulthood, the trends of lower rates in adult and middle-aged cohorts is almost universal and precedes the increase in TBI seen in the elderly population (Bruns and Hauser 2003; Cassidy *et al.* 2004).

In the USA the incidence rate for TBI in 2003 is reported as follows (Brown *et al.* 2008 p. S3):

- 15–24 years: 917.5/100 000.
- 45–64 years: 327.3/100 000.
- >65 years: 524.3/100 000.

In the UK, 15–24 year olds are over-represented in the head-injured population (Royal College of Surgeons of England, 1999). The elderly population experiences an increased incidence of TBI relative to many younger age groups (Giannoudis *et al.* 2009). This high incidence is attributed to motor vehicle accidents and falls and may be due to a combination of sensory and motor decline, deconditioning, and cognitive impairments or impairments of consciousness. The risk of TBI in the elderly increases particularly over the age of 65 years, and individuals older than 85 years are at greatest risk of TBI (Greenwald *et al.* 2003; Bruns and Hauser 2003). The TBI incidence in those aged 80 years or older was 173/100 000 population in Olmsted County. In those older than 74 years, the TBI incidence was 275/100 000 in France, 235/100 000 in San Diego and 100/100 000 population in Australia (Bruns and Hauser 2003).

## GENDER DISTRIBUTION

Males are at higher risk of TBI than females, with the highest male-to-female (M/F) ratios typically occurring in adolescence and young adulthood. Of those who suffer a traumatic brain injury, 68% are male (BSRM 1998). Baldo *et al.* (2003) identified that the highest number of hospitalised cases occurred in those aged 16–25 years; 61% were male and 39% female. Andersson *et al.* (2003) state the rate as 59% male and 41% female.

In the USA, a national sample of A&Es reported that the M/F ratio was 1.5:1 and 1.7:1. TBI incidence in females

exceeded TBI incidence in males in the elderly population (Langlois *et al.* 2006). In the USA the high M/F ratio is mainly the result of interpersonal violence and motor vehicle collisions during adolescence and young adulthood. The M/F ratio can approach or exceed 3–4:1. By contrast, there is approximate unity or inversion of the gender ratios at the extremes of age, particularly in the elderly.

## RACE AND ETHNICITY

In the USA and South Africa socio-economic factors, including violence, play a major role in TBI (Cassidy *et al.* 2004; Greenwald *et al.* 2003; Nell and Brown 1991).

Generally, TBI from violence occurs in men, non-white, living alone, less educated and unemployed when injured (Greenwald *et al.* 2003). Of those people with a violence-related injury, 80% have a history of substance abuse (Bogner *et al.* 2001). In adolescents and young adults, males and ethnic minorities are at increased risk of TBI due to violence and MVAs (Bruns and Hauser 2003).

## MECHANISM OF INJURY

In Westernised society, the mechanisms of head injury show similarity in causative factors; road traffic accidents being the most prevalent followed by falls and violence (Cassidy *et al.* 2004; Greenwald *et al.* 2003; Kraus and McArthur 1996). In general, TBI from assaults and MVAs have greater severities than do all other aetiologies combined (Bruns and Hauser 2003).

In the UK, falls (22–43%) and assaults (30–50%) are the most common causes of mild head injury (NICE 2003). Overall, falls predominate as a cause of injury in children and elderly, regardless of race and gender. Heskestad *et al.* (2009) report a high incidence of falls (882/100 000 in the over 90 age group).

In the USA, MVAs account for ± 50% of TBIs. Assaults account for ± 20%. Firearms are the third leading cause of TBI and work-related TBI is estimated at 45–50%. The work-related incidence of TBI in military personnel is 37/100 000 and 15/100 000 for civilians (Dawodu 2003). According to Mauritz *et al.* (2008) in Europe, violence-related head injury occurred more frequently in middle income people.

In Australia, road traffic accidents (40%), sports or recreation (25%), and falls (21%) account for the majority of TBIs. The high incidence of recreation-related TBI is attributed to the region's climate, coastline and rural setting.

Bicycles are used to improve the health of the nation, both for commuting to work and for leisure. The incidence of bicycle-related injuries in the USA is 0.3/100 000 population (Rivara and Sattin 2011). Bicycle injuries account for 0.25 deaths and 8.8/100 000 admissions per year. Pedestrian injuries account for 39% of RTAs and 10–20% of injuries are related to sport (Palmer 1998).

Sport is a leading cause of head injury, particularly mild traumatic brain injury (Langlois *et al.* 2006). In the USA it is estimated that per annum there are between 1.6 million and 3.8 million sports-related injuries (Langlois *et al.* 2006). Sports injuries occur from sports such as rugby, athletics, contact sports (boxing, karate, taekwondo), winter sports (skiing, snowboarding and ice hockey) and leisure activities (trampolining, horseback riding and use of all-terrain vehicles) (Cassidy *et al.* 2004; Levy *et al.* 2007; Ruedl *et al.* 2011). Women's sports generating head injuries include basketball, lacrosse and soccer. Men's football generates over 250 000 head injuries per annum. In the UK, the incidence of TBI in rugby is reported as 0.6–8/1000 per athlete game hours and taekwondo was 7–15.5/1000 athlete exposures for men and 2.5–9/1000 for women (Cassidy *et al.* 2004). The incidence of trauma in snowboarding and alpine skiing is increasing (4–8/1000 skier days); 52% of these injuries are injuries to the brain (Ackery *et al.* 2007; McBeth *et al.* 2009). The mortality rate from alpine skiing is 8% (Sulheim *et al.* 2006).

Morrell *et al.* (1998) and Slaughter *et al.* (2003) report that 87% of people in prison have had a head injury. Williams *et al.* (2010) state that 65% of adult offenders have had a head injury; 16% a moderate to severe head injury and 48% a mild head injury.

It must also be noted that personnel involved in war and terrorist attacks are at risk of suffering head injuries (Mallonee *et al.* 1996).

## SEASONAL VARIATION

Engberg and Teasdale (1998) found a seasonal variation of head injury, the lowest incidence (4–6%) in January–February and the highest incidence (12%) in July. The majority of injuries for snowboarding occur from January–March, in the afternoon, as a result of worsening snow conditions and poor visibility (McBeth *et al.* 2009).

## PREDISPOSITION

Patients with a predisposition to sustaining a head injury are those who have had a previous head injury (Dawodu 2008; Thompson and Mauk 2011).

## USE OF ALCOHOL

Alcohol is a contributory factor in head injury (Brown *et al.* 2008; Greaves *et al.* 2001; Kay and Teasdale 2001). In the UK, alcohol may be involved in an estimated 65% of adult head injuries (NICE 2003), whereas in the USA about 50% of people who sustain TBI are intoxicated at the time of injury (Agency for Healthcare Research and Quality 2004). In 2000 in the USA alcohol related MVAs resulted in 16 653 deaths and more than 300 000 injuries (Greenwald *et al.* 2003). Rosso *et al.* (2007), in an Austrian study, report that 67% of patients were drunk when injured. Only 1% of snowboarders and skiers had consumed large quantities of alcohol (McBeth *et al.* 2009).

## HEAD INJURY MORTALITY

TBI is estimated to be the primary cause of death in one third to one half of all traumatic deaths (Bruns and Hauser 2003). In most Westernised societies deaths from road traffic accidents are falling (Palmer 1998). Approximately half of all TBI deaths occur at the scene, during transport in the ambulance, or during the emergency medical phase of treatment, before hospital admission. Up to half of deaths due to trauma are as a result of head injuries and these account for most of the permanent disability (Jennett 1996). Variation in mortality rate ranges between 19–46% depending on the country under study (Basso *et al.* 2001). NICE (2003) reports a death rate of 6–10/100 000 population per annum. It adds that less than 0.2% of A&E attenders died from head injury. Greaves *et al.* (2001) report 9/100 000 as the mortality rate for head injuries. This accounts for 1% of all deaths and 15–20% of deaths between the ages of 5–35 years (Palmer 1998). The highest mortality in the USA is between the ages of 15–25 years at 32.8/100 000; the mortality rate in the elderly (>65 years) is 31.4/100 000 (Dawodu 2003).

Studies in Europe demonstrate a mortality rate from TBI of 10/100 000 per annum (Servadei *et al.* 2002; Thurman and Guerrero 1999). In Denmark case fatality within and outside the hospital was 5.4% of the population (Engberg and Teasdale 2001). In Germany the mortality rate has decreased from 27.2/100 000 population in 1972 to 9.0/100 000 in 2000 (Steudel *et al.* 2005).

Elderly patients (>64 years) have a worse mortality rate and functional outcome than patients in other age ranges (Giannoudis *et al.* 2009; Kotwica and Saracen 2010; Susman *et al.* 2002).

## CONCLUSION

Consequences of traumatic brain injuries can be costly in terms of quality of life and society (Brown *et al.* 2008;

Langlois *et al.* 2006, Yates *et al.* 2006). The Royal College of Surgeons of England (1999) recommends further research into the epidemiology of head injuries.

Knowledge of epidemiological facts is important to understand the mechanism of injury, types of injury, predisposition and seasonal variation as well as mortality in order to prepare appropriate primary prevention programmes, manage patients in A&E, plan services and attempt to decrease the incidence and prevalence of head injury in society.

# Chapter 11
# Prevention of Head Injuries

*Nadine Abelson-Mitchell*

School of Nursing and Midwifery, Faculty of Health, Education and Society, Plymouth University, Devon, UK

## INTRODUCTION

Health promotion and disease prevention are worldwide strategies. The responsibility for the prevention of head injuries is shared by all persons in all communities. Health professionals involved in the management of patients with neurotrauma need to be knowledgeable regarding the prevention of head injuries and are expected to pro-actively promote the health of the nation, rather than be reactive, in order to decrease the burden on the health services, families, societies and the economy (DH 1999).

The provision of a quality health service and the need for preventive measures in the early stages of medical care, and throughout all phases of recovery of the head injured patient, have been recognised (Bruns and Hauser 2003). The Nursing and Midwifery Council (NMC 2008: p. 2) states that nurses need to '. . . act as an advocate for those in your care, helping them to access relevant health and social care, information and support'. . .'Work with others to protect and promote the health and wellbeing of those in your care, their families and carers, and the wider community'. It can be seen that within this definition primary prevention of disease is included.

In order to devise primary prevention strategies and to plan appropriate interagency, intersectoral and interprofessional services and resources for patients with brain injury, it is essential to have valid, reliable and up-to-date epidemiological data (Abelson-Mitchell 2008; Maas *et al.* 2008; Rivara 2008; Tennant 2005). The epidemiological data reveal an urgent need for primary prevention strategies to be developed and implemented (Abelson-Mitchell 2008) (see Chapter 10).

Internationally, governments need to pay attention to neurotrauma as a major health problem. In the UK, primary prevention of accidents forms part of the strategy for *Saving Lives. Our Healthier Nation* (DH 1999). Limited regional and national primary prevention programmes have been introduced in the UK (Jennett 1996); an excellent example is the Department of Transport website (Department of Transport 2007).

Reports from Denmark, Germany, the USA and Brazil describe positive outcomes after the implementation of primary prevention programmes that focus on the prevention of RTAs, sports injuries, falls, drinking and driving, decreasing violence and domestic abuse (Baldo *et al.* 2003; Engberg and Teasdale 2001; Salvarani *et al.* 2009; Steudel *et al.* 2005). Kleiven *et al.* (2003) conclude that in Sweden, despite a number of national preventive strategies, the incidence of head injury has not been reduced – except perhaps for milder cases.

## RECOMMENDATIONS

There are numerous recommendations regarding primary prevention of head injuries. Basso *et al.* (2001) recommend

*Neurotrauma: Managing Patients with Head Injuries*, First Edition. Edited by Nadine Abelson-Mitchell.
© 2013 Blackwell Publishing Ltd. Published 2013 by Blackwell Publishing Ltd.

that a comprehensive worldwide campaign be initiated which meets the needs of developed and developing countries to decrease the incidence, prevalence and mortality of head injuries. Strategies for primary prevention of head injuries that take into account age, gender, ethnicity and socio-economic status tailored to local/regional conditions must be an outcome when planning hospital-based or community-based health services (Jennett 1996; Kleiven *et al.* 2003; Thurman *et al.* 1999).

Recommendations have been proposed in relation to the following:

- Road traffic accidents.
- Sports injuries.
- Older people.
- Interpersonal violence.

## ROAD TRAFFIC ACCIDENTS (RTAs)

Primary prevention programmes have led to a reduction in the number of RTA-associated head injuries and can decrease the risk of serious head injury or death by 85% (Dawodu 2003; Ruedl *et al.* 2011). The evidence is that helmets help to limit the extent and severity of the head injury in the event of an accident (Cassidy *et al.* 2004; Greenwald *et al.* 2003; Liu *et al.* 2009; Rivara and Sattin 2011; Steudel *et al.* 2005). Mayrose (2008) reports that using motorcycle helmets decreases the risk of brain injury by 65%.

Seatbelts in passenger cars reduce fatality by 45% and when combined with airbags, driver fatality can be reduced by 80% (Greenwald *et al.* 2003). When considering prevention of deaths due to RTAs, factors other than seatbelts and helmets, such as the introduction of safety legislation for cars, bicycle lanes, bicycle paths and passenger and pedestrian airbags, are important (Nakamura *et al.* 2002; Rivara and Sattin 2011; Ruedl *et al.* 2011). Steudel *et al.* (2005) report a decrease in TBI as a result of the introduction of legislation regarding airbags, air assisted braking systems, legislation regarding helmets and compulsory seatbelts.

### Alcohol consumption

Legislation regarding alcohol consumption and alcohol limits must be introduced and enforced. Acceptable blood alcohol limits vary from country to country (Drive and Stay Alive Inc. 2011; Nickson 2010) (see Table 11.1).

### Speed limits

*Think speed, think road safety.*

No-one is exempt from head injury, be they the drivers or passengers in motor vehicles or pedestrians. 'Stop speed-

**Table 11.1** Worldwide acceptable blood alcohol content (BAC) levels.

| BAC limit (%) | Country |
| --- | --- |
| 0.00 | Estonia, Japan, Malta, Romania, Slovakia, Czech Republic, Hungary, Saudi Arabia |
| 0.02 | Norway, Poland, Sweden |
| 0.04 | Lithuania |
| 0.05 | Austria, Belgium, Bulgaria, Chile, Croatia, Cyprus (North), Denmark, Finland, France, Germany (Germany is 0.03 if in an accident), Greece, Ireland, Israel, Italy, Latvia, Macedonia, Netherlands, Serbia/Montenegro, Portugal, Slovenia, South Africa, Spain, Turkey |
| 0.08 | UK, Ireland, Luxembourg, Malta, Switzerland, USA (all 50 states) |
| 0.09 | Cyprus (South) |

(Drinkdriving.org 2011; Nickson 2010)

ing' is the message for the community before it kills or maims. Individual countries set their own speed limits, therefore before driving it is essential to know the specific legislation regarding speed limits.

### Tips to limit road traffic accidents

- Take responsibility.
- Observe the rules of the road.
- Take additional precautions in bad weather, e.g. snow or ice.
- Drive within the speed limit.
- Wear a seatbelt.
- Wear appropriate head gear.
- Stop those who have consumed alcohol/recreational drugs from driving.
- Be alert and concentrate on the activity of driving.
- Do not drive when tired.
- Do not undertake other activities whilst driving, e.g. use of mobile phones/eating.
- Review the system of driving license renewal particularly in the elderly population (Department of Transport 2011).

(Traumaticbraininjury.com)

## Car design

Various organisations are responsible for scientifically testing the design of cars. Suggestions include safer car design that protects pedestrians, includes crumple zones, side airbags and bonnet airbags, that absorb the crash energy (Crandall *et al.* 2002; Elliott 2011; Euro NCAP no date; SafetyNet 2009).

## Road design

Attention needs to be paid to road design to decrease mortality and morbidity related to traffic accidents (European Campaign for Safe Road Design 2011) as:

- 'Half a million (people were) killed on EU roads in the last decade.
- Safe road design could cut annual death rates and injuries by 50 000.
- Road crashes cost annual €160bn (2% of EU GDP).
- Europe's new 10-year plan must incorporate safe road design.'

Road traffic accidents tend to take place outside built up areas, on single carriageways and national roads as well as roads with low traffic flow. Some authorities have produced road signs denoting areas with high accident rates (Kent and Medway Safety Camera Partnership 2011; Road Safety Partnership Gloucestershire County Council 2011).

It is essential for drivers to heed and take extra care in areas designated as high risk areas.

## ACTION REGARDING THE USE OF PRESCRIPTION, OVER THE COUNTER AND ILLICIT DRUGS

Polypharmacy and use of recreational drugs contribute to the incidence of head injury (Weinstein *et al.* 1994). Measures need to be introduced to limit the number of drugs people are consuming. In particular, head injured patients are at risk of polypharmacy as well as the use of recreational drugs. Substance abuse post-injury also needs to be prevented.

### Tips to limit drug use

- Implement drug campaigns to decrease use and availability of illicit drugs.
- Responsible self-administration of medication.
- Use a weekly pill dispenser to ensure accurate dosage of prescribed medication.
- Regular review of prescription and over the counter medication.
- Monitor medication for drug interactions.

**Table 11.2**   Speed limits in the UK.

| Vehicle | Miles per hour (km per hour) | | | |
|---|---|---|---|---|
| | **Built-up areas*** | **Single carriageways** | **Dual carriageways** | **Motorways** |
| **Cars and motorcycles** (including car derived vans up to 2 tonnes maximum laden weight) | 30 (48 km/h) | 60 (97 km/h) | 70 (113 km/h) | 70 (113 km/h) |
| **Cars towing caravans or trailers** (including car derived vans and motorcycles) | 30 (48 km/h) | 50 (80 km/h) | 60 (97 km/h) | 60 (97 km/h) |
| **Buses and coaches** (not exceeding 12 metres in overall length) | 30 (48 km/h) | 50 (80 km/h) | 60 (97 km/h) | 70 (113 km/h) |
| **Goods vehicles** (not exceeding 7.5 tonnes maximum laden weight) | 30 (48 km/h) | 50 (80 km/h) | 60 (97 km/h) | 70** (113 km/h) |
| **Goods vehicles** (exceeding 7.5 tonnes maximum laden weight) | 30 (48 km/h) | 40 (64 km/h) | 50 (80 km/h) | 60 (97 km/h) |

(Farlam 2011, 'Road speed limits in the United Kingdom', adapted from www.smartdriving.co.uk/Driving/Defensive Driving/Speed/UK_Speed_Limits.hmtl)
*The 30 mph limit usually applies to all traffic on all roads with street lighting unless signs show otherwise.
**60 mph (96 km/h) if articulated or towing a trailer.

## PREVENTION OF SPORTS INJURIES

Head injuries in sport, as well as their sequelae, are a major concern (Thurman 1998). Responsible participation in sport is to be encouraged provided suitable protection is available. Use of protective helmets when cycling, horse riding, skating, abseiling, skiing, snowboarding and roller-blading are also said to be beneficial (Davidson 2005; Lippi and Mattiuzzi 2004; McCrory 2002a, 2002b; Sulheim *et al.* 2006). It is important to ensure that helmets fit correctly and are secured in place. The use of padded headgear for rugby union football does not reduce the incidence of head injury (McIntosh *et al.* 2009). The introduction of new rules of engagement in karate has decreased the incidence and distribution of injuries (Macan *et al.* 2006). The prevention of injuries from contact sports such as soccer, baseball, boxing and rugby should be included in primary prevention programmes (Andersen *et al.* 2004; Bloom *et al.* 2004; Browne and Lam 2006; McCrory 2002b).

### Tips to limit sports injuries

- Use safety gear.
- Wear protective helmets/clothing.
- Ensure players are physically fit by undertaking a pre-match health assessment.
- Do not play sport if alcohol has been consumed.
- Time out in matches has been recommended.

## CARE OF OLDER PEOPLE

Care of older people in the community is multi-faceted and may involve interagency, intersectoral and interprofessional working. The number of elderly in the population is increasing as is the number of falls in the elderly population (Coronado *et al.* 2005; Kannus *et al.* 2007; Kiefer 2008; Maas *et al.* 2008).

It is important to ascertain, when possible, whether elderly people are taking anticoagulants. The use of anticoagulants may promote bleeding in people who have had a head injury and may have an effect on the extent of injury and final outcome (Reynolds *et al.* 2003).

### Tips for preventing falls

- Managing mobility issues:
  - Appropriate assessment of mobility needs.
  - Use of mobility aids.
  - Stairlift if appropriate.
- Prevention measures for falls in the home are essential:
  - No slippery surfaces.
  - No loose fitting carpets.
  - Use of handrails.
  - Use of mobility aids in the home, e.g. walking stick, frame.
  - Limit number of steps and number of times person must go up and down stairs.
  - Don't leave parcels on floor as trip hazard.
  - Appropriate support in the home.
- Prevention measures for falls in public are essential:
  - Repair of damaged pavements/drain covers/roads, etc.
  - Appropriate lighting.
  - Appropriate support outside the home.
- Managing polypharmacy.
- Prevention, management and education for dementia and cognitive decline.
- Poor vision:
  - Assess visual acuity and visual fields on a regular basis.
  - Use of spectacles and other visual aids.

(Traumaticbraininjury.com)

## INTERPERSONAL VIOLENCE

Recent developments within the United Kingdom, and internationally, suggest that interpersonal violence be included in primary prevention programmes. In the USA, programmes focusing on gun control are important in view of the high levels of gun ownership (Dawodu 2003; Thurman *et al.* 1999).

### Tips to limit interpersonal violence

- Avoid high risk areas where possible.
- Know your neighbours and neighbourhoods.
- Ensure guns and keys for gun safe are stored in a locked space.
- Keep the weapon(s) unloaded.
- Ammunition to be stored separately.
- Educate population regarding gun management and safe practice.

(Traumaticbraininjury.com)

## CONCLUSION

Health professionals may need to advise patients, families and communities regarding prevention of neurotrauma based on the knowledge provided in this chapter. People need to take responsibility, take precautions and consider the potential consequences of their actions. Primary health-care needs to focus on primary prevention of neurotrauma. Head injury is preventable, provided that governments take note of prevention strategies and tailor-made primary prevention programmes are developed for specific countries, regions and communities and implemented in an appropriate manner.

A worldwide, age-orientated, multimedia plan should be developed. The key target areas should be: young men with particular regard to RTAs; the use of protective clothing and equipment for occupational and sporting activities; avoidance of alcohol when driving; and interpersonal violence. Campaigns amongst people of working age should relate to: safety at work; building safety; safety at home; reducing risk in low income families and ethnic minorities (Dawodu 2008). Prevention of head injury in older people is essential.

It is the responsibility of all health professionals to undertake research into the effectiveness of prevention programmes (Rivara 2008), develop primary prevention programmes, introduce them and engage the community in order to decrease morbidity and mortality within local communities.

In the words of CL Osborn: 'Society is more likely to take action against the ravages of traumatic brain injury if it understands how pernicious, pervasive, and huge the problem is' (Faul *et al.* 2010: p. 2).

### Activity 11.1

**Scenario**

Drinking and driving is dangerous, preventing sports injuries, interpersonal violence and falls is essential.

**Questions**
- Are you actively involved in the community?
- Do you belong to school groups, social groups, cultural or religious groups?

- How much are you doing individually and collectively to reduce disease and to maintain the health of your family, patients and community?
- When last did you commit to decreasing head injuries within the community by offering to be involved in health promotion?
- What risk reducing strategies have you introduced within the community?

### Activity 11.2

Perform a community assessment in your local area to establish the possible epidemiology of head injuries.

### Activity 11.3

With your manager's permission, based on Activity 11.2, prepare a plan for an age-specific prevention programme.

Introduce the programme within the community, perhaps through a voluntary or charitable organisation.

### Activity 11.4

Develop a primary prevention programme for patients and families in the unit.

Introduce the programme in the unit.

### Activity 11.5

Compile a primary prevention pamphlet for patients in the unit.

## Activity 11.6

### Scenario

Charles, 18 years old, Steven, 19 years old, and Chris, 17 years old, were 'tombstoning' (jumping off a cliff into the sea) off Plymouth Sound. They thought the water was deep enough.

Charles dived into the water and hit his head on a rock. He had a fractured base of skull with a CSF leak from his right ear. His GCS was 5/15. He was in hospital for 6 weeks. He then attended a rehabilitation centre for 4 months. He is now going back home to live with his parents and the doctor has told him he is lucky to be alive.

The others received no injuries but they have told you they will go back to 'tombstoning' when the weather improves.

### Exercise

Prepare a primary prevention programme for presentation at schools.

# Chapter 12
# Applied Anatomy and Physiology

*Nadine Abelson-Mitchell*

School of Nursing and Midwifery, Faculty of Health, Education and Society, Plymouth University, Devon, UK

## INTRODUCTION

In-depth knowledge and understanding of anatomy and physiology enables health professionals to make informed decisions regarding practice. Providing patients, families, carers and the community with relevant knowledge enables them to make informed lifestyle choices. It is for this reason that this section includes such detail.

## THE NERVOUS SYSTEM

The nervous system comprises the central nervous system (CNS) and the peripheral nervous system (PNS).

The CNS includes:

- The brain.
- The spinal cord.

The PNS includes:

- Cranial nerves.
- Spinal nerves.
- Autonomic nervous system:
  - Sympathetic nervous system.
  - Parasympathetic nervous system.

The spinal cord and spinal nerves are not discussed in the text.

## THE SCALP

The scalp is described as it is the outside covering of the head and provides protection to the underlying structures.

The scalp consists of five layers:

- *Skin.*
- *Subcutaneous connective tissues.* Blood vessels are found in this fibrous layer. The connective tissue holds the vessels open thus profuse bleeding occurs when the scalp is damaged.
- *Aponeurotic layer.*
- *Loose sub-aponeurotic layer.*
- *Periosteum over the skull bone.*

The mnemonic to remember the five layers of the scalp is *SCALP.*

### Blood supply to the scalp

Five pairs of arteries, all originating from the external carotid artery, supply blood to the scalp. These are:

- The supratrochlear artery.
- The supraorbital artery.
- The superficial temporal artery.
- The occipital artery.
- The posterior auricular artery.

## Venous drainage

Venous drainage of the scalp is via the supratrochlear vein and supraorbital vein that join to form the facial vein. The superficial temporal vein joins the maxillary vein to become the retromandibular vein. The anterior division of the retromandibular vein and the facial vein join to become the common facial vein that empties blood into the internal jugular vein. The external jugular vein is formed by the posterior auricular vein and the posterior division of the retromandibular vein, and the occipital vein ends in the sub-occipital venous plexus.

---

### Implications for practice

A cut sustained by knocking the head at low velocity against a sharp edge, without any loss of consciousness or other neurological symptoms, is a scalp laceration and not a brain injury (though there may be grey areas between the two).

The scalp is very vascular and one can get significant blood loss from a scalp wound.

Ensure the scalp is checked:

- For bleeding, as the fibrous layer holds vessels open and clotting is prolonged.
- For any lacerations or damage.
- For brain tissue, if brain tissue is seen within a wound, this must indicate that there is a depressed skull fracture with a tear of the dura mater.
- For undetected lacerations as these may become infected and result in brain infections such as meningitis or abscesses.
- For evidence of a fracture; when repairing a wound, gently palpate the underlying skull with a gloved finger. This may reveal a fracture.

---

The head includes the face and the cranium. The face consists of 14 bones but will not be described further.

---

### Implications for practice

Head injury is often associated with face trauma. Fractures of the middle third of the face, in which the bones of the face separate from the cranium (Le Fort fractures), and fractures of the mandible may compromise the airway. It is important to ensure a patent airway at all times.

---

## THE SKULL

The skull is the skeleton of the head and is a box enclosing the brain. A series of eight flat bones are united and interlocked by sutures.

### Anterior aspect of the skull

The anterior aspect of the skull is viewed when the head is seen from the front (Figure 12.1).

This view includes:

- The frontal bone that is smooth and convex and forms the supra-orbital margins of the eye orbits. Between the two orbits is the glabella.
- The nasal region.
- The maxilla.
- The mandible.

---

### Implications for practice

The glabella tap is used when testing for Parkinson's disease. This may be relevant for patients who develop Parkinson's-like symptoms post-neurotrauma.

---

### Superior aspect of the skull

The superior aspect of the skull is oval in form. It is broadened posteriorly by the parietal eminences.

The bones of the superior aspect of the skull are:

- Frontal bone.
- Parietal bone.
- Occipital bone.

This view forms the calvaria or skullcap (Figure 12.2). On the inner aspect of the calvaria there are grooves for the meningeal arteries. There are also grooves for the superior sagittal sinus. Its margins mark the attachment of the falx cerebri.

---

### Implications for practice

A fracture of the skull may damage the middle meningeal artery and cause an extradural haematoma.

---

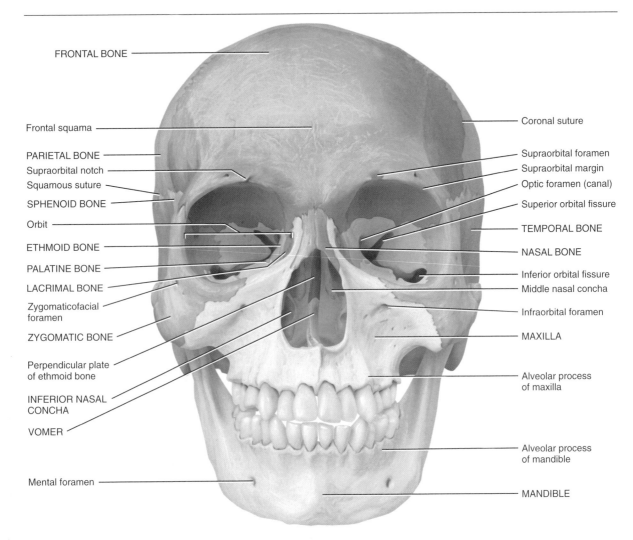

**FRONTAL BONE**

Frontal squama

**PARIETAL BONE**
Supraorbital notch
Squamous suture
**SPHENOID BONE**
Orbit
**ETHMOID BONE**
**PALATINE BONE**
**LACRIMAL BONE**
Zygomaticofacial foramen
**ZYGOMATIC BONE**
Perpendicular plate of ethmoid bone
**INFERIOR NASAL CONCHA**
**VOMER**
Mental foramen

Coronal suture
Supraorbital foramen
Supraorbital margin
Optic foramen (canal)
Superior orbital fissure
**TEMPORAL BONE**
**NASAL BONE**
Inferior orbital fissure
Middle nasal concha
Infraorbital foramen
**MAXILLA**
Alveolar process of maxilla
Alveolar process of mandible
**MANDIBLE**

**Figure 12.1** Anterior view of the skull. From *Principles of anatomy and physiology: Organisation, support and movement, and control systems of the human body*. Tortora, G.J. & Derrickson, B. Copyright © 2011 John Wiley & Sons, Inc. For a colour version of this figure, please refer to the plate section.

**Sutures of the skull**

The coronal suture separates the frontal and the two parietal bones. The sagittal suture separates the two parietal bones and lies in the midline. It ends anteriorly at the coronal suture. The lambdoid suture separates the parietal bones from the occipital bones. The lambdoid suture extends to form the parietomastoid and the occipitomastoid sutures. There are a number of anatomical variants. The most common (in 8% of adults) is that the frontal bone is in two parts, separated by a metopic suture.

The fontanelles are not described as they close within two years of birth.

**Posterior aspect of the skull**

The posterior aspect is round in outline.

It is modified by the parietal eminences and the mastoid process infero-laterally. In its centre is the lambdoid suture. The external occipital protuberance protrudes from the median line of the occipital bone (Figure 12.3).

**Lateral aspect of the skull**

The lateral aspect of the skull is partly face and partly cranium (Figure 12.4).

The cranial portion consists of the temporal fossa, external acoustic meatus and mastoid regions. The facial por-

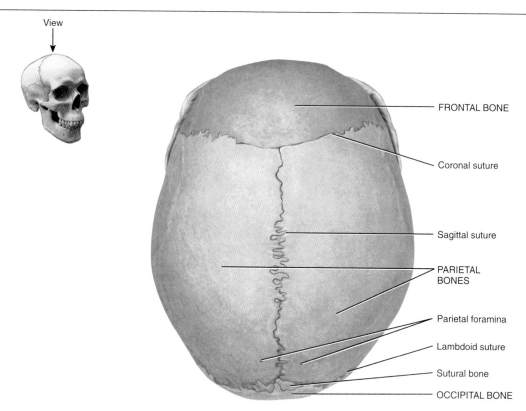

**Figure 12.2** Superior and right lateral view of the skull. From *Principles of anatomy and physiology: Organisation, support and movement, and control systems of the human body*. Tortora, G.J. & Derrickson, B. Copyright © 2011 John Wiley & Sons, Inc. For a colour version of this figure, please refer to the plate section.

tions are the zygomatic arch, infratemporal fossa and lateral aspect of the maxilla and mandible. The medial sagittal section of the skull shows the locations and structures within the skull (Figure 12.5).

**Base of the skull**

The base of the skull is divided into three anatomical sections (±¹/₃ each) (Figure 12.6):

- Anterior fossa.
- Middle fossa.
- Posterior fossa.

**Anterior section**

The anterior section houses the frontal lobes of the brain. It extends from the alveolar arch of the maxilla and includes the hard palate and the pterygoid plates up to the internal nasal passages/openings. The anterior cranial fossa is limited posteriorly by the border of the lesser wing of the sphenoid bone and the groove of the optic chiasm. Its floor

is formed by the orbital plates of the frontal bone, the cribriform plate (for passage of CN I) of the ethmoid bone and the lesser wing and forepart of the sphenoid bone. In the midline anteriorly attached to the falx cerebri, is the crista galli of the ethmoid bone.

> **Implications for practice**
>
> In patients with anterior fossa damage and/or a fracture:
>
> - Injuries of the frontal lobe of the brain may result in personality, IQ, memory and mood changes.
> - Fractures of the base of the skull in the anterior cranial fossa may cause:
>   - Damage to CN I (olfactory nerve) – anosmia, changes in smell and taste.
>   - CSF leakage from the nose (CSF rhinorrhoea). This may result in air entry into the skull causing an aerocele.

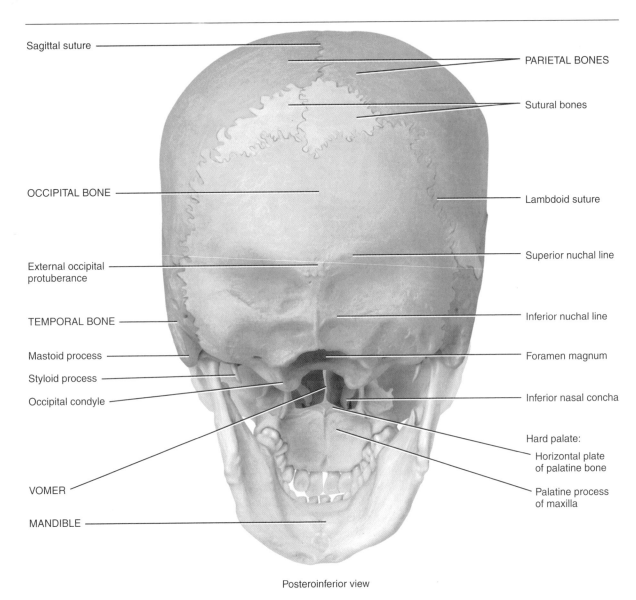

Posteroinferior view

**Figure 12.3** Posterior view of the skull. From *Principles of anatomy and physiology: Organisation, support and movement, and control systems of the human body.* Tortora, G.J. & Derrickson, B. Copyright © 2011. John Wiley & Sons, Inc. For a colour version of this figure, please refer to the plate section.

## Middle section

The middle cranial fossa extends from the nasal openings to the mastoid processes on either side of the foramen magnum. This is composed of the sphenoid bone, temporal bone and the occipital bone.

The *sphenoid bone* is posterior to the alveolar margin of the maxilla and consists of the pterygoid process with a medial and lateral plate. The greater wing of the sphenoid has a vertical and horizontal portion formed by the crest of the sphenoid. In the lateral plate of the pterygoid process are the foramen ovale and foramen spinosum. The body of the sphenoid is just anterior to the foramen magnum.

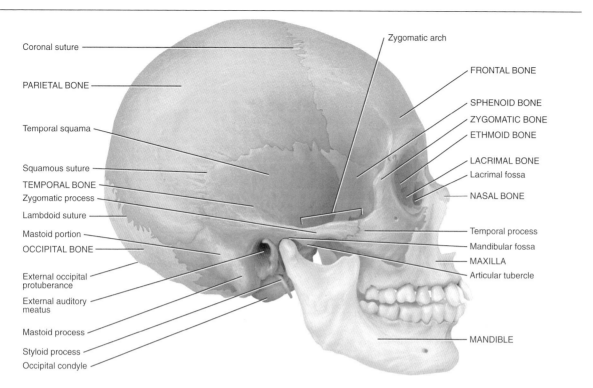

**Figure 12.4** Lateral view of the skull. From *Principles of anatomy and physiology: Organisation, support and movement, and control systems of the human body*. Tortora, G.J. & Derrickson, B. Copyright © 2011. John Wiley & Sons, Inc. For a colour version of this figure, please refer to the plate section.

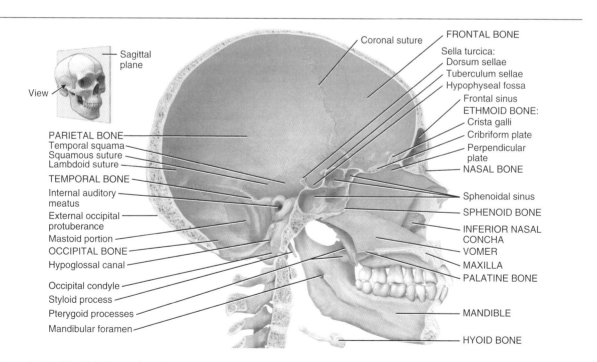

**Figure 12.5** Medial view of sagittal section of the skull. From *Principles of anatomy and physiology: Organisation, support and movement, and control systems of the human body*. Tortora, G.J. & Derrickson, B. Copyright © 2011. John Wiley & Sons, Inc. For a colour version of this figure, please refer to the plate section.

The *temporal bone* is divided into different portions:

- *The petrous bone* stretches from the foramen lacerum to the styloid process. It has various appertures namely, the auditory tube, carotid foramen for passage of the internal carotid artery, jugular foramen for passage of the internal jugular vein, CN IX, CN X and CN XI.
- The *squamous* part is thin and flat and forms the anterior and superior part of the temple. It includes the zygomatic process and the temporo-mandibular joint.
- The *mastoid* portion is found posterior and inferior to the external auditory meatus and contains the mastoid air cells, as well as the internal auditory meatus – the passageway for the facial nerve (CN VII) and the vestibulochochlear nerve (CN VIII) and the stylomastoid foramen the passageway for the facial nerve (CN VII) and stylomastoid artery.

The middle cranial fossa extends from the posterior limits of the anterior cranial fossa (posterior border of the lesser wings of the sphenoid) to the superior angles of the petrous portion of the temporal bone.

The bones of the fossa are:

- Body and greater wings of the sphenoid.
- Squamous portion of temporal bone.
- Anterior surface of the petrous portion of the temporal bone.
- Sphenoidal angle of the parietal bone.

The fossa is continuous across the midline and includes:

- The chiasmic groove that leads to the optic canal for the passage of the optic nerve (CN II) and the ophthalmic artery.
- Anteriorly the superior orbital fissure transmits vessels and nerves into the orbit.
- The sella tursica lining the hypophyseal fossa for the pituitary gland.
- Lateral to the sella tursica is the groove for the internal carotid artery.

The lateral portions of the middle fossa are deep and house the temporal lobes of the brain.

Other foramina in the middle cranial fossa include:

- Foramen rotundum – passageway for maxillary division of CN VII.
- Foramen ovale – passageway for branch of CN V and accessory meningeal artery.

- Foramen spinosum – passageway for middle meningeal artery.
- Foramen lacerum – passageway for ascending pharyngeal artery.

---

**Implications for practice**

Fractures of the base of the skull in the temporal region may cause deafness either through damage to the middle ear or sensorineural deafness as a result of damage to CN VIII (auditory nerve).

Fractures involving the sella tursica may be associated with pituitary gland injury.

---

**Posterior section**

The posterior cranial fossa extends to include the whole of the occipital bone and the occipital condyles as well as the borders of the foramen magnum. The posterior fossa is large and deep and accommodates the cerebellum, pons variola and medulla oblongata.

The fossa is formed by:

- The dorsum sella of the sphenoid bone.
- The petrous portion of the temporal bone. The superior angle of the petrous temporal forms the anterior limit of the fossa and gives rise to the tentorium cerebelli.
- The occipital bone. The transverse groove in the occipital bone houses the transverse sinus and the posterior limit of the posterior fossa.

The foramen magnum is at the centre of the base of the skull. The following pass through the foramen magnum:

- Meninges.
- Spinal cord.
- Ascending rootlets of the accessory nerve (CN II).
- Vertebral arteries.
- Anterior and posterior spinal arteries.
- Ligaments passing between the occiput and the axis.

Anteriorly to the foramen magnum, the basilar portion of the occipital bone, fused with the base of the sphenoid,

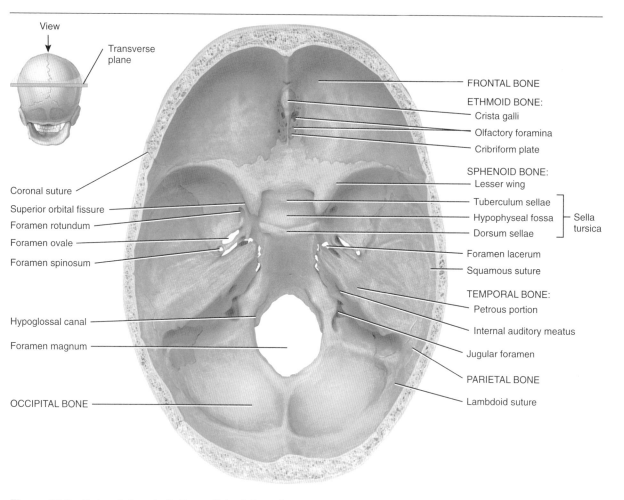

View
Transverse plane

FRONTAL BONE

ETHMOID BONE:
Crista galli
Olfactory foramina
Cribriform plate

SPHENOID BONE:
Lesser wing
Tuberculum sellae
Hypophyseal fossa
Dorsum sellae
— Sella tursica

Foramen lacerum
Squamous suture

TEMPORAL BONE:
Petrous portion
Internal auditory meatus

Jugular foramen

PARIETAL BONE

Lambdoid suture

Coronal suture
Superior orbital fissure
Foramen rotundum
Foramen ovale
Foramen spinosum

Hypoglossal canal
Foramen magnum

OCCIPITAL BONE

**Figure 12.6**   Base of the skull. From *Principles of anatomy and physiology: Organisation, support and movement, and control systems of the human body*. Tortora, G.J. & Derrickson, B. Copyright © 2011. John Wiley & Sons, Inc. For a colour version of this figure, please refer to the plate section.

supports the pons variola and medulla oblongata. Posteriorly to the foramen magnum the occipital crests separate the cerebellae fossae and allow attachment to the falx cerebelli and holds the occipital sinus.

The posterior fossa includes:

- Jugular foramen for passageway of cranial nerves.
- Internal acoustic meatus for the passage of the facial and vestibular cochlear nerves as well as the labyrinthine artery.

Implications for practice

Patients with a posterior fossa fracture may present with:

- CSF leaks or blood draining from the external auditory meatus.
- Injury to the brain stem.
- Raised intracranial pressure.

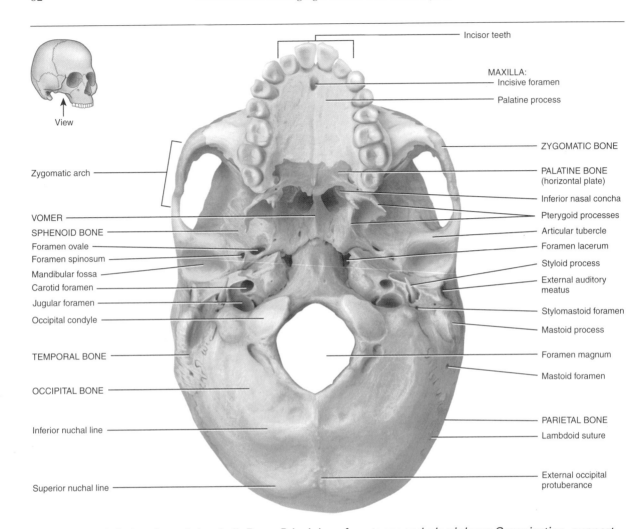

**Figure 12.7**   Inferior view of the skull. From *Principles of anatomy and physiology: Organisation, support and movement, and control systems of the human body.* Tortora, G.J. & Derrickson, B. Copyright © 2011. John Wiley & Sons, Inc. For a colour version of this figure, please refer to the plate section.

## The cranium

The content of the cranium consists of the following structures:

- Meninges.
- Brain.
- System of blood vessels.
  - Arterial supply.
  - Venous drainage.

### *The meninges*

The meninges cover the brain and spinal cord and consist of three layers (Figure 12.8):

- Dura mater.
- Arachnoid mater.
- Pia mater.

### *Dura mater*

This is the outermost layer. The dura mater (referred to as the dura) is a thick, dense, fibrous layer that encloses and protects the brain and spinal cord. It extends along the cranial nerves and spinal nerves when they leave the cranium or spine, and becomes continuous with their sheath.

The cranial dura is two-layered. There is a periosteal and meningeal layer. The meningeal layer forms duplications

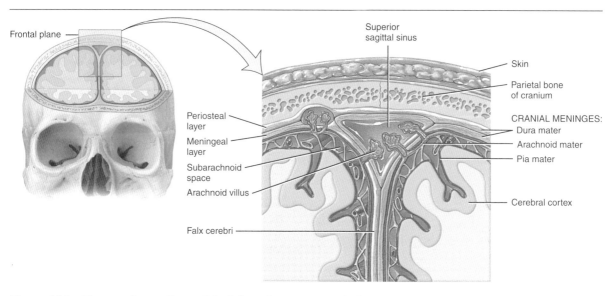

**Figure 12.8**   The meninges. From *Principles of anatomy and physiology: Organisation, support and movement, and control systems of the human body.* Tortora, G.J. & Derrickson, B. Copyright © 2011. John Wiley & Sons, Inc. For a colour version of this figure, please refer to the plate section.

which are prolonged between the parts of the brain, i.e. the falx cerebri, falx cerebelli, tentorium cerebelli and the diaphragma sella. Between these duplications the venous channels and venous sinus are formed.

### THE FALX CEREBRI

The falx cerebri is a sickle shaped duplication of the dura. It occupies the longitudinal central fissure in the midline and separates the two cerebral hemispheres. Anteriorly it is attached to the crista galli of the ethmoid bone. Posteriorly it is attached to the internal occipital protruberance and becomes continuous with the tentorium cerebelli. The superior sagital venous sinus is contained within its superior aspect. The inferior margin of the falx cerebri arches over the corpus callosum and contains the inferior sagital venous sinus.

### TENTORIUM CEREBELLI

The tentorium cerebelli separates the cerebellum from the cerebral hemispheres. The tentorium cerebelli is attached at the circumference to the edge of the groove for the transverse sinus on the inner surface of the occipital bone. The anterior margin arches around the

brain stem and attaches to the anterior clinoid process behind the optical canal. The falx cerebri ends along its median ridge.

### FALX CEREBELLI

The falx cerebelli separates the two cerebellar hemispheres. It is attached to the internal occipital crest and to the inferior aspect of the tentorium cerebelli. It contains the occipital sinus.

### DIAPHRAGMA SELLA

The diaphragma sella lines the cavity in which the pituitary gland is found.

#### Arachnoid mater

This is the middle layer. The arachnoid mater (referred to as the arachnoid) is a delicate, transparent membrane composed of collagenous and elastic fibres that is covered on its inner surface by squamous epithelial cells. The arachnoid loosely invests the brain and, except for the deep longitudinal cerebral fissure, does not dip down into its sulci. The arachnoid layer is separated from the pia mater by the sub-arachnoid space that contains CSF. The sub-arachnoid space is crossed by trabeculae of the pia mater and arachnoid. The arachnoid bridges over intervals between the brain and forms cisterns. In these cisterns large quantities of CSF are located. Arachnoid granulations are tuft-like collections of highly folded arachnoid which project through the dura mater into the dural sinuses. It is through their thin membrane that CSF is passed into the blood.

*Pia mater*

This is the innermost layer. This layer is delicate, friable and is a vascular membrane. The pia mater follows the contours of the brain and cannot be separated from the brain. It sends prolongations into the brain as septae along the perivascular spaces.

---

**Implications for practice**

Bleeding between the periosteum and the dura will result in an extradural (epidural) haematoma

Bleeding between the dura and the arachnoid will result in a subdural haematoma.

Bleeding beneath the arachnoid is a subarachnoid haemorrhage.

---

**Implications for practice**

Blockage to CSF flow can be caused in several ways:

1 **Communicating hydrocephalus**
   There is a structural blockage in CSF flow, for example post-head injury or from an anatomical cause. There may also be overproduction of CSF. The arachnoid granulations are not blocked. This may lead to ↑ICP requiring treatment.
2 **Non-communicating hydrocephalus**
   The arachnoid granulations are blocked, for example with blood post-trauma or as a result of a sub-arachnoid bleed and there is limited or no drainage of the CSF. This may lead to ↑ICP requiring treatment.

---

**STRUCTURE OF THE BRAIN**

The brain contains 10 billion neurones, weighs 1.5 kgs (3.5 lbs) and comprises 2% of the total body weight (Figures 12.9, 12.10, 12.11).

Embryologically, the brain is divided into three sections:

- Forebrain.
- Midbrain.
- Hindbrain.

These sections are further divided as follows:

- **Forebrain.**
  Cerebral hemispheres ⎤
  Lateral ventricles    ⎬ Known as the Telencephalon
  Basal nuclei          ⎦
  Thalamus       ⎤
  Hypothalamus   ⎬ Diencephalon
  3rd ventricle  ⎦
- **Midbrain.**
  Cerebral peduncles     ⎤
  Corpora quadrigemina   ⎬ Mesencephalon
  Cerebral aquaduct      ⎦
- **Hindbrain.**
  Cerebellum   ⎤
             ⎬ Metencephalon
  Pons         ⎦
  Medulla oblongata    Myelencephalon
  4th ventricle

**The forebrain**

*Cerebrum*

There are two cerebral hemispheres separated by a longitudinal cerebral fissure. The surface of the cerebrum is enlarged by the presence of gyri and sulci. The cerebrum is composed of grey matter on the outside and white matter on the inside and is responsible for the integration of the motor and sensory functions. The two hemispheres are connected by the corpus callosum that consists of a head, a neck and a tail.

In addition to neurones (nerve cells) the grey matter also contains glial cells which have specific functions (Table 12.1).

The white matter consists of three types of fibres:

- Association fibres that connect the cortical parts of the same cerebral hemispheres.
- Commisural fibres that connect the two cerebral hemispheres.
- Projection fibres that join the cortex with lower centres via the internal capsule.

The internal capsule is the pathway for motor function. It consists of white matter and extends from the cortex via the thalamus to the brain stem. In cross-sectional dissection the internal capsule looks like a 'butterfly' (Figure 12.10).

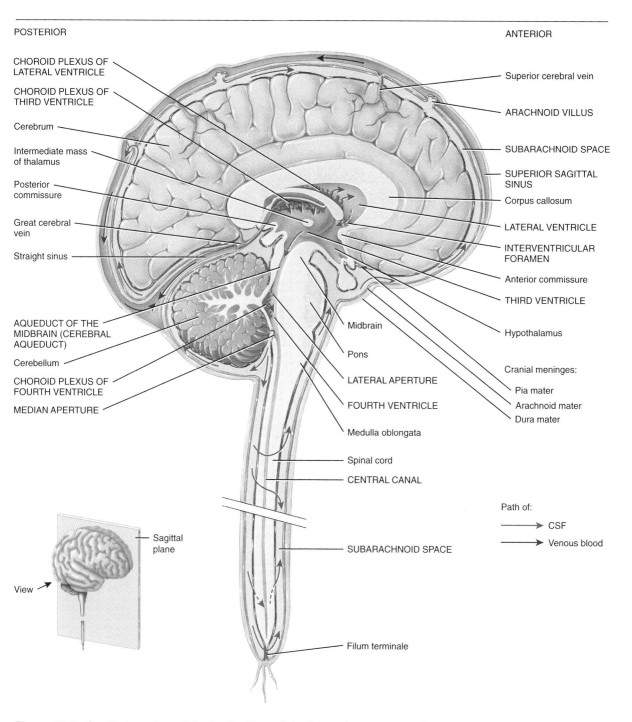

POSTERIOR

ANTERIOR

CHOROID PLEXUS OF LATERAL VENTRICLE

CHOROID PLEXUS OF THIRD VENTRICLE

Cerebrum

Intermediate mass of thalamus

Posterior commissure

Great cerebral vein

Straight sinus

AQUEDUCT OF THE MIDBRAIN (CEREBRAL AQUEDUCT)

Cerebellum

CHOROID PLEXUS OF FOURTH VENTRICLE

MEDIAN APERTURE

Sagittal plane

View

Midbrain

Pons

LATERAL APERTURE

FOURTH VENTRICLE

Medulla oblongata

Spinal cord

CENTRAL CANAL

SUBARACHNOID SPACE

Filum terminale

Superior cerebral vein

ARACHNOID VILLUS

SUBARACHNOID SPACE

SUPERIOR SAGITTAL SINUS

Corpus callosum

LATERAL VENTRICLE

INTERVENTRICULAR FORAMEN

Anterior commissure

THIRD VENTRICLE

Hypothalamus

Cranial meninges:

Pia mater

Arachnoid mater

Dura mater

Path of:

CSF

Venous blood

**Figure 12.9** Sagittal section of the brain. From *Principles of anatomy and physiology: Organisation, support and movement, and control systems of the human body*. Tortora, G.J. & Derrickson, B. Copyright © 2011. John Wiley & Sons, Inc. For a colour version of this figure, please refer to the plate section.

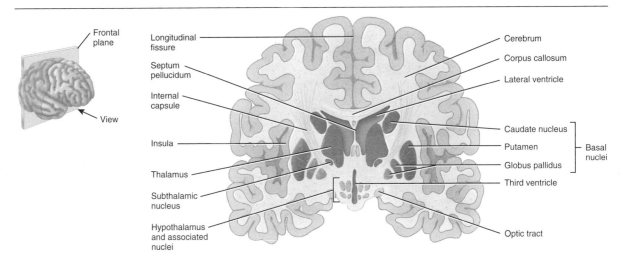

**Figure 12.10**   Anterior section of the brain. From *Principles of anatomy and physiology: Organisation, support and movement, and control systems of the human body.* Tortora GJ & Derrickson B. Copyright © 2011. John Wiley & Sons, Inc. For a colour version of this figure, please refer to the plate section.

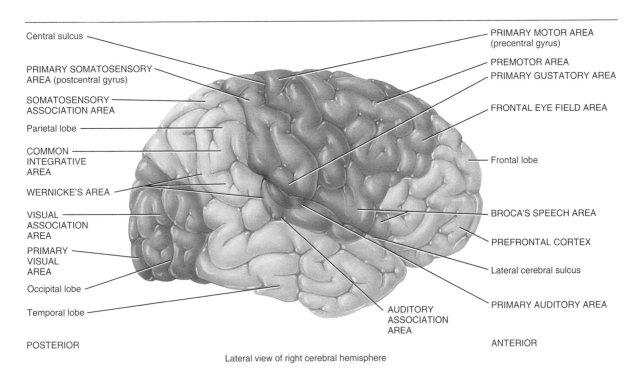

**Figure 12.11**   Functional areas of the brain. From *Principles of anatomy and physiology: Organisation, support and movement, and control systems of the human body.* Tortora, G.J. & Derrickson, B. Copyright © 2011. John Wiley & Sons, Inc. For a colour version of this figure, please refer to the plate section.

**Table 12.1** Functions of neuroglia.

| Structure | Function |
| --- | --- |
| Astrocytes | Act as cleaner for brain debris |
| | Transport nutrients to neurones |
| | Involved in cell metabolism |
| Oligodendrocytes | Form myelin sheaths |
| Ependymal cells | Line surface of brain |
| | Form part of blood brain barrier (BBB) |
| Microglia | Involved in immune system |

(Scribd.com 2011)

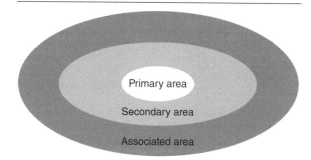

**Figure 12.12** Graphic demonstrating primary, secondary and association areas of cerebrum. For a colour version of this figure, please refer to the plate section.

The cerebrum is divided into lobes.

All areas of function in the cerebrum comprise a primary area related to the particular function, for example vision in the occipital lobe, a secondary area where there is some activity related to the function and an association area responsible for some further activity (Figure 12.12). The closer the injury to the primary area, the more severe the deficit (Scribd.com 2011).

The two frontal lobes are responsible for subconsciousness, thought, intelligence, morals, memory, personality and mood. Located in the posterior area of the frontal lobe, anterior to the deep central sulcus, is the motor area containing the motor homunculus. On the left side of the brain the inferior area of the frontal lobe, just superior to the lateral sulcus, is the area of speech.

*Parietal lobe*

The anterior portion of the parietal lobe is the sensory area. Each part of the body is represented within the motor and sensory homunculus with the left side of the body being represented on the right side of the brain and vice versa. The body is represented in an upside down pose with areas of anatomical and physiological importance being allocated larger areas of representation, for example lips and tongue compared to abdominal muscles. This representation can be shown, pictorially, as a homunculus (from the Latin for 'little human'; Figure 12.13). From various parts of the body fibres travel via specific motor or sensory tracts in the spinal cord to the motor or sensory homunculus for these stimuli to be interpreted.

*Temporal lobe*

The superior portion of the temporal lobe, inferior to the sulcus, is the cortical area of hearing and smell. The temporal lobe also plays a part in memory.

*Occipital lobe*

The occipital lobe is responsible for vision.

*The limbic system* (Figure 12.14)

*Structure*

The limbic system, the emotional brain, is found on the inner border of the cortex located in the telecephalon and diencephalon (Swenson 2006: p.1).

The limbic system comprises the following structures:

- The amygdala found in the anterior temporal lobe is involved in the co-ordination of behaviour as well as autonomic and endocrine response to environmental stimulation. The amygdala decides what memories are stored and where they are to be stored.
- The hippocampus, found in the medial aspect of the temporal lobe, forms the medial wall of the lateral ventricle. It is involved in explicit memory (recall of facts and events), short term memory, long term memory and cognitive mapping. It is not involved in working and procedural memory or memory storage learning (Boeree 2009).
- The limbic cortex is involved in motivation, mood, judgement and insight:
  - The fornix involves input from hippocampus to mammillary bodies and septal nuclei.
  - The mammillary body is involved in memory.
  - The limbic lobe comprises:
    - The parahippocampus gyrus concerned with spatial memory.
    - The cingulate gyrus involved in cognition and attention.

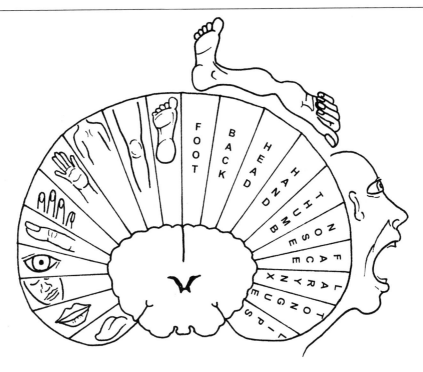

**Figure 12.13**   Picture of homunculus.

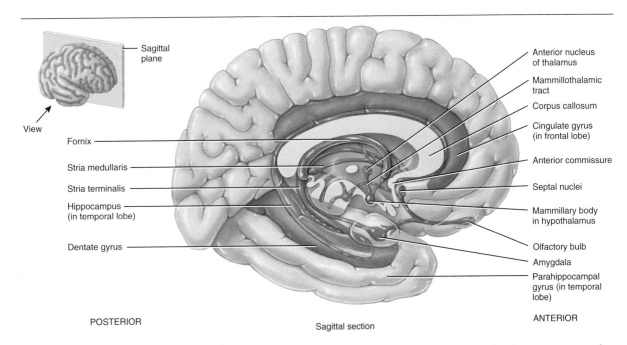

**Figure 12.14**   The limbic system. From *Principles of anatomy and physiology: Organisation, support and movement, and control systems of the human body.* Tortora, G.J. & Derrickson, B. Copyright © 2011. John Wiley & Sons, Inc. For a colour version of this figure, please refer to the plate section.

- The dentate gyrus involved in the regulation of happiness and management of memories.
- The septal nuclei provide critical connections.

These areas link with the hypothalamus, thalamus and cerebral cortex.

*Function*

The limbic system is responsible for recognising a person's previous experience in determining emotional responses, memory and learning (Boeree 2009). It is also involved in survival instincts, 'flight and fright', fear and rage, as well as pleasurable feelings relating to sexual responses and eating (Bailey 1987).

---

**Implications for practice**

1. The limbic system is of particular importance in rehabilitation and recovery as it is responsible for emotional control, memory and learning.
2. Damage to the limbic system from hypoxia or cell damage may result in:
   - Difficulty with abstract reasoning.
   - Mood disturbances or agitation.
   - Out-of-control emotions.
   - Extreme violence.
   - Suicide.
   Patients demonstrating these types of behaviour will need to be monitored closely and may need a behaviour modification programme and in extreme circumstances medication.
3. Clinically, the patient's emotional responses may be determined by their previous experience stored within their long or short-term memory. The recall and response to these memories may be stimulated by a current environmental stimulus. It is therefore important to establish whether there are certain activities or events known to the patient or family that will set off these strong emotional responses. Once the professionals have this knowledge it may be possible to avoid replicating situations that spark strong emotional responses such as fear, anxiety and rage. Alternatively, memories, that on recall spark positive responses, can be used within the rehabilitation programme to elicit positive emotional responses such as happiness and pleasure.

---

*Art vs Academic*

The right and left sides of the brain are responsible for different functions. The 'right' side of the brain is the 'artistic' side and the 'left' side of the brain is the 'academic' side.

*Left side (academic)*
- Analysis.
- Language.
- Logic.
- Linearity.
- Numbers.
- Sequencing.

*Right side (arty)*
- Colour.
- Creativity.
- Daydreaming.
- Dimensions.
- Images.
- Imagination.
- Intuitiveness.
- Music.
- Rhythm.

Most people have developed their right or left side of the brain as a dominant side. Thus they are good at academic activities or they are artistic. Balance is achieved when both sides function equally.

---

**Implications for practice**

Loss of function of either side of the brain will need re-organisation and training. When preparing rehabilitation programmes it is important to involve both the right and left side functions of the brain in therapeutic activities.

---

*Hypothalamus*

The hypothalamus is responsible for hormonal control, water balance, temperature control and appetite.

---

**Implications for practice**

Damage to the hypothalamus may result in:

- Diabetes insipidus.
- Hyperpyrexia.
- Changes in appetite.

## Thalamus

The thalamus is a relay system, a low level information processor and a gate-keeper that blocks or transmits impulses. The thalamus is responsible for emotional control.

## Brain stem

Anatomically the brain stem is the pons variola and medulla oblongata.

## Midbrain

The Reticular Activating System (RAS) is found in the midbrain. The RAS is a network of granular nerve cells that resembles a bunch of grapes. The RAS is responsible for maintaining the state of wakefulness, i.e., a level of consciousness.

There are two components to RAS:

- Bulboreticular formation found in the midbrain, pons variola and medulla oblongata.
- Non-specific thalamic nuclei.

Reticular fibres may be ascending fibres (ARAS) or descending fibres (DRAS). Both ascending and descending fibres go to the:

- Thalamus.
- Caudate nucleus.
- Limbic system.
- Neocortex.

Some of the descending fibres (DRAS) go down the spinal cord to the dorsal roots.

There are three primary sources of input to the RAS:

1. Homeostasis:
   The body's metabolic processes maintain homeostasis. The body's internal environment is controlled by the hypothalamus and reticular nuclei, the limbic system and the cortex.
2. Sensoristasis:
   Sensory information from the external environment as there is a cortical urge for curiosity. Sensations go via the reticular formation because all sensory tracts connect to the reticular tracts and form collateral connections. Information comes from specific thalamic nuclei via non-specific thalamic nuclei and the bulboreticular system.

3. The subsystem for organising, regulating and verifying activities and behaviour. RAS can be modified by primary and secondary projection areas.

## Pons variola

The pons variola is responsible for respiration and cardiovascular function.

## Medulla oblongata

The medulla oblongata is responsible for respiration.

## Pituitary gland

The vascular pituitary gland is a pea-sized structure located on the sella tursica in the pituitary fossa. The pituitary gland is responsible for hormonal control, fluid balance and body homeostasis.

The pituitary gland has two lobes:

- Anterior pituitary.
- Posterior pituitary.

The pituitary gland produces the hormones listed in Table 12.2.

## Blood supply

The blood supply is from the internal carotid artery. The pituitary arteries branch into numerous arteries and form a pituitary portal system to transfer blood and hormones.

## Venous drainage

Venous drainage from the anterior pituitary is via the adenohypophyseal veins and drainage from the posterior pituitary is via the neurohypophyseal veins. Both the adenohypophyseal veins and the neurohypophyseal veins form the confluent pituitary vein that drains into the cavernous sinuses.

---

### Implications for practice

1. Traumatic injury to the pituitary may result in loss of pituitary function and hypopituitarism.
2. Lesions may suppress or increase production of hormones thus affecting other bodily functions.
3. The stress reaction is controlled by the pituitary gland, in particular ACTH causing cortisol release.

## Implications for practice

Lesions or damage to the ADH-producing cells in the pituitary gland may result in neurogenic or central diabetes insipidus. It is essential that this is monitored as the patient can dehydrate very quickly as there is no re-absorption of $H_2O$ in the renal tubules.

### Diagnosis

Urine osmolality: <200 mOsmol/kg in the presence of polyuria (>3 L/day)

Urine SG: <2001

Serum osmolality: $Na^+$ <135 mmol/L or 135 mEq/L usually <130 mmol/L

Water deprivation test:
The water deprivation test involves fluid restriction for 4–18 hours. During this time the urine osmolality and patient weight is monitored. This is continued until 2–3 consecutive samples vary by <30 mOsm/kg (or <10%). ADH is then administered and the response noted. If there is a good response to the ADH administration diabetes insipidus is confirmed.

### Clinical features

- Incessant thirst.
  - If the patient is awake they will drink anything to try and quench their thirst – tap water, flower water, etc.
  - If unconscious, the patient will show signs and symptoms of severe dehydration.
- Excessive pale coloured urine.

### Treatment
Vasopressin (Oxytocin).

## *Cerebellum*

The cerebellum is found in the posterior fossa. It consists of grey matter on the outside and white matter on the inside. The white matter forms a tree like structure called the Arbovitae (tree of life). The cerebellum is responsible for fine co-ordination and involuntary movement. The cranial nerves are also attached to the cerebellum.

## *Cranial nerves*

There are 12 cranial nerves that emerge from the brain stem. Each nerve has a particular function. This may be purely motor, purely sensory or both (Table 12.4).

**Table 12.2** Hormones of the pituitary gland.

| Lobe | Hormone | Target organ |
|---|---|---|
| Posterior | ADH | Acts on renal tubules causing $H_2O$ to be released in response to the level of dissolved ions in the blood |
| | Oxytocin | Acts on uterine muscle to cause contractions |
| Anterior | Growth Hormone | Stimulates protein anabolism and growth in bones and muscles |
| | TSH | Thyroid to stimulate production of thyroxine |
| | FSH/LH/ICSH | Testes/Ovaries |
| | Prolactin | Breast – milk production |
| | ACTH | Adrenal cortex to stimulate production of cortisol |
| | MSH | Stimulates pigmentation of skin |

## Implications for practice

Damage/Disease of the cerebellum results in changes in fine motor movement and co-ordination.

**Table 12.3** Clinical manifestations of cerebellar disease.

| Manifestation | Mnemonic |
|---|---|
| Vertigo | V |
| Ataxia | A |
| Nystagmus | N |
| Intension tremor | I |
| Slurred speech | S |
| Hypotonia | H |

A mnemonic to remember the names of the cranial nerves is:

On old Olympus towering top a Fin and German viewed a hop.

A mnemonic to remember the function (sensory, motor or mixed (both)) of the cranial nerves is:

Some say marry money but my brother says bad business marries money.

**Table 12.4** Cranial nerves.

| Cranial nerve number | Cranial nerve Name | Function | Exit point from skull | Test | Abnormality |
|---|---|---|---|---|---|
| I | Olfactory (sensory) | Sense of smell | Cribriform plate | Smell coffee or cloves. Test each nostril separately | Anosmia (unable to smell) |
| II | Optic (sensory) | Visual acuity Visual fields | Optic foramen | Use Snellen chart or newspaper Check optic disc, vessels and periphery of retina | Blindness Decreased visual activity Altered visual fields, e.g. homonymous hemianopia; bilateral hemianopia |
| III | Oculomotor (motor) CNIII/CNIV/CNVI are tested together | Supply muscles of eye | Superior orbital fissure | Follow examiner's finger, one eye at a time Up, down, sideways Check size, shape and equality of pupils Check pupillary response: Direct light reflex Consensual light reflex See Fig. 18.2 | Ptosis Cannot look up/down or medially |
| IV | Trochlear (motor) | Supply muscles of eye | Superior orbital fissure | | Diplopia Cannot look down or laterally |
| V | Trigeminal (mixed) | Superficial sensation to the cornea, the mucosa of the nose and mouth and the skin of the face and forehead. In addition the motor fibres supply the muscles of mastication | V1 Superior orbital fissure V2 Foramen rotundum V3 Foramen ovale | Check sensitivity of both sides of face with hot and cold objects, light touch and pinprick Check corneal reflex with a wisp of cotton wool Palpate muscles when jaw is clamped Check jaw jerk – tap middle of chin with reflex hammer while mouth slightly open. Should be sudden slight movement of mouth | Loss of face sensation Introduction of infection in eye No corneal reflex No response |
| VI | Abducens (motor) | Supply muscles of eye | Superior orbital fissure | Check for nystagmus (jerky movement of eyeball when looking laterally) | Cannot look laterally |

| Cranial nerve number | Cranial nerve Name | Function | Exit point from skull | Test | Abnormality |
|---|---|---|---|---|---|
| VII | Facial (mixed) | Movement and sensation of tongue | Stylomastoid foramen | Test ability to wrinkle forehead, frown, smile and raise eyebrows<br><br>Identify taste of salt or sugar on both sides of the tongue anteriorly | Asymmetry<br>Lesion in nucleus for taste sensation or sensory fibres of the facial nerve<br>Dry mouth, reduced tears<br>Loss of taste (anterior ⅔ of tongue) |
| VIII | Acoustic (sensory) | Cochlear branch<br>Vestibular branch | Internal acoustic meatus | Examine outer ear<br>Examine ear canal with otoscope<br>Test hearing on both sides, e.g. clock for air conduction and tuning fork for bone conduction<br>Caloric tests | Altered hearing:<br>Deafness<br>Tinnitus<br><br>(Usually undertaken for brain death)<br>Vertigo, nystagmus |
| IX | Glossopharyngeal (mixed) | Sensory fibres supply mucosa of soft palate, tonsils and adjacent areas | Jugular foramen | Use tongue depression to check for gag reflex | Loss of taste (posterior ⅓ of tongue)<br>No gag reflex |
| X | Vagus (mixed) | Supplies motor fibres to the pharynx, larynx and soft palate | Jugular foramen | Check ability to swallow and speak clearly with no hoarseness<br>Say 'ah' to check symmetry of vocal cords and symmetry of movement of the soft palate | Dysphagia<br>Hoarseness<br>Loss of cough reflex |
| XI | Accessory (motor) | Movement of trapezius and sternocleidomastoid muscles | Jugular foramen | Check strength of trapezius muscle on both sides – shrug shoulders<br>Palpate sternocleidomastoid muscles for strength | Weakness in shrugging shoulders |
| XII | Hypoglossal (motor) | Muscles of tongue | Hypoglossal canal | Ask patient to stick out tongue and look for atrophy or tremor and test movement from side to side against a tongue depressor | Tongue atrophy<br>Deviation of tongue to affected side<br>Fasciculation |

## Blood supply to the brain

The brain is a vital organ and receives 20% of the blood supply. Grey matter receives six times more blood than white matter. The amount of blood in the brain at any given time is 750 mls/minute.

In order to understand the blood supply to the brain it is necessary to describe cardiac physiology.

---

**Explaining cardiac physiology**

$$CO = SV \times HR$$

Where CO is an end product of the stroke volume [amount of blood pumped out per ventricle per contraction (70 mls)] multiplied by the heart rate.

$$CO = 10 - 15 \text{ mls of blood goes to the brain per cardiac cycle}$$

$$BP = CO \times TPR$$

Where blood pressure is an end product of the cardiac output (amount of blood pumped out per ventricle per minute) multiplied by the total peripheral resistance (the resistance of the blood vessels throughout the body).

---

Implications for practice

If the blood pressure drops below 80 mm Hg, hypoxia of the brain can occur; below 60 mm Hg, anoxia can occur; below 40 mm Hg, cerebral death occurs.

---

### *Determinants of blood supply to brain*

- Carotid arteries.
- Vertebral arteries.
- Circle of Willis.

### *Circulation of the brain*

The blood supply to the brain varies for the left and right sides of the brain and is as follows.

Blood leaves the left side of the heart via the ascending aorta. The aortic arch gives rise to the right brachiocephalic artery, which divides to form the right subclavian artery and the right common carotid artery. The left common carotid artery and the left subclavian artery arise directly from the aortic arch.

Each subclavian artery gives rise to a vertebral artery that runs via the transverse foramen of the cervical vertebra. The vertebral arteries join to form the basilar artery. This supplies the posterior portion of the cerebrum, cerebellum, pons and inner ear and joins the Circle of Willis (Figures 12.15 and 12.16).

Each common carotid artery divides into an external carotid artery and internal carotid artery.

The external carotid artery forms the superficial temporal and the maxillary artery and supplies blood to structures of the head including the dura mater and arachnoid mater but not the brain.

The internal carotid artery enters the cranium via the carotid foramen near the sella tursica. The internal carotid artery divides to form the anterior cerebral artery that supplies the frontal lobes and cerebrum, and the middle cerebral artery that goes towards the temporo-parietal cerebrum.

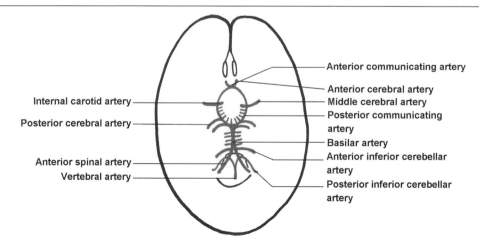

**Figure 12.15**  The Circle of Willis. For a colour version of this figure, please refer to the plate section.

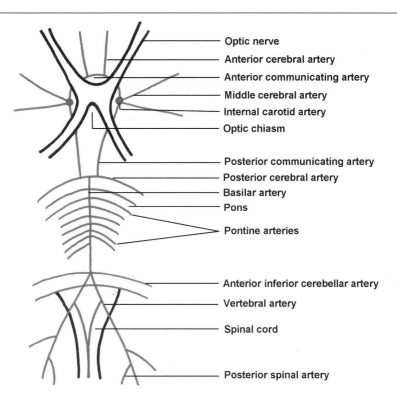

**Figure 12.16**  Diagrammatic representation of the Circle of Willis. For a colour version of this figure, please refer to the plate section.

These arteries link up to the basilar artery that has formed from the joining of the two vertebral arteries over the pons variola. The basilar artery gives rise to the tranverse arteries, anterior inferior cerebellar artery and the posterior cerebral artery on either side of the brain to supply the temporal and occipital lobes. The Circle of Willis includes the branches of the internal carotid artery, the anterior cerebral arteries, the anterior communication arteries, the posterior cerebral arteries and the posterior communicating arteries to form a complete arterial circle that enables free flow of blood within the cerebral circulation.

---

Implications for practice

Atheromatous plaques and narrowing of vessels from hypertension and other pathology may affect blood flow in the cerebral circulation, therefore the left side of the Circle of Willis may not enable blood flow to the right side and vice versa.

---

*Cerebral blood flow*

**Explaining cerebral blood flow**

**CPP is calculated as follows:**

$CPP = MAP - ICP$

Cerebral perfusion pressure is the mean arterial blood pressure minus the intracranial pressure.

$MAP = (systolic - diastolic)/3 + diastolic$

e.g.    Systolic        144 mm Hg
        Diastolic       90 mm Hg
        ICP             15 mm Hg

**Calculation:**

$MAP = (144 - 90) = 54/3 = 18 + 90 = 108$

$CPP = 108 - 15 = 93$ mm Hg

**Cerebral blood flow (CBF)**

**CBF = CPP (MAP − ICP)/CVR where:**
CPP = cerebral perfusion pressure
MAP = mean arterial blood pressure
ICP = intracranial pressure
CVR = cerebrovascular resistance

Factors affecting cerebral blood flow:

*Extracerebral factors:*
- Blood pressure.
- Cardiac function.
- Blood viscosity.

*Intracerebral factors:*
- Arterial disease.
- ↑ Intracranial pressure.
- Space occupying lesion.

In the normal brain, cerebral blood flow (CBF) is maintained by an autoregulatory mechanism which allows the brain to maintain a constant cerebral blood flow despite large variations in blood pressure.

---

**Types of autoregulation:**

1. **Pressure controlled myogenic mechanism**
   MAP = 60–150 mm Hg
   < 60 mm Hg                    ↓CBF
   >150 mm Hg                    ↑CBF
   Operates with MAP = 40 mm Hg
2. **Chemical metabolic regulation**
   a. $PaCO_2$
      High  →  vasodilation      →  ↑ Blood flow
      Low   →  vasoconstriction  →  ↓ Blood flow
   b. $O_2$
      ↓    vasodilation
      ↑    vasoconstriction
   c. $H^+$ (pH)
      ↓    vasodilation
      ↑    vasoconstriction
3. **Neurogenic regulation**
   a. Sympathetic stimulation → vasoconstriction
   b. Parasympathetic simulation → vasodilation

---

Factors affecting autoregulation include:

1. MAP
2. ICP > 40 to 50 mm Hg
3. Local or diffuse injury or ischaemia
4. Vasomotor paralysis where there is no autoregulation.

---

**Implications for practice**

Autoregulation does not work at the extremes of blood pressure. Thus at a very low blood pressure, cerebral blood flow will fall.

Autoregulation also fails in the injured or diseased brain when cerebral blood flow is directly proportional to cerebral perfusion pressure.

---

*Blood brain barrier (BBB)*
Within the brain the endothelial cells form a semi-permeable membrane that controls the flow of fluid and substances between the brain and the bloodstream. Astrocytes surrounding blood vessels of the brain form a tight protection and may be responsible for the transport of electrolytes through the BBB. Certain substances are allowed through the BBB, for example anaesthetic gases and alcohol, while other substances are not, such as hormones (Nair and Peate 2009).

---

**Implications for practice**

1. In head injury, maintaining cerebral blood flow is vital. This necessitates
   - Maintaining the mean arterial pressure.
   - Evacuating any haematoma.
   - Controlling raised intracranial pressure.
   - Maintaining normal $PaO_2$.
   - Maintaining normal $PaCO_2$.
2. Trauma to the carotid or vertebral arteries may cause a reduction of blood flow to the brain and may present as a stroke.
3. Due to diseases, such as atherosclerosis, patients may present with interruption of the blood supply to the brain, for example cerebro-vascular accident.

---

*Venous drainage*
Blood drains from the face, scalp and the brain via the superior sagittal sinus, the inferior sagittal sinus, straight sinus, transverse sinus, into the confluence of sinuses where they all meet. The blood then enters the sigmoid sinus and thereafter flows into the internal jugular vein (Figure 12.17).

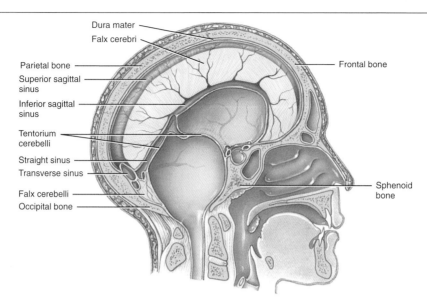

**Figure 12.17** Venous drainage. From *Principles of anatomy and physiology: Organisation, support and movement, and control systems of the human body.* Tortora, G.J. & Derrickson, B. Copyright © 2011 John Wiley & Sons, Inc. For a colour version of this figure, please refer to the plate section.

---

### Implications for practice

As blood from the face drains via the brain to the internal jugular vein it is important that lesions on the face, such as pimples, are managed with clean hands and aseptic equipment to prevent a venous sinus thrombosis from occurring.

### Cerebrospinal fluid (CSF) (Figures 12.18 & 12.9)

Cerebrospinal fluid (CSF) is a clear fluid produced by the choroid plexus of the lateral and fourth ventricle; 500 mls of CSF is produced per day. The total volume of CSF is changed ± three times per day. Normally there is 150 mls in circulation at any one time. The CSF passes from the lateral ventricles through the Foramen of Munro to the third ventricle through the Aqueduct of Sylvius to the fourth ventricle. From the fourth ventricle some of the CSF goes via the Foramen of Magendie to the central canal and some goes through the Foramen of Lushka to the subarachnoid space. Arachnoid villi within the subarachnoid space absorb the CSF which enters the venous circulation (Table 12.5).

### Intracranial pressure (ICP)

#### Definition

Intracranial pressure is the pressure exerted within the skull. The normal ICP ranges between 0 and 15 mmHg (50–150 mm CSF). ICP is maintained in a steady state of equilibrium by the factors that determine ICP.

#### Determinants of ICP

Factors affecting ICP are:

- Integrity of the skull.
- Brain size.
- CSF flow.
- Blood supply and venous drainage.

#### The Monro–Kellie hypothesis

The skull is a rigid box and cannot increase its volume. Within the skull the brain takes up 80% of the available space, CSF accounts for 10% of available space and blood supply accounts for the final 10% of available space. If the volume of the brain increases (e.g. due to cerebral oedema), the volume of blood or CSF must decrease if the ICP is to be maintained within normal limits.

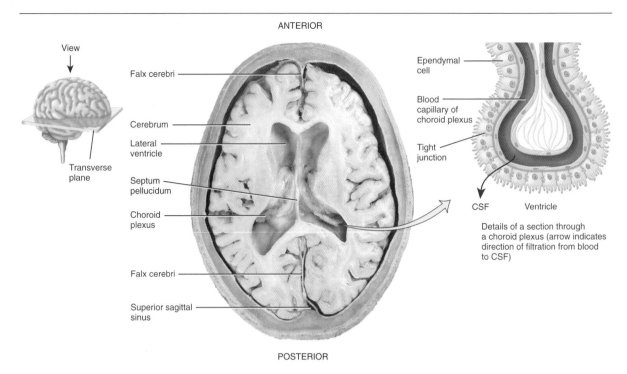

**Figure 12.18** Cerebrospinal fluid circulation. From *Principles of anatomy and physiology: Organisation, support and movement, and control systems of the human body*. Tortora, G.J. & Derrickson, B. Copyright © 2011 John Wiley & Sons, Inc. For a colour version of this figure, please refer to the plate section.

**Table 12.5** Properties of cerebrospinal fluid.

| Property | Value |
|---|---|
| Colour | Clear and watery |
| Pressure | 0–15 mmHg |
| Specific gravity | 1005–1008 |
| Reaction | Alkaline, pH 7.4 |
| Protein | 40 mg % |
| Glucose | 50–75 mg % |
| Chlorides | 720–750 mg % |
| Cells | <3 lymphocytes |
| Calcium | 5.3–5.6 mg % |
| Sulphates | 0.6 mg % |
| Potassium | 12–17 mg % |
| Urea | 15–40 mg % |
| Inorganic sulphates | 1.5–2.1 mg % |
| Cholesterol | Trace |
| Creatinine | Trace |
| Bicarbonate | 50–75 (volume of $CO_2$ per 100 mls) |
| Red blood cells | Nil |

The compensatory mechanisms include:

1. Displacement of CSF to the spinal subarachnoid space and peri-optic subarachnoid space.
2. Compression of the dural sinuses.
3. Decreased production of CSF.
4. Vasoconstriction of the cerebral vasculature.

The relationship of change in volume to change in pressure is called *compliance*. If all compensatory mechanisms are exhausted this will affect compliance.

Factors influencing compliance include:

1. Amount of volume increased.
2. Time frame for accommodation.
3. Size of intracranial compartment.

Beyond a certain level, decompensation may occur resulting in raised ICP.

### *ICP wave form*

Within the waveform there are three peaks (Figure 12.19):

P1  The percussion wave originates from an arterial pulsation and is peaked.

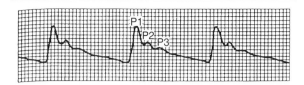

**Figure 12.19**    Intracranial pressure wave forms.

## Implications for practice

- Performing regular neurological observations to determine any signs and symptoms of ↑ICP is essential to manage patients with neurotrauma.
- If the patient presents with ↑ICP do not perform a lumbar puncture as this could lead to coning.

## The motor pathways

There are two pathways in the brain concerned with motor function:

1. The pyramidal motor pathway.
2. The extrapyramidal motor pathway.

### *The pyramidal motor pathway*

The pyramidal system is responsible for voluntary motor movement and is made up of upper motor neurones, lower motor neurones and internuncial neurones. The lower motor neurones and internuncial neurones form part of the reflex arc.

The pyramidal motor pathway commences in the Betz cells of the motor cortex in the parietal lobe. The motor area of the parietal cortex is represented by the motor homunculus (see Figure 12.12). The motor area is divided into the primary motor area, the secondary motor area and the associated motor area depending on the extent of function in that area. The fibres of the pyramidal motor system travel via the internal capsule to the pons variola and medulla oblongata to supply the face, eyes, mouth and pharynx. Other fibres go directly to the medulla oblongata. Of the fibres that go via the medulla oblongata to the pyramids 85% decussate or cross over to supply the opposite side of the body. Once the fibres decussate they then go via the corticospinal tracts. From there the fibres travel to the internuncial neurone, anterior motor neurone and thence to the effector organ where the motor response occurs.

A positive Babinski response is when the sole of the foot is stroked with the end of a patella hammer, the big toe extends upwards.

A positive cremaster response is when the inside of the thigh is stroked, the scrotum on the same side rises.

Clonus occurs when the foot is dorsiflexed and the stimulus is maintained, the result is that the foot moves backwards and forwards until such time as the stimulus is removed.

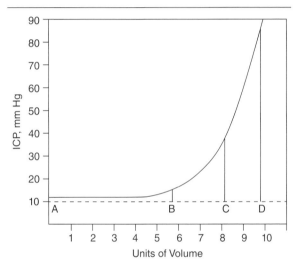

From point A to just before B, the ICP remains constant although there is addition of volume (compliance is high). At point B, even though the ICP is within normal limits, compliance begins to change, as evidenced by the slight rise in volume (low compliance). From points C to D, ICP rises significantly with each minute increase in volume (compliance is lost).

**Figure 12.20**    Pressure volume curve.

P2 This is known as the tidal wave. It terminates in a dicrotic notch and is a reflection of compliance. With ↑ICP there is a progressive rise in P2.

P3 The dicrotic wave follows the dicrotic notch.

## Implications for practice

1. Damage to the pyramidal motor system can present as either an upper or lower motor neurone lesion. Upper motor neurone lesions occur in the brain or spinal cord. Lower motor neurone lesions can occur in the anterior horn cells of the spinal cord but usually occur distal to that, for example in the nerve root where it emerges from the spinal cord or in a peripheral nerve.
2. To ensure appropriate diagnosis and management of the patient, it is important to differentiate between upper and lower motor neurone lesions (Table 12.6).

**Table 12.6** Differences between upper and lower motor neurone lesions.

| Upper motor lesion | Lower motor lesion |
| --- | --- |
| Spastic paralysis | Flaccid paralysis |
| Hyperreflexia | Hyporeflexia |
| Babinski response | No Babinski response |
| Cremaster response | No cremaster response |
| Abdominal reflexes | No abdominal reflexes |
| Clonus | Absence of clonus |
| No atrophy | Atrophy present |

### The extrapyramidal system

The extrapyramidal system consists of the basal ganglia in addition to nuclei in other regions of the brain, and is responsible for somatic motor function, involuntary movement, adjusting body posture, fine movement and co-ordination. The basal ganglia are made up of grey matter (see Figure 12.10).

The basal ganglia are:

- Globus pallidus.
- Substantia nigra.
- Caudate nucleus.
- Thalamus.
- Amygdala.
- Putamen.

The fibres of the extrapyramidal system originate in the deep motor cortex and then travel to the basal ganglia in the cerebral hemispheres via the internal capsule. From the basal ganglia fibres of the extrapyramidal system go to the cerebellum where control of the extrapyramidal system is based.

The fibres then traverse the spinal cord in different tracts, namely:

- The vestibular tract.
- The reticulospinal tract.
- The propriospinal tract.

Thereafter the fibres are directed to the internuncial neurone, anterior motor neurone and effector organ.

## Implications for practice

Damage to the extrapyramidal system does not cause paralysis. It results in loss of voluntary movement, chorea, athetosis and Parkinson's tremor with slowed movement, tremors and rigidity of muscles.

### The autonomic nervous system (ANS)

The ANS maintains homeostasis within the body, regulating the automatic and involuntary functions such as the heart, blood vessels and lungs.

The neurotransmitter involved in parasympathetic control is acetylcholine that tends to have a relaxing, slowing down effect on the body in contrast to norepinephrine, the neurotransmitter for the sympathetic nervous system that normally speeds things up.

### Functions of the autonomic nervous system

The ANS is responsible for the bodies' responses to internal and external alterations in body function (Table 12.7).

### Parasympathetic nervous system

The parasympathetic nervous system has a craniosacral outflow. The pre-gangliotic fibres emerge through cranial nerves III, VII, IX and X as well as sacral spinal nerves II and III or III and IV. These emerge as the splanchnic nerves. The synapse of pre- and post-gangliotic fibres occurs on the wall of the organ being innervated.

**Table 12.7** Effects of SNS and PNS on the body.

| Body organ | SNS | PNS |
| --- | --- | --- |
| Cell | ↑ Metabolism | – |
| Lungs | Dilates bronchioles | Constricts bronchioles |
| Pupils | Dilates pupils | Constricts pupils |
| Heart | ↑ Heart rate | ↓ Heart rate |
| Blood vessels | Dilates blood vessels in heart/muscle Constricted blood vessels in non-essential organs and skin | – |
| Liver | ↑ Release of glucose | – |
| Gastrointestinal system | ↓ Peristalsis Constriction of sphincters | ↑ Peristalsis Dilates sphincters |
| Bladder | Involuntary control | Voluntary control |
| Skin | Vasoconstriction, hairs stand up | |

(Nair and Peate 2009: p. 255)

The pre-ganglionic fibres synapse with cells in the following ganglia:

- Cranial nerve III – the ciliary ganglion responsible for muscles constricting the pupil, the muscles constricting the lens and accommodation.
- Cranial nerve VII – The sphenopalatine ganglion is responsible for the lachrymal gland that secretes tears as well as the submandibular ganglion that produces saliva.
- Cranial nerve IX – otic ganglion.
- Cranial nerve X – ganglia in walls of the viscera of the respiratory tract, gastrointestinal tract and cardiovascular system.

*Sympathetic nervous system*

The sympathetic chains are found on either side of the spine close to the midline and join over the coccyx (Figure 12.21). The pre-ganglionic fibres may reach the ganglion via a synapse at the same level, by travelling up or down.

The post-ganglionic fibres leave the sympathetic chain as the grey ramus communicans and are distributed through the anterior and posterior rami of the spinal nerves (Figure 12.22).

Sympathetic chains occur on the following ganglia:

- Cervical 3.
- Thoracic 11 and 12.
- Lumbar 4.
- Sacral 4 and 5.

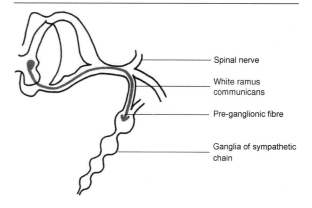

**Figure 12.21** Sympathetic nervous system showing the pre-ganglionic fibre.

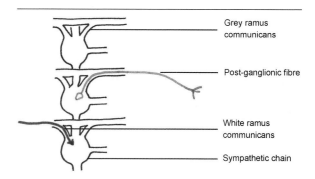

**Figure 12.22** Sympathetic nervous system showing the post-ganglionic fibre.

## ADDITIONAL CONCEPTS RELATED TO NEUROPHYSIOLOGY

### Neuroplasticity

Previously it was thought that neuroplasticity was only a feature of brain development in neonates and young children of less than 3 to 4 years of age. Extensive and continuing research has shown that this is not the case. Provided the brain is constantly challenged, involved in stimulation and new experiences, neuroplasticity can take place throughout life.

### What is neuroplasticity?

Neuroplasticity occurs throughout the brain and refers to changes in the structure of the brain that enable the brain to be re-moulded and change over one's lifetime in response to external stimuli, experience and activity. The principle of neuroplasticity is that the brain is incredibly malleable, adaptable and responsive and can lay down new pathways or re-arrange existing pathways throughout life to aid learning and memory through experience (Hell and Ehlers 2008). All neurones act independently but, when trying to acquire new skills, many neurones will be involved in the work and act simultaneously to process the neural information. It is this process that gives the brain its plasticity. Reverberation occurs when the stimulus bounces from the first neurone to the next neurone and back again. It creates a 'neural echo' and it is this neural echo that allows the neuroplasticity process to begin. There are numerous ways in which the brain can rebuild damaged connections, establish new connections or strengthen connections:

- Functional map expansion: this occurs when the cells surrounding the damaged area change their shape and perform the functions of the damaged neurones.
- Compensatory masquerade: when damage occurs alternate pathways respond to changes.
- Homologous region adoption: this allows another part of the brain to take over the function of the part that has been damaged.
- Cross model re-assignment: this allows sensory input such as sight to be replaced by another one such as touch, e.g. the use of Braille.
- Synaptic pruning: this occurs by deleting old connections or by allowing others to just fade away if they are not efficient or not often used, whilst those that are used are made more dense.
- Synaptic reformation.

### Neuroplasticity and learning

Research has shown that the structure and chemistry of neural networks can change as a result of external stimuli.

---

**Top tips**

1. 'Use it' or 'lose it'.
2. Exercise the brain as well as the body.
3. Remember 'practice makes perfect'.

---

**Implications for practice**

1. Consider whether:
   - Skills that have been lost can be relearned.
   - Deterioration and degeneration of brain cells can be prevented.
   - The effects of brain damage can be reversed.
   - New skills can be developed.
2. Throughout the patient's journey, it is therefore important to introduce activities or interventions that can either form new neural synapses, strengthen neural connections that are present or change the cortical structure of the brain (Westerberg and Klingberg 2007).
3. Develop activities that the patient can undertake using all parts of the body.
4. Do not neglect the injured part as this will result in compensation by other parts and will not encourage neuroplasticity, e.g. hand tapping exercises; hand crawling up wall exercises and brushing hair.

---

## ACID-BASE BALANCE

### Introduction

In order for practitioners to be able to aid decision making and manage head injury patients effectively, it is necessary to understand the fundamental principles of acid-base balance. If you follow these easy steps it will make acid-base balance theory easy to understand and apply in practice.

### Definition

The body is designed to operate within a very narrow pH range of 7.35–7.45. Acid-base balance is the process that maintains the pH of the body tissues in order to maintain a chemical environment that will allow all body systems to work optimally.

Body Cell                          Plasma

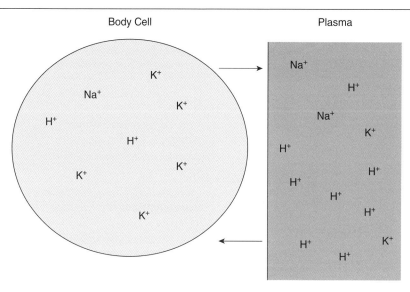

**Figure 12.23** Simple ion exchange.

### Ways of maintaining acid-base balance

There are four ways of maintaining acid-base balance:

1. Simple ion exchange.
2. Use of buffering systems, namely haemoglobin (Hb) in the red blood cell (RBC) and phosphoric acid ($HPO_4$) in urine.
3. Respiratory control.
4. Selective re-absorption of ions by the kidney.

#### Simple ion exchange (Figure 12.23)

The body uses simple ion exchange to maintain acid-base balance. This takes place in all cells in the body including the RBC, lungs and the kidney. Simple ion exchange involves the exchanging of positive ions for other positive ions across a membrane. It may be a positively charged ion of another substance, e.g. $K^+$, $Mg^+$ or $H^+$. Ions exchange across a membrane until such time as the number of charges on each side are equivalent. The same process occurs for negatively charged ions such as $HCO_3^-$ $Cl^-$ within the body. Negative ions are not able to exchange for positive ions and positive ions cannot exchange for negative ions.

#### Haemoglobin buffering system (Figure 12.24)

The haemoglobin buffering system, otherwise known as the chloride shift, occurs via red blood cells (RBC), plasma and body cells. The buffering system refers to the fact that a substance can be added to the RBC and haemoglobin and taken away from the RBC and haemoglobin without altering the structure of the cell itself.

In a RBC there is carbon dioxide ($CO_2$) and water ($H_2O$), potassium hydroxide (KOH) and haemoglobin. The process is as follows:

- $CO_2$ diffuses from the body cell via the plasma into the RBC. $H_2O$ is an end product of activities within the cell. Under the influence of the catalyst, carbonic anhydrase, the $CO_2$ and $H_2O$ combine to form carbonic acid ($H_2CO_3$). At the same time within the cell, there is oxyhaemoglobin ($HbO_2$). When the haemoglobin releases oxygen to travel via the plasma to the body cells, potassium hydroxide (KOH) is also released.
- The $H_2CO_3$ combines with potassium hydroxide (KOH) to form $H_2O$ and potassium bicarbonate ($KHCO_3^-$). The $KHCO_3^-$ separates to form $K^+$ and $HCO_3^-$. In the meantime within the plasma there is naturally occurring sodium chloride ($NaCl_2^-$). The active sodium pump keeps the sodium within the plasma. The sodium pump does not allow the sodium to exchange with the potassium in the red blood cell. The $Na^+$ separates from the $Cl_2^-$. The $Cl_2^-$ is then able to enter the red blood cell and combine with $K^+$ to form $K^+Cl_2^-$. The $HCO_3^-$ released from the $KHCO_3^-$ enters the plasma to combine with sodium to form $NaHCO_3^-$. This is the chloride shift. The chloride shift occurs because positive ions can only be exchanged for positive ions and negative ions can only be exchanged for negative ions. Therefore the bicarbonate ions are exchanged for the chloride ions until such time as the negative ions within the RBC equate with the negative ions in the plasma.

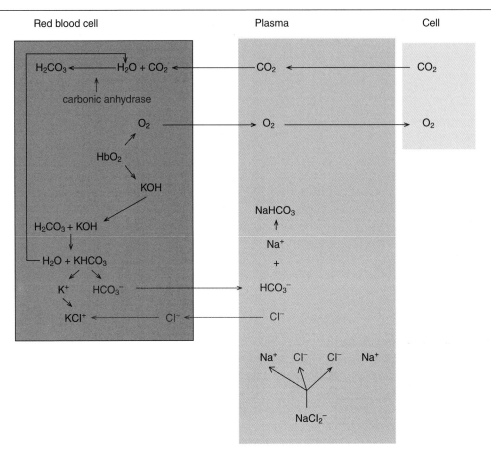

**Figure 12.24**  Haemoglobin buffering system.

***Respiratory control*** (Figure 12.25)

It is in this format that the RBC now travels to the lungs ($KCl_2$ in the RBC and $NaHCO_3^-$ in the plasma).

There are three ways in which $CO_2$ reaches the lungs, namely:

- Via the chloride shift that involves the RBC and accounts for 88–90% of the $CO_2$ reaching the lungs.
- $CO_2$ dissolved in plasma accounts for 3–5%.
- Carboxyhaemoglobin ($HbCO_2$) accounts for 8–10%.

In the lungs the RBC once again becomes the carbon dioxide factory as follows:

- The $O_2$ level in the alveolar cell is higher than that in the RBC.
- The $O_2$ starts to diffuse into the RBC to form oxyhaemoglobin.

- At the same time the $KCl_2$ in the RBC separates into $K^+$ and $Cl_2^-$.
- In the plasma, the $NaHCO_3$ separates into $Na^+$ and $HCO_3^-$. The $HCO_3^-$ moves into the cell and the $Cl_2^-$ moves out of the RBC into the plasma. The reverse of the chloride shift.
- In the RBC the $K^+$ combines with the $HCO_3^-$ to form KOH and $CO_2$.
- The $CO_2$ level in the RBC is higher than that in the alveolar cell. The $CO_2$ starts to diffuse from the RBC to the alveolar cell and into the atmosphere. An excellent way of getting rid of $CO_2$ and maintaining the acid-base balance within the normal range.
- The RBC now travels to the rest of the body and the process begins again.

***Selective re-absorption from the kidney*** (Figure 12.26)

Within the kidney tubules the process of eliminating acid products involves simple ion exchange of $H^+$ and $K^+$. The

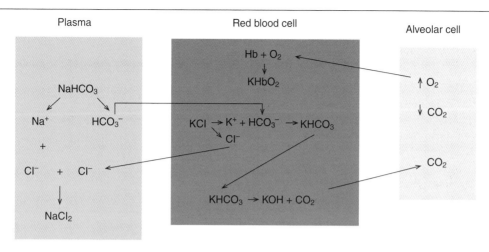

**Figure 12.25** Respiratory control.

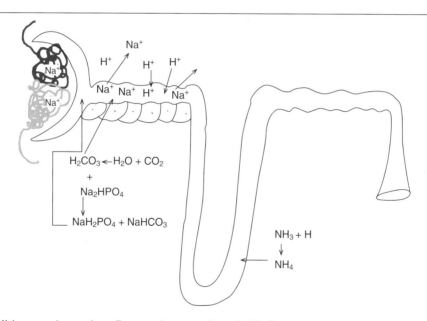

**Figure 12.26** Kidney reabsorption. For a colour version of this figure, please refer to the plate section.

hydrogen phosphate ($HPO_4^-$) is a buffer found in the kidneys. Within the glomerular filtrate $CO_2$ plus $H_2O$ combine to form $H_2CO_3$. This $H_2CO_3$ (a weak acid) combines with disodium hydrogen phosphate ($Na_2HPO_4$) to form sodium di-hydrogen phosphate ($NaH_2PO_4$) (a stronger acid). This is then excreted in the urine. In addition, within the kidney tubules ammonia ($NH_3$) combines with additional $H^+$ ions to form ammonium salts ($NH_4$) that are excreted in the urine. These processes assist the body to maintain a urine pH of 5.5–8.

## SUMMARY

It is the above physiological processes that help maintain the bodies' normal pH. The body is able to compensate should the pH alter. If the body is not able to compensate sufficiently for changes in pH due to illness or injury this

## Implications for practice

In summary:

pH < 7.35 is an acidosis and pH > 7.45 is an alkalosis.
Raised $pCO_2$ indicates a respiratory acidosis.
Lowered $pCO_2$ indicates a respiratory alkalosis.
Lowered $HCO_3^-$ indicates a metabolic acidosis.
Raised $HCO_3^-$ indicates a metabolic alkalosis.

In a primary metabolic acidosis, the body will try to compensate by creating a respiratory alkalosis. This occurs quickly.

In a primary respiratory acidosis, the body will try to compensate by creating a metabolic alkalosis.

In addition, mixed pictures can occur, for example the shocked patient who is hypoventilating may have a combined respiratory and metabolic acidosis.

will be reflected in the patient's clinical presentation and arterial blood gas sample. When examining an arterial blood gas sample it is important to establish the pH, $PaCO_2$ and $PaO_2$ as well as the cause of the problem. This may occur at a respiratory level or metabolic level. Management of the patient will depend on the severity of the acidosis or alkalosis.

## CONCLUSION

A good knowledge of anatomy and physiology and the practical implications of pathophysiology will enable the health profession to provide safe, effective care as well as provide patients with accurate information based on scientific evidence fundamental to making appropriate lifestyle choices.

## Quiz

**Anatomy and physiology of the nervous system**

1. THE SCALP
    a. What are the names of the five layers of the scalp?
    b. What are the purposes of each layer?
    c. Why is a scalp laceration likely to bleed profusely?
    d. Why is a patient who has a scalp laceration that becomes infected likely to develop a brain abscess thereafter?

2. THE SKULL
    a. How would you describe the superior aspect of the skull?
    b. How would you describe the lateral aspect of the skull?
    c. How would you describe the posterior aspect of the skull?
    d. How would you describe the inferior aspect of the skull?
    e. How would you describe the sutures of the skull?
    f. What are the purposes of the sutures?
    g. If the sutures do not develop normally, what condition may arise?
    h. Examine the base of the skull and state the path for the following:
        i. spinal cord
        ii. internal jugular vein
        iii. internal carotid artery
        iv. meningeal artery
        v. vagus nerve

3. THE MENINGES
    a. The meninges consist of _____ layers.
    b. How would you describe each layer of the meninges?
    c. How would you describe the falx cerebri and the falx cerebelli?

4. THE VENOUS DRAINAGE OF THE BRAIN
    a. Describe the venous drainage of the brain using the following table:
       NAME     LOCATION     FUNCTION
    b. How would you differentiate between the two groups of sinuses?
    c. Draw a schematic representation of the venous drainage of the brain.

5. THE NEURONE
    a. What is the definition of the term 'neurone'?
    b. How would you describe the basic structure of each part of a neurone?
    c. What are the functions of each part of a neurone?
    d. List four types of neuroglia that are to be found in the CNS.

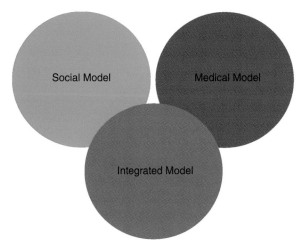

**Figure 2.1**  Model of neurotrauma management.

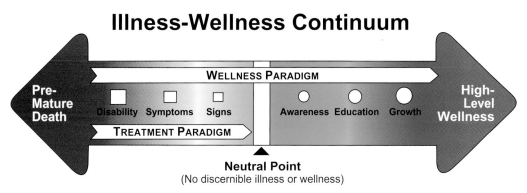

**Figure 2.3**  Illness–wellness continuum. www.thewellspring.com. Travis, Copyright © 2004, 1988, 1972 JW Travis. Reproduced with permission.

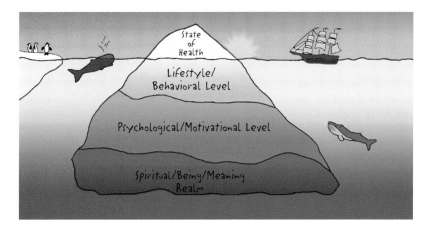

**Figure 2.4**  The Iceberg Model. www.mywellnesstest.com/IcebergModel.asp. Travis © 1978, 1988, 2004 JW Travis. Reproduced with permission.

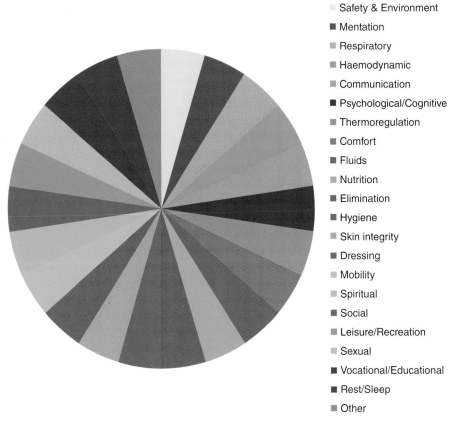

**Safety & Environment**
**Mentation**
**Respiratory**
**Haemodynamic**
**Communication**
**Psychological/Cognitive**
**Thermoregulation**
**Comfort**
**Fluids**
**Nutrition**
**Elimination**
**Hygiene**
**Skin integrity**
**Dressing**
**Mobility**
**Spiritual**
**Social**
**Leisure/Recreation**
**Sexual**
**Vocational/Educational**
**Rest/Sleep**
**Other**

**Figure 3.1**  Needs Approach Model.

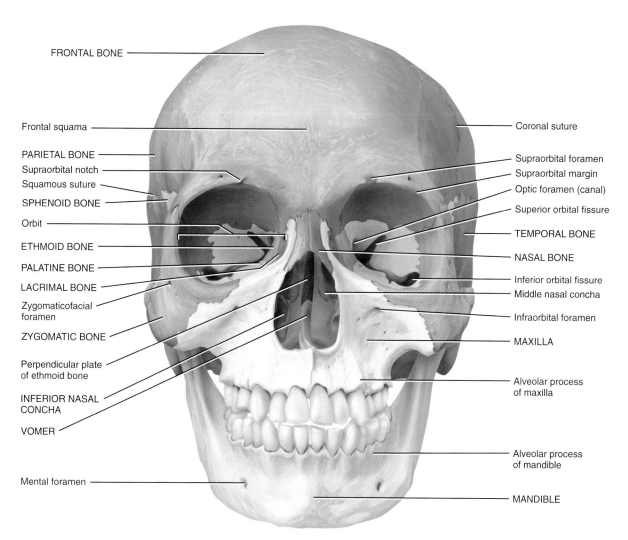

FRONTAL BONE

Frontal squama

PARIETAL BONE

Supraorbital notch

Squamous suture

SPHENOID BONE

Orbit

ETHMOID BONE

PALATINE BONE

LACRIMAL BONE

Zygomaticofacial foramen

ZYGOMATIC BONE

Perpendicular plate of ethmoid bone

INFERIOR NASAL CONCHA

VOMER

Mental foramen

Coronal suture

Supraorbital foramen

Supraorbital margin

Optic foramen (canal)

Superior orbital fissure

TEMPORAL BONE

NASAL BONE

Inferior orbital fissure

Middle nasal concha

Infraorbital foramen

MAXILLA

Alveolar process of maxilla

Alveolar process of mandible

MANDIBLE

**Figure 12.1** Anterior view of the skull. From *Principles of anatomy and physiology: Organisation, support and movement, and control systems of the human body.* Tortora, G.J. & Derrickson, B. Copyright © 2011 John Wiley & Sons, Inc.

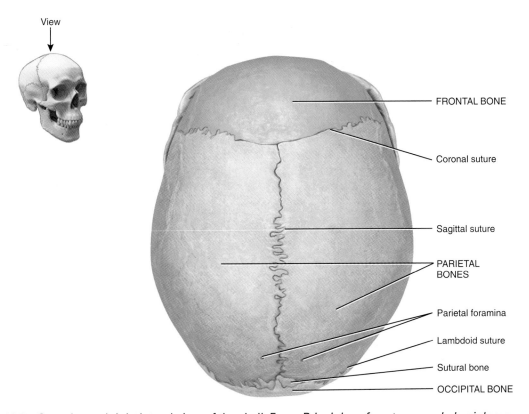

View

FRONTAL BONE

Coronal suture

Sagittal suture

PARIETAL BONES

Parietal foramina

Lambdoid suture

Sutural bone

OCCIPITAL BONE

**Figure 12.2** Superior and right lateral view of the skull. From *Principles of anatomy and physiology: Organisation, support and movement, and control systems of the human body.* Tortora, G.J. & Derrickson, B. Copyright © 2011 John Wiley & Sons, Inc.

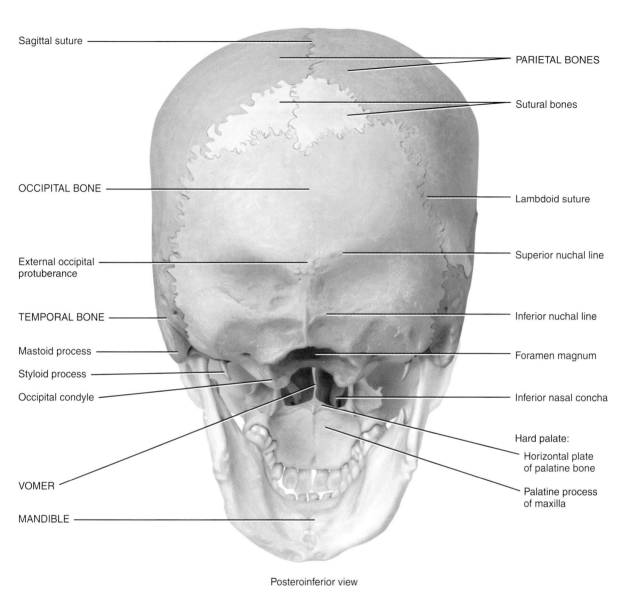

Sagittal suture

PARIETAL BONES

Sutural bones

OCCIPITAL BONE

Lambdoid suture

External occipital protuberance

Superior nuchal line

TEMPORAL BONE

Inferior nuchal line

Mastoid process

Foramen magnum

Styloid process

Occipital condyle

Inferior nasal concha

Hard palate:

Horizontal plate of palatine bone

VOMER

Palatine process of maxilla

MANDIBLE

Posteroinferior view

**Figure 12.3** Posterior view of the skull. From *Principles of anatomy and physiology: Organisation, support and movement, and control systems of the human body.* Tortora, G.J. & Derrickson, B. Copyright © 2011. John Wiley & Sons, Inc.

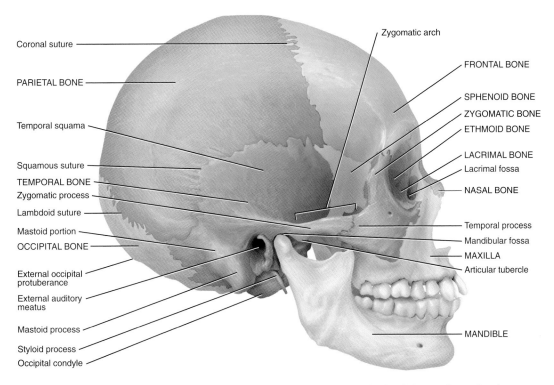

**Figure 12.4** Lateral view of the skull. From *Principles of anatomy and physiology: Organisation, support and movement, and control systems of the human body.* Tortora, G.J. & Derrickson, B. Copyright © 2011. John Wiley & Sons, Inc.

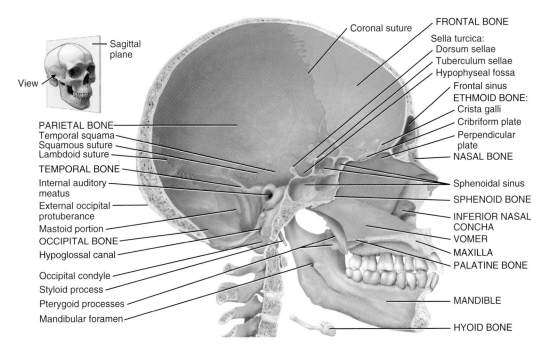

**Figure 12.5** Medial view of sagittal section of the skull. From *Principles of anatomy and physiology: Organisation, support and movement, and control systems of the human body.* Tortora, G.J. & Derrickson, B. Copyright © 2011. John Wiley & Sons, Inc.

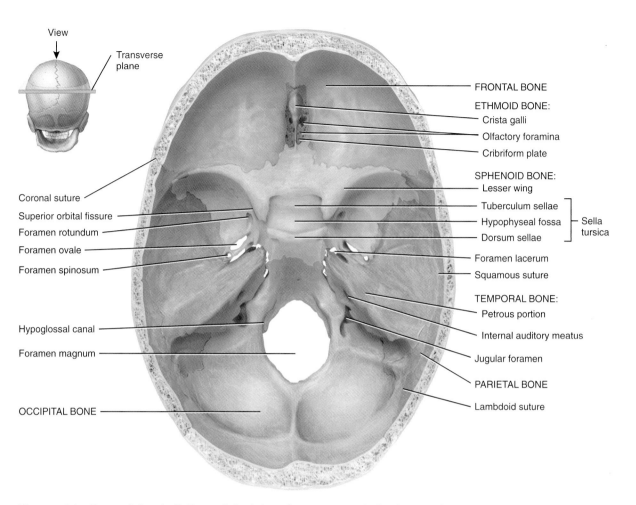

**Figure 12.6** Base of the skull. From *Principles of anatomy and physiology: Organisation, support and movement, and control systems of the human body.* Tortora, G.J. & Derrickson, B. Copyright © 2011. John Wiley & Sons, Inc.

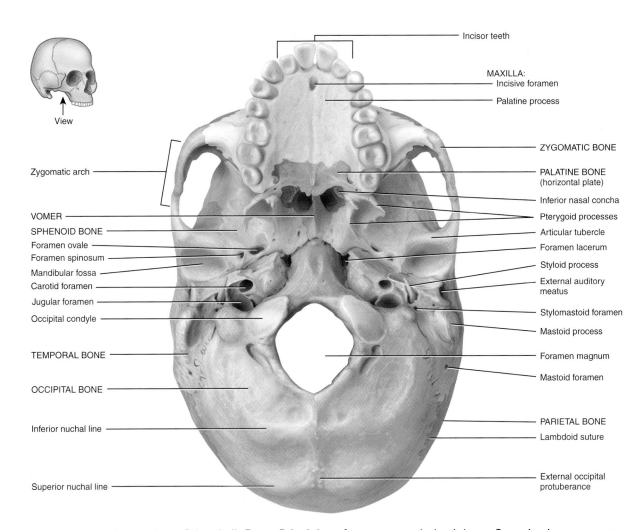

**Figure 12.7** Inferior view of the skull. From *Principles of anatomy and physiology: Organisation, support and movement, and control systems of the human body.* Tortora, G.J. & Derrickson, B. Copyright © 2011. John Wiley & Sons, Inc.

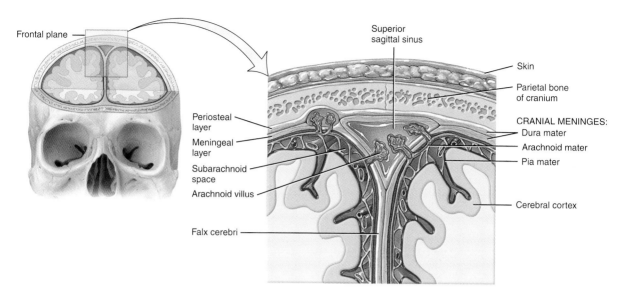

**Figure 12.8** The meninges. From *Principles of anatomy and physiology: Organisation, support and movement, and control systems of the human body*. Tortora, G.J. & Derrickson, B. Copyright © 2011. John Wiley & Sons, Inc.

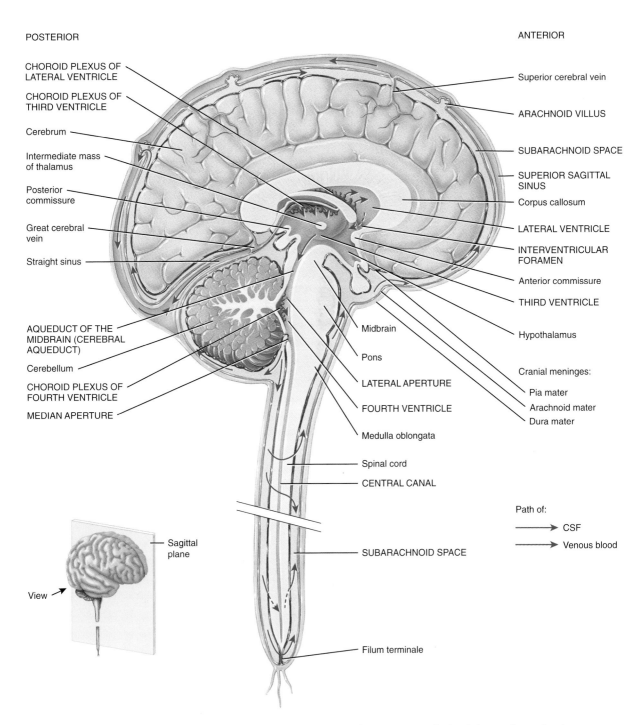

POSTERIOR

ANTERIOR

CHOROID PLEXUS OF
LATERAL VENTRICLE

CHOROID PLEXUS OF
THIRD VENTRICLE

Cerebrum

Intermediate mass
of thalamus

Posterior
commissure

Great cerebral
vein

Straight sinus

AQUEDUCT OF THE
MIDBRAIN (CEREBRAL
AQUEDUCT)

Cerebellum

CHOROID PLEXUS OF
FOURTH VENTRICLE

MEDIAN APERTURE

Superior cerebral vein

ARACHNOID VILLUS

SUBARACHNOID SPACE

SUPERIOR SAGITTAL
SINUS

Corpus callosum

LATERAL VENTRICLE

INTERVENTRICULAR
FORAMEN

Anterior commissure

THIRD VENTRICLE

Hypothalamus

Midbrain

Pons

LATERAL APERTURE

FOURTH VENTRICLE

Medulla oblongata

Cranial meninges:

Pia mater

Arachnoid mater

Dura mater

Sagittal
plane

View

Spinal cord

CENTRAL CANAL

SUBARACHNOID SPACE

Path of:

CSF

Venous blood

Filum terminale

**Figure 12.9** Sagittal section of the brain. From *Principles of anatomy and physiology: Organisation, support and movement, and control systems of the human body*. Tortora, G.J. & Derrickson, B. Copyright © 2011. John Wiley & Sons, Inc.

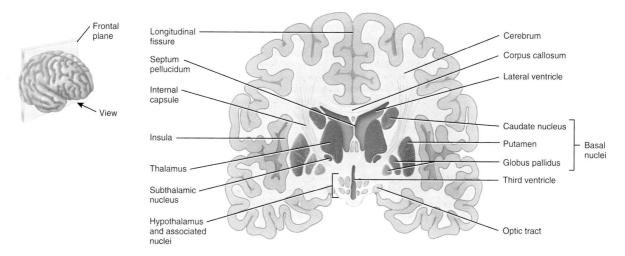

**Figure 12.10** Anterior section of the brain. From *Principles of anatomy and physiology: Organisation, support and movement, and control systems of the human body.* Tortora GJ & Derrickson B. Copyright © 2011. John Wiley & Sons, Inc.

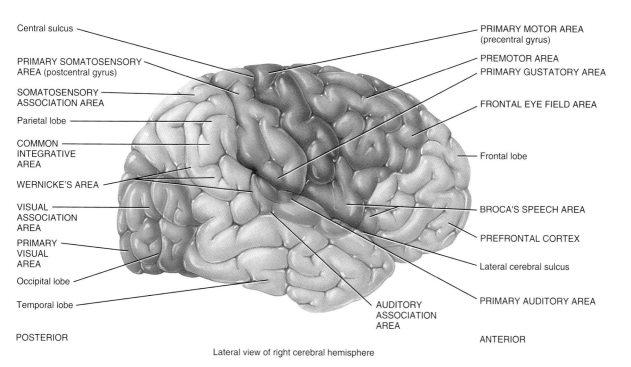

**Figure 12.11** Functional areas of the brain. From *Principles of anatomy and physiology: Organisation, support and movement, and control systems of the human body.* Tortora, G.J. & Derrickson, B. Copyright © 2011. John Wiley & Sons, Inc.

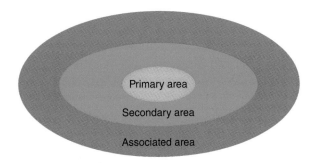

Figure 12.12 Graphic demonstrating primary, secondary and association areas of cerebrum.

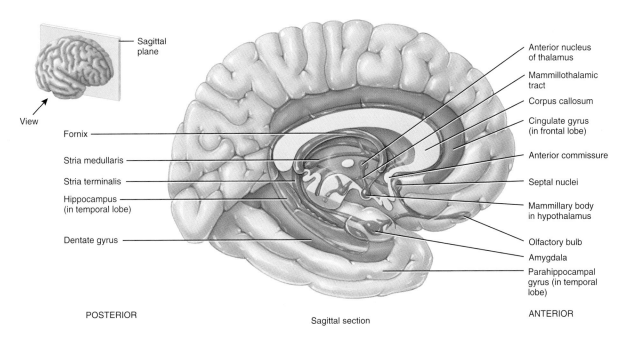

Figure 12.14 The limbic system. From *Principles of anatomy and physiology: Organisation, support and movement, and control systems of the human body.* Tortora, G.J. & Derrickson, B. Copyright © 2011. John Wiley & Sons, Inc.

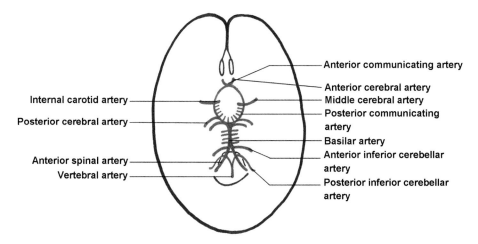

**Figure 12.15** The Circle of Willis.

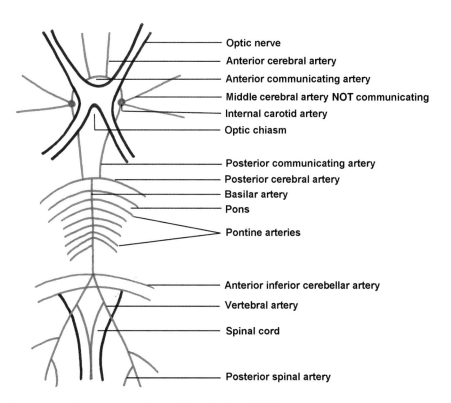

**Figure 12.16** Diagrammatic representation of the Circle of Willis.

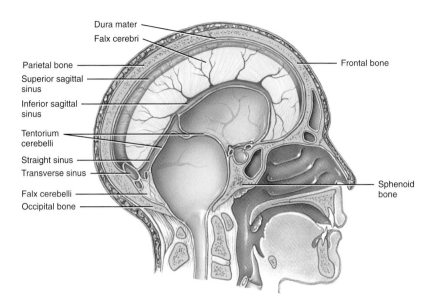

Figure 12.17 Venous drainage. From *Principles of anatomy and physiology: Organisation, support and movement, and control systems of the human body.* Tortora, G.J. & Derrickson, B. Copyright © 2011 John Wiley & Sons, Inc.

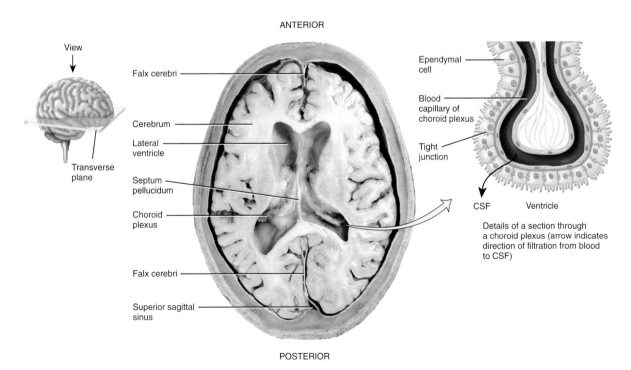

Figure 12.18 Cerebrospinal fluid circulation. From *Principles of anatomy and physiology: Organisation, support and movement, and control systems of the human body.* Tortora, G.J. & Derrickson, B. Copyright © 2011 John Wiley & Sons, Inc.

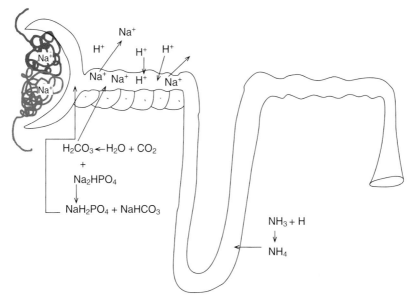

**Figure 12.26** Kidney reabsorption.

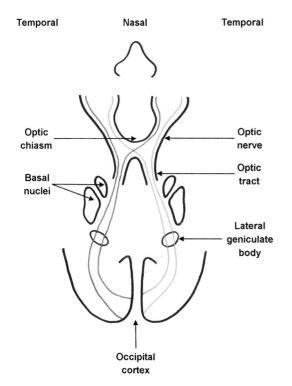

**Figure 18.2** Diagram of optic chiasm.

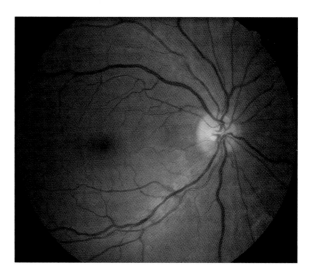

**Figure 18.3** Normal appearance of optic disc.

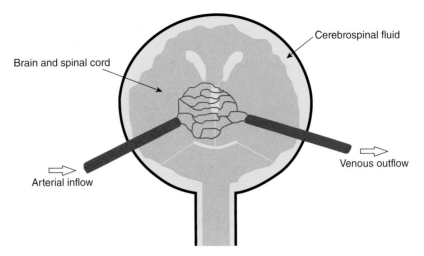

**Figure 22.7**   Schematic diagram showing the contents of the cranium according to the Monro–Kellie doctrine. With kind permission from Derriford Hospital, Plymouth Hospitals NHS Trust.

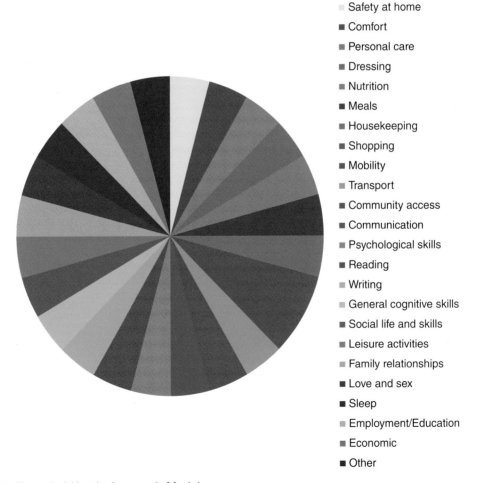

- Safety at home
- Comfort
- Personal care
- Dressing
- Nutrition
- Meals
- Housekeeping
- Shopping
- Mobility
- Transport
- Community access
- Communication
- Psychological skills
- Reading
- Writing
- General cognitive skills
- Social life and skills
- Leisure activities
- Family relationships
- Love and sex
- Sleep
- Employment/Education
- Economic
- Other

**Figure 27.2**   Extended Needs Approach Model.

6. THE BRAIN
   a. What is the position of the grey matter and white matter in the:
      i. cerebrum?
      ii. cerebellum?
   b. Draw a view of the brain from a side view and label all structures.
   c. Draw a sagittal section of the brain and label all structures.
   d. Using the following table, describe the parts of the cerebrum, their location and function:
      PART     LOCATION     FUNCTION
   e. Using the following table, describe the parts of the cerebellum, their location and function:
      PART     LOCATION     FUNCTION
   f. Using the following table, describe the parts of the midbrain, their location and function:
      PART     LOCATION     FUNCTION
   g. Using the following table, describe the parts of the hindbrain, their location and function.
      PART     LOCATION     FUNCTION

7. THE ARTERIAL SUPPLY TO THE BRAIN
   a. How would you describe the arterial supply of the brain using the following table?
      NAME     LOCATION     FUNCTION
   b. Draw a schematic diagram to represent the Circle of Willis.
   c. What is the function of the Circle of Willis?

8. CEREBROSPINAL FLUID (CSF)
   a. What is the definition of CSF?
   b. What are the functions of CSF?
   c. How would you describe the production of CSF?
   d. How would you describe the contents of CSF?
   e. What is normal CSF pressure?
   f. How would you describe the flow of CSF?
   g. How would you describe the absorption of CSF?

9. THE CRANIAL NERVES
   a. How many cranial nerves are there?
   b. What is the name and function of each cranial nerve?

10. THE MOTOR SYSTEM
   a. Define the following terms
      i. pyramidal motor system
      ii. extrapyramidal motor system
      iii. upper motor neurone
      iv. lower motor neurone
      v. reflex arc
   b. How would you differentiate between the pyramidal and extrapyramidal motor systems?
   c. How would you describe the pyramidal motor system?

11. THE AUTONOMIC NERVOUS SYSTEM
   a. What two systems make up the autonomic nervous system?
   b. How would you describe the sympathetic nervous system in terms of its structure, function, and location?
   c. How would you describe the parasympathetic nervous system in terms of its structure, function, and location?
   d. What are the outflows of the:
      i. sympathetic nervous system
      ii. parasympathetic nervous system

12. THE PITUITARY GLAND
   a. How would you describe the location of the pituitary gland?
   b. List the hormones found in the following pituitary glands:
      i. posterior pituitary gland
      ii. anterior pituitary gland
   c. What are the functions of each hormone listed?

13. ACID-BASE BALANCE
   a. State the normal arterial blood gas values.
   b. How does the body maintain homeostasis?
   c. Describe respiratory acidosis.
   d. Describe metabolic acidosis.

# Chapter 13
# Investigations

*Nadine Abelson-Mitchell*

School of Nursing and Midwifery, Faculty of Health, Education and Society, Plymouth University, Devon, UK

There are numerous investigations that need to be undertaken in order to maintain quality care for patients with neurotrauma. These investigations are related not only to the nervous system but to other systems that maintain body homeostasis. Specific investigations are mentioned in the various chapters of this book. Details of the investigations that need to be considered, throughout the patient's journey, are included in this chapter.

The investigations have been divided into five sections:

1. Central nervous system:
   - CT scan.
   - MRI scan.
   - Cervical spine CT or x-rays (see Chapter 21).
   - Thoraco-lumbar spine CT or x-rays (see Chapter 21).
   - Skull x-ray.
   - EEG.

2. Cardiac:
   - Electrocardiograph.
   - Haemoglobin and full blood count.
   - Clotting (see Chapter 21).
   - Blood group and cross-match blood (see Chapter 21).

3. Respiratory:
   - Blood gases.
   - Chest x-ray.

4. Renal:
   - Urea and electrolytes.

5. Miscellaneous:
   - Blood sugar (see Chapter 3).
   - Abdominal ultrasound/FAST (see Chapter 21).
   - Pregnancy test (if appropriate).
   - Other blood tests as indicated.

For ease of reference the investigations have been tabulated (see Table 13.1).

**Table 13.1**  Investigations.

| Name of investigation | Computerised tomography (CT scan) |
|---|---|
| **Definition** | A CT scan is a specialised x-ray that combines a series of x-ray slices, taken at 3 mm intervals, at many different angles to produce cross-sectional images of the skull and cranial contents. Each slice can be viewed individually or in 3D. The CT images are reviewed and stored as electronic files. |
| **The investigation** 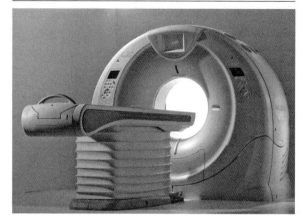 **Figure 13.1**  CT scanner. Reproduced with kind permission from Toshiba Medical Systems Ltd. | The CT scanner is shaped like a large doughnut standing on its side (Figure 13.1). The patient lies on a narrow table, that slides into the 'doughnut hole', called a gantry, that may be fitted with a special cradle to hold the patient's head firmly. Straps and pillows may be used to secure the patient in position. CT scans are painless and take only a few minutes to complete. The preparation time is often more than the scan time. During a CT scan, the patient is exposed to much more radiation than when undergoing a standard x-ray, but the benefits of the CT scan outweigh the potential risks. |
| **During the CT scan** | As the x-ray tube rotates around the head, the table slowly moves through the gantry. The machine makes clicking and whirring noises while rotating. While the table is moving the patient may need to hold their breath to prevent the images from blurring. The patient is alone in the room but a technologist, who communicates with the patient via intercom, is in an adjoining room. Reassure the patient throughout the procedure. |
| **Contrast material** | IV radio-contrasts for CT scans are generally iodine-based. Images may be taken without radio-contrast (pre-contrast) or with contrast (post-contrast). Contrast may be used to highlight specific structures/lesions. When the contrast is injected the patient may feel a warm sensation in the pelvic region and abdomen. The patient may also have a desire to micturate. After a few seconds this sensation passes. |
| **Reason for doing investigation** | To diagnose the extent of the head injury. To establish the integrity of the patient's skull. To determine whether there are any fractures, pneumocele, extradural, subdural, subarachnoid or intracranial bleeds or damage to the skull and brain. To determine signs of cerebral oedema or ↑ICP/ hydrocephalus. |

*(Continued)*

**Table 13.1** (*Continued*)

| Name of investigation | Computerised tomography (CT scan) |
| --- | --- |
| **Pre-investigation management** | Patient needs to be relatively stable before moving to CT, e.g. secure the airway.<br>Patient needs to be able to lie still. May need anaesthetising if they cannot/will not. If patient suffers from claustrophobia doctor may arrange for sedation.<br>Consent to perform CT scan needed, particularly if contrast to be used.<br>Check if patient had contrast administered previously and reaction to contrast.<br>Check if patient pregnant.<br>No need to be nil per mouth.<br>Take usual medications, unless otherwise instructed.<br>Report if patient on Metformin.<br>Change into a gown, if required.<br>Contra-indication:<br>• Allergy to contrast medium. |
| **Post-investigation management** | Wait for a short time in the radiology department to ensure no adverse side effects, if contrast material used.<br>Encourage the patient to increase their fluid intake to rid the body of contrast medium.<br>If no sedation used, resume usual activities immediately after the scan.<br>If sedation used, do not drive or operate machinery until effects have worn off.<br>Care of IV site – remove cannula, cover with plaster for 30–60 min, observe for any bleeding or swelling. Report if present. |
| **Results** | See Figures 13.2, 13.3, 13.4 and 13.5. |

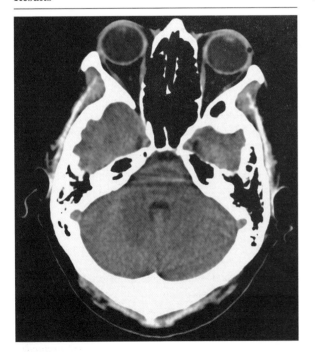

**Figure 13.2** Normal CT scan.

**Table 13.1** (*Continued*)

| Name of investigation | Computerised tomography (CT scan) |
|---|---|

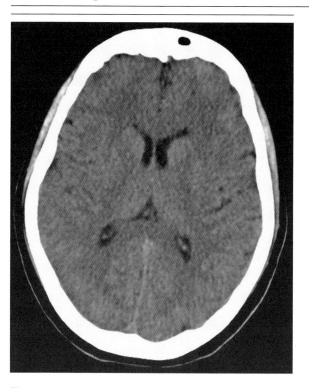

**Figure 13.3** Normal CT scan.

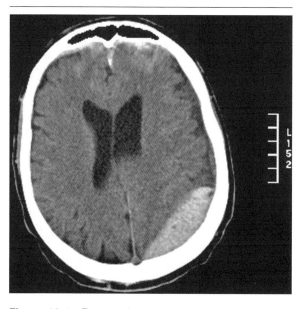

**Figure 13.4** Extraparietal bleed.

(*Continued*)

**Table 13.1** (*Continued*)

| Name of investigation | Computerised tomography (CT scan) |
|---|---|

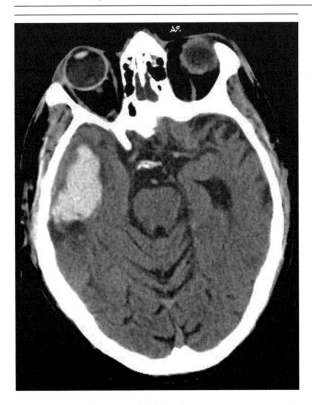

**Figure 13.5** Intracranial bleed.

| Name of investigation | MRI scan |
|---|---|

**Definition**

Non-invasive technique used to create detailed 3D high resolution images of the brain and skull structures using a magnetic field and radio waves.

**The investigation**

The MRI machine looks like a tunnel that has an opening on both ends (see Figure 13.6). The patient lies down on a movable table that slides into the opening of the tunnel.

A painless procedure that usually takes about an hour.

During the MRI scan, a repetitive tapping, thumping noise can be heard. Earplugs may be provided or the patient may be asked to bring some music with them to try and obliterate the noise.

As movement can result in blurred images the patient must keep very still.

IV contrast may be injected into the arm veins to enhance the appearance of certain structures.

For a functional MRI (fMRI) the patient may need to perform a number of small tasks, e.g.
- Tapping thumb against fingers.
- Rubbing a block of sandpaper.

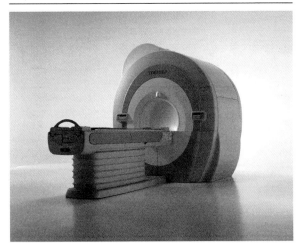

**Figure 13.6** MRI scanner. Reproduced with kind permission from Toshiba Medical Systems Ltd.

**Table 13.1** (*Continued*)

| Name of investigation | MRI scan |
|---|---|
| | • Answering simple questions.<br>• Reading.<br>• Eating.<br>The patient is alone in the room but a technologist, who communicates with the patient via intercom, is in an adjoining room. Reassure the patient throughout the procedure. |
| **Reason for doing investigation** | To establish the integrity of the patient's skull.<br>To determine whether there are any fractures, pneumocele, extradural, subdural, subarachnoid or intracranial bleeds, ↑ICP or damage to the skull and brain. |
| **Pre-investigation management** | Consent to perform MRI scan is required.<br>Check if patient allergic to contrast or had contrast previously.<br>Check if any reaction to contrast.<br>Check if patient is pregnant.<br>No need to be nil per mouth.<br>Take usual medications, unless otherwise instructed.<br>If patient suffers from claustrophobia doctor may arrange for sedation.<br>Remove all clothing containing metal, e.g. buttons or fasteners.<br>Remove all metal containing objects, e.g. jewellery, hairpins, spectacles, dentures and hearing aids.<br>Change into a gown, if required.<br>Contra-indication:<br>• Presence of pacemaker.<br>• Tell radiologist if metal or electronic devices present in body, also aneurysm clips, metallic ocular foreign bodies.<br>• Check if any kidney or liver disease present (may not be able to use contrast, e.g. Gadolinium). |
| **Post-investigation management** | If contrast used, nursing mothers should not breastfeed for 36–48 hours after an MRI.<br>Increase fluid intake provided this is within management plan.<br>The contrast may cause an allergic reaction.<br>Care of IV site – remove cannula, cover with plaster for 30–60 min, observe for any bleeding or swelling. Report if present. |

(*Continued*)

**Table 13.1** (*Continued*)

| Name of investigation | MRI scan |
| --- | --- |
| **Results** | See Figures 13.7 and 13.8. |

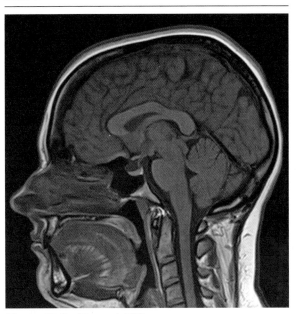

**Figure 13.7**   Normal MRI scan.

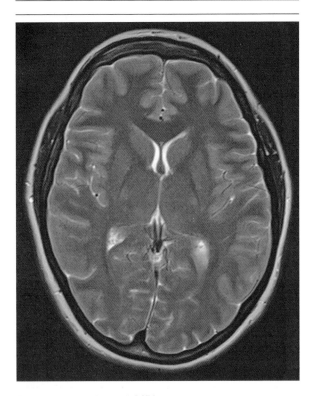

**Figure 13.8**   Normal MRI scan.

**Table 13.1**   (*Continued*)

| Name of investigation | Skull x-ray |
| --- | --- |
| **Definition** | The taking of an x-ray of the skull. |
| **The investigation** | An x-ray of the skull taken from various views. |
| **Reason for doing investigation** | To establish the integrity of the patient's skull. <br> To determine whether there are any fractures or pneumoceles. |
| **Pre-investigation management** | Explain procedure to patient. <br> Reassure patient throughout procedure. |
| **Special precautions** | Check if patient is pregnant, particularly in the first trimester of pregnancy. <br> Bleeds and underlying damage may not be detected by the use of a skull x-ray. |
| **Post-investigation management** | No special management. <br> Reassure patient. |
| **Results** | A fractured skull or underlying brain damage may result in CNS compromise and↑ICP (see Figure 13.9). |

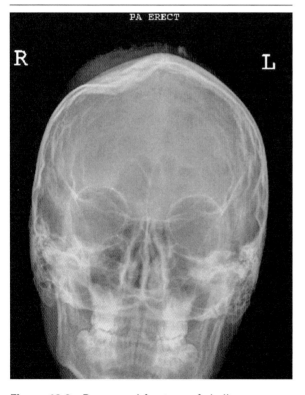

**Figure 13.9**   Depressed fracture of skull.

(*Continued*)

**Table 13.1** (*Continued*)

| Name of investigation | Electroencephalogram (EEG) |
| --- | --- |
| **Definition** | Non-invasive technique.<br><br>To detect and record electrical brain activity small electrodes (flat metal discs) are attached to the scalp with special adhesive, using a 'cap' or wire. |
| **The investigation** | Painless procedure.<br><br>An EEG usually takes 30–60 minutes.<br><br>The head is measured and marks are made on the scalp where the electrodes will be attached (see Figure 13.10). The electrodes are connected with wires to an EEG machine that records brain waves.<br><br>During the test the patient will be instructed to:<br>• Lie quietly.<br>• Open/close eyes.<br>• Hyperventilate.<br>• Undertake various tasks, e.g. reading, arithmetic calculations. |

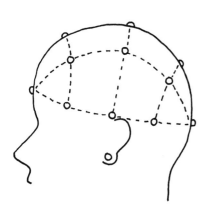 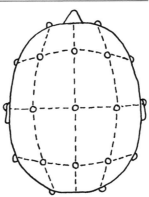

**Figure 13.10**    EEG electrode application.

| | |
| --- | --- |
| **Reason for doing investigation** | To detect:<br>• Seizures.<br>• Encephalitis.<br>• Brain death. |
| **Pre-investigation management** | Follow specific instructions, e.g. sleep deprivation or medication.<br>Wash hair prior to test.<br>Avoid caffeine six hours before the test. |
| **Post-investigation management** | Remove the electrodes or cap.<br>If no sedative used, return to normal activities.<br>If sedative used, rest and no driving for the remainder of the day. |

**Table 13.1** (*Continued*)

| Name of investigation | Electroencephalogram (EEG) |
|---|---|
| **Results** | EEG recording reflects brain activity, via electrical impulses (see Figure 13.11). |

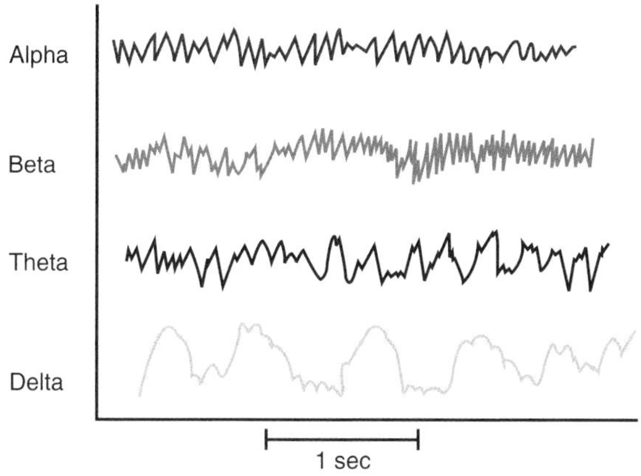

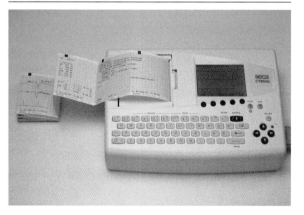

**Figure 13.11** EEG brain activity. From *Principles of anatomy and physiology. Organisation, support and movement, and control systems of the human body.* Tortora, G.J. & Derrickson, B.H. Copyright © 2011 John Wiley and Sons, Inc.

| Name of investigation | Electrocardiograph (ECG) |
|---|---|
| **Definition** | A recording of the heart rhythm. |
| **The investigation** | May be performed using 12 lead ECG with printout, via Bluetooth or telemetry depending on the equipment available (see Figure 13.12). |

**Figure 13.12** ECG machine. With kind permission from SECA Ltd, UK. Copyright © 2012 SECA.

(*Continued*)

**Table 13.1**  (*Continued*)

| Name of investigation | Electrocardiograph (ECG) |
| --- | --- |
| **Reason for doing investigation** | To ensure an acceptable heart rhythm.<br>To assess possible damage to heart post-trauma.<br>To detect associated cardiac problems. |
| **Pre-investigation management** | Explain procedure to patient.<br>Maintain patient's dignity and respect throughout procedure.<br>Ensure ECG leads are placed in correct position (see Figure 13.13).<br>Minimise electrical interference.<br>Record ECG.<br>Refer ECG to appropriate person for interpretation. |

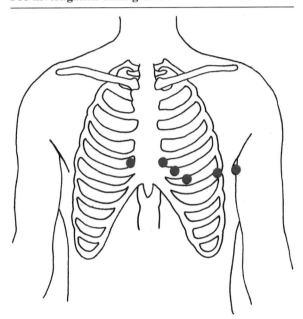

**Figure 13.13**   Correct placement of ECG leads.

| | |
| --- | --- |
| **Special precautions** | Take precautions when using electricity. |
| **Post-investigation management** | Remove leads.<br>Clean patient. |
| **Results** | Management of the patient will be determined by the interpretation of the ECG.<br>Clinically the patient may present with normal rhythm, tachycardia of various origins, bradycardia or other forms of arrhythmia. The cause of the arrhythmia will determine the management of the problem (see Figures 13.14 and 13.15). |

**Table 13.1** (*Continued*)

| Name of investigation | Electrocardiograph (ECG) |
| --- | --- |

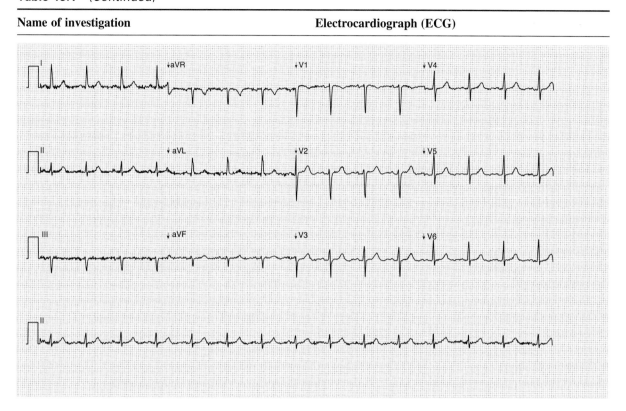

**Figure 13.14** Normal ECG.

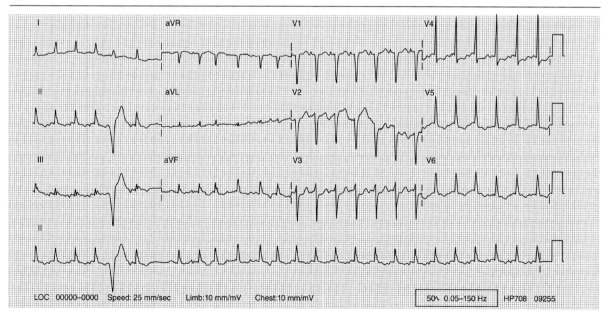

**Figure 13.15** Sinus tachycardia.

(*Continued*)

**Table 13.1**   (*Continued*)

| Name of investigation | Full blood count |
| --- | --- |
| **Definition** | The taking of a venous blood sample to interpret haematology values. |
| **The investigation** | The taking of a venous blood sample. |
| **Reason for doing investigation** | To establish the patient's cardiovascular and haematological function post trauma as reflected in the full blood count. |
| **Pre-investigation management** | Explain procedure to patients.<br>Select site to perform procedure. |
| **Special precautions** | Maintain principles of infection control regarding body fluids. Venous blood samples must only be taken by someone trained in this technique. |
| **Post-investigation management** | On completion of procedure compress site for five minutes. Ensure there is no haematoma or blood loss from site. |
| **Results** | Some units have their own machines to measure full blood counts, others need to send the sample to the laboratory and await the results (see Table 13.2).<br>1. Alteration in the oxygen carrying capacity of the blood may affect cerebral perfusion.<br>2. An increase in the white cell count will demonstrate an infection. It is important to locate the site of infection such as a respiratory infection, urinary tract infection, wound infection or infection within the CNS, e.g. brain abscess or meningitis.<br>3. Additional investigations relating to the cardiovascular and haematological system may need to be undertaken in patients who have polytrauma such as the INR (international normalised ratio) or prothrombin time as well as partial thromboplastin times. The results of these tests will reflect any abnormality in the clotting mechanism. |
| Name of investigation | Chest x-ray |
| **Definition** | The taking of an x-ray of the chest. |
| **The investigation** | A chest x-ray. |
| **Reason for doing investigation** | To establish the patients respiratory functioning in terms of the chest and lung structure as well as heart size (Figure 13.16). To determine whether there are any fractures, pneumothorax (Figure 13.17), haemothorax or damage to underlying structures in the chest. |
| **Pre-investigation management** | Explain procedure to patient.<br>Reassure patient throughout procedure. |
| **Special precautions** | Check whether there is any possibility of the patient being pregnant, particularly in the first trimester of pregnancy. |
| **Post-investigation management** | Reassure patient. |

**Table 13.1** *(Continued)*

| Name of investigation | Chest x-ray |
| --- | --- |
| **Results** | Respiratory compromise, fractured ribs, a pneumothorax or haemothorax may result in hypoxia that will have a direct effect on cerebral perfusion. In trauma a chest drain will usually be inserted if there is any pneumothorax. |

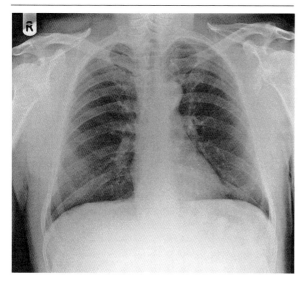

**Figure 13.16** Normal chest x-ray.

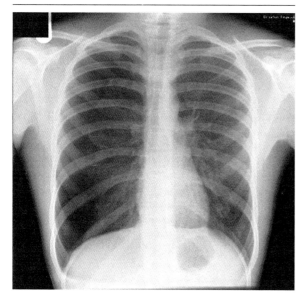

**Figure 13.17** Pneumothorax.

*(Continued)*

**Table 13.1**  *(Continued)*

| Name of investigation | Arterial blood gases |
|---|---|
| **Definition** | The taking of an arterial blood sample to interpret blood gas values. |
| **The investigation** | Taking an arterial sample of blood. |
| **Reason for doing investigation** | To establish the patients respiratory and acid-base functioning.<br>To determine blood gas results in terms of the pH, pO2, pCO2, HCO3⁻, base excess. |
| **Pre-investigation management** | Explain procedure to patient.<br>Taking arterial blood gases is a painful procedure, although local anaesthetic may be used.<br>Reassure patient throughout the procedure.<br>Select site to perform procedure |
| **Special precautions** | Arterial blood gas samples must only be taken by someone trained in this technique. |
| **Post-investigation management** | On completion of procedure compress site for a minimum of five minutes.<br>Ensure there is no bleeding. Check pulse post-procedure.<br>Complications of arterial blood gas access sites include:<br>• Haematoma.<br>• Blood loss from site.<br>• Arterial aneurysm. |
| **Results** | Some units have their own machines to measure blood gases, others need to send the sample to the laboratory and await the results.<br>Normal blood gas values are given in Table 13.3.<br>When interpreting blood gases the results are said to be normal or may be interpreted as respiratory acidosis, respiratory alkalosis, metabolic acidosis or metabolic alkalosis (see Chapter 12).<br>Table 13.4 illustrates the differences in the values relative to a normal blood gas result. |
| **Name of investigation** | Urea and electrolytes |
| **Definition** | The taking of a venous blood sample to interpret urea and electrolyte values. |
| **The investigation** | Taking of a venous blood sample. |
| **Reason for doing investigation** | To establish the patients metabolic function as reflected in the urea and electrolyte values. |
| **Pre-investigation management** | Explain procedure to patients.<br>Select site to perform procedure. |
| **Special precautions** | Venous blood samples must only be taken by someone trained in this technique. |

**Table 13.1** (*Continued*)

| Name of investigation | Urea and electrolytes |
|---|---|
| **Post-investigation management** | On completion of procedure compress site for five minutes. Ensure there is no haematoma or blood loss from site. |
| **Results** | Some units have their own machines to measure urea and electrolyte values (Table 13.5), others need to send the sample to the laboratory and await the results. |

| Name of investigation | Urinalysis |
|---|---|
| **Definition** | The taking of a urine sample to interpret values of components of urine. |
| **The investigation** | Taking of urine sample. |
| **Reason for doing investigation** | To establish the patients kidney function as reflected in the urinalysis. To assess possibility of urinary tract infection. Specific Gravity: 1002. If this is raised, dehydration may be the cause. If lowered diabetes insipidus should be suspected. Pregnancy test. |
| **Pre-investigation management** | Explain procedure to patients. Patient to wash hands before procedure. Take catheter sample using aseptic technique or give patient specimen jar into which to pass urine. After collection of the sample ask patient to cover sample and notify nurse it has been completed. |
| **Special precautions** | Avoid contamination of sample. Patient/nurse to wash hands before and after procedure. |
| **Post-investigation management** | Sample will be tested using urinalysis or other suitable product. Specific gravity will be measured. |
| **Results** | Record and report results. |

Websites that may provide additional information include:
www.mayoclinic.com
http://www.globalrph.com/labs

**Table 13.2**   Full blood count.

| Variable | Value (normal range)* |
|---|---|
| Haemoglobin (Hb) | |
|   Male | 13–18 gms/dL |
|   Female | 12–16 gms/dL |
| Red cell count (RBC) | 3.9–5.1 L |
| Haematocrit | |
|   Male | 41–50% |
|   Female | 35–46% |
| Mean corpuscular volume (MCV) | 80–100 femtolitres |
| Mean corpuscular haemoglobin (MCH) | 27–32 picograms |
| Mean corpuscular haemoglobin concentration (MCHC) | 32–36% |
| Red cell distribution width (RDW) | 11–15 |
| Platelet count | 150 000–400 000 cmm |
| Prothrombin time | 11–16 seconds |
| INR (international normalised ratio) (prothrombin index) | 0.8–1.2 |
| White blood cell count (WBC) | 4300–10 800 cmm |
| White blood cell count differential: | |
|   Neutrophils | 1.7–6.2/L |
|   Lymphocytes | 1.0–3.4/L |
|   Monocytes | 0.2–0.8/L |
|   Eosinophils | 0.0–0.4/L |
|   Basophils | 0.0–0.1/L |

(Medicinenet.com 2012)

*Please note: different laboratories have different ranges for some of the tests. Please ensure you use the values considered within your institution.*

**Table 13.3**   Normal blood gas values.

| Variable | Value (normal range) |
|---|---|
| pH | 7.35–7.45 |
| $PaCO_2$ | 4.5–6.0 kPa (35–45 mm Hg) |
| $PaO_2$ | 10.0–13.0 kPa (70–100 mm Hg)*/** |
| $SaO_2$ | 93–98% |
| $HCO_3^-$ | 22–26 mEq/L |
| % MetHb | <2.0% |
| % COHb | <3.0% |
| Base excess | −2.0–2.0 mEq/L |
| $CaO_2$ | 16–22 ml $O_2$/dl |

(Medicinenet.com 2012)

*At sea level.

**Age dependent.

**Table 13.4** Differences in values relative to normal blood gas.

| Variable | Normal range | Respiratory acidosis | Respiratory alkalosis | Metabolic acidosis | Metabolic alkalosis |
|---|---|---|---|---|---|
| | | $CO_2 > 45$ | $CO_2 < 35$ | $HCO_3^- < 22$ | $HCO_3^- > 26$ |
| pH | 7.36–7.44 | ↓ | ↑ | ↓ | ↑ |
| $pO_2$ | 80–100 mm Hg | →↓ | ↑ | ↓ | → |
| $pCO_2$ | 35–40 mm Hg | ↑ | ↓ | ↓ | ↑ |
| Standard bicarbonate | 20–30 meq/L | ↑ | ↓ | ↓ | ↑ |
| Base excess | −2/+2 | ↑ | ↓ | ↓ | ↑ |

**Table 13.5** Normal urea and electrolyte values.

| Variable | Value (normal range)* |
|---|---|
| Serum sodium | 133–146 mmol/L |
| Serum potassium | 3.5–5.3 mmol/L |
| Serum urea | 2.5–7.8 mmol/L |
| Serum chloride | 95–108 mmol/L |
| Serum bicarbonate | 22–29 mmol/L |
| Serum phosphate | 0.8–1.5 mmol/L |
| Serum magnesium | 0.7–1.0 mmol/L |
| Ionized calcium | 1.14–1.3 |
| Serum albumin | 35–50 gm/L |
| Serum total protein | 60–80 gm/L |
| Serum creatinine | 44–80 μmol/L |
| Serum osmolality | 275–295 mmol/kg |

(Medicinenet.com 2012)

*Please note: different laboratories have different ranges for some of the tests. Please ensure you use the values considered within your institution.*

# Chapter 14
# Pharmacology for Neurotrauma Patients

*Nadine Abelson-Mitchell and Penny Franklin*

School of Nursing and Midwifery, Faculty of Health, Education and Society, Plymouth University, Devon, UK

## INTRODUCTION

Health professionals must be knowledgeable about the pharmaceutical agents utilised in the management of neurotrauma patients. It is important to understand the pharmaceutical action of the drug, doses, side effects and precautions. Knowledge of pharmaceutical agents is essential for safe practice as well as patient, family and carer education.

This discussion is limited specifically to drugs used for neurotrauma. It is important to note that, unless nurses have prescribing rights (NMC 2006), it is usually the doctor who prescribes the drugs and the nurse who administers them. The scope of practice and the level of competence of the nurse (NMC 2008) must be taken into account when accepting responsibility for administering medication to a head injured person.

When administering drugs it is important that the nurse is aware of the patient's medical and drug history, including a history of medical conditions, past, present and ongoing, and remembers to obtain a family medical history. It is important to ascertain the patient's current medication, medication taken in the last three months (that may have been stopped or amended) and a history of allergies and sensitivities.

When taking a history, often from the carer, ensure that you obtain, as fully as possible, a social history, e.g. does the patient drink alcohol and how much and was the patient using illicit substances? Also try to obtain as full as possible, lifestyle, dietary and occupational history as this might influence the pharmacological treatment of the patient.

### Special groups

Remember that patients who are elderly might process the drug differently. In the older person, aged 60 and above, perfusion to vital organs is less and so absorption, distribution, metabolism and excretion might be impaired. They generally have fewer receptor sites and sometimes also greater sensitivity to drugs. Also they are likely to have a level of hepatic and renal impairment, which again is likely to affect metabolism and excretion of the drug, and again the type of drug used, the dose and dose range might need to be adjusted accordingly.

When administering drugs to any age group it is of utmost importance to take into account the formulary guidance and safety precautions and contra-indications; in England the latest version of the British National Formulary are used (BMJ Group and the Royal Pharmaceutical Society of Great Britain 2011).

Throughout the book the drugs are presented using their generic names as in various countries drugs have different trade names, whereas the generic names are international.

In general, there are specific groups of drugs that are used in neuroscience practice.

## ANAESTHETIC AGENTS

These may be used to induce a coma, to limit oxygen requirements and decrease the metabolic rate of brain tissue.

Pharmaceutical agents that may be used:

For rapid sequence induction (RSI) intubation:

- Propofol.
- Fentanyl.
- Atracurium.

For coma induction:

- Thiopentone.

## ANALGESICS

It is important to manage the patient's pain as pain increases ICP. The analgesic selected needs to be effective without causing sedation and constipation. It is important to use an 'analgesic ladder' starting with the mildest analgesic and then progressing, if necessary, according to the patient's response. Pharmaceutical agents that may be used are:

- Paracetamol.
- Non-steroidal anti-inflammatories (NSAIDs).
- Weak opioids:
  - Codeine phosphate.
  - Tramadol.
- Morphine based drugs:
  - Oramorph.
  - Zomorph.
  - MST.
  - Oxycodone.
  - OxyContin.

## DIURETICS

Osmotic diuretics may be used to decrease the amount of tissue fluid, increase urine output and control cerebral oedema. Other diuretics may also be used. It is important to monitor and treat dehydration and electrolyte imbalance.

Pharmaceutical agents that may be used are:

- 10–20% Mannitol.
- 5% $NaCl_2$.

## ANTI-EPILEPTIC DRUGS

The use of anti-epileptic drugs remains controversial. Some doctors use anti-epileptics from the outset to prevent seizures in moderate or severe head injuries, others only introduce anti-epileptics if the patient presents with a seizure at any stage in their recovery.

Note that if anti-epileptic agents are introduced into the management programme it is important to check the regulations relating to the use of anti-epileptics and driving that apply in the country where the patient lives.

Pharmaceutical agents that may be used are:

- Phenytoin.
- Sodium valproate.

## ANTICOAGULANTS

The use of anticoagulants in neurotrauma is controversial as there is a risk of bleeding. It is important to remember that after neurotrauma the patient's clotting cascade may alter. Anticoagulants may be prescribed to prevent deep vein thrombosis (DVT).

Pharmaceutical agents that may be used are:

- Fractionated Heparin.
- Aspirin.

## ANTI-EMETICS

It is important to manage the patient's nausea and vomiting as vomiting increases intracranial pressure. Anti-emetics are known to have extrapyramidal side effects so they are used with caution.

Pharmaceutical agents that may be used are:

- Metaclopramide.
- Cyclizine.
- Ondansetron.

## LAXATIVES

It is important to prevent constipation as the valsalva manoeuvre and straining on defaecation raises ICP.

Pharmaceutical agents that may be used are:

- Laxido.
- Senna.
- Glycerine suppositories.
- Phosphate enema.

## CONCLUSION

Drug administration differs per country as there are different protocols for management of neurotrauma. Legislation regarding the prescribing of drugs and the availability of drugs also differs. For this reason a detailed section of the actual drugs used has not been included.

The reader is referred to the following websites as resources regarding drugs used in neurotrauma:

- In the UK    www.nhs.uk/medicine-guides
- In the USA   www.rxlist.com
- General      www.drugs.com

**Activity 14.1**

1. Compile a list of drugs utilised in the unit.
2. Using Table 14.1, provide details of the drugs used in the unit as an aid to teaching peers.
3. Using Table 14.1, provide details of the drugs used in the unit as an aid to teaching patients, families and carers.
4. Develop some learning material that will assist in teaching about drugs.

**Table 14.1**  List of pharmaceutical agents.

| Generic Name | Indications | Special precautions | Dosage | Side effects |
|--------------|-------------|---------------------|--------|--------------|
|              |             |                     |        |              |

**Activity 14.2**

Debate the use of drugs in behaviour modification (see Chapter 7).

**Activity 14.3**

Debate the use of drugs in the management of patients with aggressive behaviour (see Chapter 7).

# Chapter 15
# Applied Microbiology

*Nadine Abelson-Mitchell*

School of Nursing and Midwifery, Faculty of Health, Education and Society, Plymouth University, Devon, UK

## INTRODUCTION

This section only considers meningitis, encephalitis and brain abscess as a direct result of neurotrauma. It is important to remember that patients with neurotrauma are susceptible to hospital acquired infections and other infections, such as respiratory infections and urinary tract infections.

## MENINGITIS

### Definition

Inflammation of the meninges.

### Predisposing factors

Meningitis may be caused by exposure to a pre-existing infection or acquired by in-patients, who have lowered immunity, where there is exposure to pathogens.

### Causes of meningitis

- Bacterial infection.
  - Meningitis that develops post-head injury is usually caused by *Streptococcus pneumoniae* via a breach in the base of the skull. It is also possible to develop other forms of meningitis post-head injury depending on the patient's circumstances. Other forms of meningitis, including meningococcal meningitis, are not described.
- Viral infection known as:
  - Acute benign lymphocytic meningitis or acute aseptic meningitis.

### Pathophysiology

Meningitis may involve the arachnoid layer, piamater, subarachnoid space and cerebrospinal fluid. If all three layers of the meninges are involved it is known as a pachymeningitis. There is little involvement of the cortex and there may be involvement of the cranial nerves (II, III, IV, VI, VII, VIII) (see Table 15.1).

**Table 15.1** Classification of meningitis.

| Type | Causative organism | Incidence |
|------|--------------------|-----------|
| **Bacterial:** | | |
| Pneumococcal | *Streptococcus pneumoniae* (+) | Young/old |
| *Haemophilus influenzae* | *Haemophilus influenzae* (-) | 3 months to 8 years |
| Meningococcal | *Neisseria meningitidis* | Children/young adults |
| *Staphylococcus aureus* | *Staphylococcus aureus* | Neonates |
| **Viral meningitis:** | | |
| Mumps | | |

*Neurotrauma: Managing Patients with Head Injuries*, First Edition. Edited by Nadine Abelson-Mitchell.
© 2013 Blackwell Publishing Ltd. Published 2013 by Blackwell Publishing Ltd.

## Clinical features of meningitis

Symptoms may develop rapidly or over a period of time. There may be evidence of cerebrospinal fluid leakage from the ear, nose or mouth.

The adult patient may present with the following:

- Non-specific symptoms:
  - Listlessness/difficult to wake up.
  - Fever.
  - Anorexia.
  - Vomiting/diarrhoea.
- Classic symptoms:
  - Headache.
  - Photophobia.
  - Fever (90% of patients).
  - Decreasing level of consciousness.
  - Stiff neck (85% of patients).
  - Signs of a meningeal irritation:
    - Kernig's sign: the patient is unable to straighten the knee when the hip is fixed at a 90° angle.
    - Brudzinski's sign: the patient flexes their neck when the hip or knee are flexed.
  - Generalised convulsions.
  - Raised intracranial pressure.
  - Cranial nerve dysfunction.

## Investigations

- It is essential to take a detailed history and perform a physical examination.
- A lumbar puncture will be undertaken to obtain CSF.
- If meningitis is present the appearance of the CSF will be as follows (see Table 15.2)
- Undertake a chest x-ray to exclude signs of a chest infection.
- Perform blood culture.
- Take nose and throat swabs.
- Undertake routine blood sampling.
- CT scan.

## Treatment

- Admit patient to unit where appropriate supportive care is available, e.g. ICU/HDU/Ward.
- Nurse in a quiet, darkened room.
- Ensure adequate airway and ventilation.
- Monitor cardiac function.
- Monitor fluid intake/elimination.
- Establish IV line.

- Administer medication as per doctors' orders:
  - Antibiotics.
  - Dexamethasone.
  - Analgesics.
  - Antipyretics.

## Relevant nursing diagnoses

Nursing diagnoses of relevance to patients with meningitis, encephalitis and brain abscess include:

- Need for safe, therapeutic environment.
- Alteration in cerebral function.
- Potential increase in intracranial pressure.
- Increasing neurological deficit.
- Presence of behavioural disturbance.
- Alteration in respiratory function.
- Inability to maintain airway.
- Alteration in thermoregulation.
- Fluid volume deficit/overload.
- Alteration in nutritional status.
- Inability to attend to self-care needs.
- Altered psychological status.

See Chapter 22 for Nursing Care Plan.

## Complications

There may be no complications after meningitis but complications that might occur include:

- Headaches.
- Seizures.
- Hydrocephalus.
- Cranial nerve deficits:
  - Blindness.
  - Deafness.
- Paresis or paralysis.
- Complications of bed rest such as pressure sores and DVT.

## Prognosis/outcome

The outcome after meningitis will depend on the cause of the meningitis as well as rapidity of onset. In patients with the rapid onset meningitis the death rate may be as high as 90%.

## ENCEPHALITIS

## Definition

Inflammation of the brain substance.

## Pathophysiology

Encephalitis involves inflammation of the brain. Raised intracranial pressure and destruction of brain matter are features of encephalitis. There may be involvement of the cranial nerves (II, III, IV, VI, VII, VIII).

## Clinical features of encephalitis

- Nausea and vomiting.
- Headache.
- Fever.
- ↓ Level of consciousness.
- Signs of meningeal irritation:
  - Kernig's sign: The patient is unable to straighten the knee when the hip is fixed at a 90° angle.
  - Brudzinski's sign: The patient flexes their neck when the hip or knee are flexed.
- Cerebral oedema.
- ↑ Intracranial pressure ++++.
- Cranial nerve dysfunction.
- Temporal lobe herniation.

## Investigations

- It is essential to take a detailed history and perform a physical examination.
- A lumbar puncture will be undertaken to obtain cerebrospinal fluid provided there is NO papilloedema present.
- If encephalitis is present the appearance of the CSF will be as in Table 15.2.
- CT scan.
- MRI scan.
- Undertake routine bloods.

## Treatment

Modalities of treatment include the use of various pharmaceutical agents:

- Antiviral agents such as Acyclovir.
- Dexamethasone.
- Phenytoin.
- Furosemide.
- Cimetidine.

- Symptomatic treatment:
  - Antipyretics.

## Complications

There may be no complications after encephalitis but complications that might occur include:

- Neurological deficits.
- Personality disorders.
- Psychosis.
- Dementia.
- Cranial nerve deficits.
- Paralysis/Paresis.
- Complications of bed rest such as pressure sores and deep vein thrombosis.

## BRAIN ABSCESS

### Introduction

Brain abscesses, although uncommon, may be life threatening and require urgent medical attention (Honda and Warren 2009).

### Definition

Bacterial infection of the brain that is circumscribed to form an abscess. The area is walled off and contains white

**Table 15.2** Appearance of CSF.

| Value | Meningitis | | Encephalitis |
| --- | --- | --- | --- |
| | **Bacterial** | **Viral** | **Viral** |
| Appearance | Cloudy | Clear | Clear |
| Glucose | ↓ | → | → |
| White blood cell count | Polymorphonucleocytes | Mononuclear | Mononuclear |
| Protein | ↑ | → | ↑ |
| Culture | Positive | Negative | ++ |

blood cells, bacteria and fluid that forms an intraparenchymal collection of pus (Muzumdar *et al.* 2010: p. 136).

## Classification

There are various classifications used for brain abscesses:

1. According to location
2. According to cause.

## Causes of brain abscess

- Bacterial infection of the brain caused by:
  - Penetrating injury.
  - Brain surgery.
  - Distant infections spread by blood to brain tissue, e.g. bacterial endocarditis. Haematological spread from distant focus accounts for 25% of infected patients (Brook 2011).
  - Continuous suppurative focus, for example sinusitis/mastoiditis. This accounts for 45–50% of infected patients.

## Pathophysiology

Trauma accounts for 10% of brain abscesses and the incidence of brain abscess from trauma is increasing (Muzumdar *et al.* 2010). Infective agents may include *Staphylococcus aureus* including MRSA, *Streptoccocus pneumoniae*, *Haemophilus influenzae*, Enterobacteriaceae, *Clostridium*, *Pseudomonas* and others.

Bacteria enter the brain and start to grow in the brain tissue. This causes an area of cerebritis (7–14 days) (brain inflammation) with related oedema. As the infection expands it causes further destruction of the brain matter, liquification (2–3 weeks) and abscess formation with a fibrotic capsule (Bernardini 2004). This space occupying lesion may result in increased intracranial pressure. The abscess may erupt thus spreading the infective agent.

## Clinical features of brain abscess

The adult patient may present with the following symptoms depending on the size and location of the abscess:

- Headache*.
- Alteration in level of consciousness.
- Nausea and vomiting.
- Fever*.
- Seizure.

---

*Suggestive of brain abscess but may not always be present (Tseng and Tseng 2006).

- Focal neurological deficit*, for example.
  - Speech difficulties.
  - Difficulties with vision.
  - Paresis or paralysis.
- Raised intracranial pressure.
- Cranial nerve dysfunction.

## Investigations

- It is essential to take a detailed history and perform a physical examination.
- Undertake an x-ray of the chest to look for signs of infection.
- CT scan to detect number, size and location of abscesses that will demonstrate enhancement rings.
- MRI scan with contrast.
- Perform blood culture.
- Undertake full blood count.

## Treatment

- Seek cause of brain abscess.
- Manage ↑ ICP if present.
- Drainage of abscess to identify causative organism:
  - CT guided needle aspiration.
  - Craniotomy.
- Confirm causative organism.
- Commence intravenous antibiotics immediately.
- Use of corticosteroid remains controversial although it may be used to reduce cerebral oedema (Brook 2011).
- Supportive care.
- Repeated imaging to determine that the abscess size is decreasing.
- Check the Department of Transport regulations as the patient may not be able to drive post-surgery because of the risk of seizures.

## Complications

There may be no complications after a brain abscess but complications that might occur include:

- Rupture of the brain abscess may cause extradural empyema.
- Headaches.
- Seizures.
- Neurological deficit.
  - Paresis.
  - Paralysis.
- Return of abscess.

**Prognosis/outcome**

Recovery from a brain abscess is normally good. The outcome after a brain abscess depends on prompt diagnosis and management of the infective agent (Tseng and Tseng 2006). Only 10% of brain abscesses are fatal (NHS Choices 2010). If a brain abscess ruptures, the mortality rate is 5–15% (Brook 2011).

**CONCLUSION**

Early diagnosis and management of meningitis, encephalitis and brain abscesses results in improved outcomes for these patients. Therefore health professionals need to have the knowledge to detect and report these conditions swiftly.

# Section 3
# FEATURES OF NEUROTRAUMA

## INTRODUCTION

This section introduces the reader to the background knowledge necessary to provide multidisciplinary quality care to patients with neurotrauma. Vital aspects of management, such as the classification of neurotrauma, raised intracranial pressure and patient assessment, are described. Patient assessment is described in detail to enable the health professional to conduct a comprehensive examination of the CNS in all settings.

---

### Key objectives

On completion of this section you should be able to achieve the following:

- Define head injury.
- Classify head injuries.
- Differentiate between primary and secondary injury.
- Describe the maintenance of normal intracranial pressure.
- State normal values for intracranial pressure.
- List the causes of raised intracranial pressure.
- Manage a patient with raised intracranial pressure.
- Undertake an assessment using the Glasgow Coma Scale.
- Conduct a comprehensive neurological assessment of a patient.
- Record and report findings.

---

### Ethical/legal considerations

Debate the ethical issues related to this section.

Consider and apply the legal and ethical issues highlighted in these chapters to neurotrauma practice:

- Data Protection Act 1998.
- Freedom of Information Act 2000.
- Patient dignity and respect.
- Confidentiality.
- Substance abuse.
- Social practices.

# Chapter 16
# Classification of Traumatic Brain Injury

*Zuhair Noori[1] and Nadine Abelson-Mitchell[2]*

[1]Croydon Healthcare Trust, London, UK
[2]School of Nursing and Midwifery, Faculty of Health, Education and Society, Plymouth University, Devon, UK

## INTRODUCTION

It is important to understand the basis for classifying neurotrauma. More importantly, it is essential to be able to maintain quality of care and promote recovery based on the classification systems.

There are numerous ways in which TBI can be classified namely:

- Primary and secondary brain injury.
- Open and closed head injury.
- Severity of injury.

## PRIMARY AND SECONDARY BRAIN INJURY

Brain damage, following trauma, is classified as primary injury or secondary injury. Primary injury occurs at the time of impact. Secondary injury is further brain damage caused by later reaction of the brain to the primary injury or as a result of other extracranial causes.

### Primary injury

The primary injury occurs at the instance of the impact and is the result of physical and chemical changes in the brain (see Table 16.1). Sometimes a primary injury is so severe that it will inevitably be fatal.

### Secondary brain injury

Secondary brain injury is a delayed reaction of the brain to the initial insult, and may persist from a few minutes to up to two weeks. In secondary brain injury neurochemical mediators that influence brain function are affected (see Table 16.2).

### Case study

The death of the actress, Natasha Richardson, who was injured in a skiing accident, is a vivid example of how secondary brain damage can occur. She had a bump to her head. At the time of injury, there were no symptoms whatsoever apart from the cognition of impact. She was normal for a period, and then died suddenly from secondary brain changes some hours later.

Secondary injury may be classified as those of intracranial origin (see Table 16.3) and extracranial causes (see Table 16.4) such as hypoxia, hypotension, increased intrathoracic pressure, anaemia and inappropriate management.

*Neurotrauma: Managing Patients with Head Injuries*, First Edition. Edited by Nadine Abelson-Mitchell.
© 2013 Blackwell Publishing Ltd. Published 2013 by Blackwell Publishing Ltd.

**Table 16.1**  Types of primary injuries.

| Type of injury | Explanation |
| --- | --- |
| Skull fractures may be:<br>  Simple linear<br>  Depressed<br>  Compound | A break in the bone.<br><br>A force, severe enough to fracture the skull, is likely to injure the brain. The complications of a skull fracture can cause secondary brain injury, such as extradural haematoma or infection, thus the presence of a skull fracture may be a marker of a brain injury. |
| Concussion | Brief impairment of awareness, i.e. dazed, memory loss, and actual loss of consciousness. |
| Contusion of the brain | Bruising of the brain tissue caused by the direct impact of the skull overlying the region or indirectly or on the opposite side (contracoup).<br><br>Typically localised to the inferior and lateral surfaces of the temporal and frontal lobes. |
| Laceration | Linear disruption of brain tissue. |
| Traumatic axonal injury/<br>Diffuse axonal injury | Due to disruption of the brain structures, nerve fibres are stretched and pulled apart. The effects might present later on as secondary injury. |
| Intracerebral haematoma | An immediate reaction on impact, which causes rupture of the blood vessels and accumulation of a blood clot that displaces brain tissues around it. Some of the immediate epidural haematomas can also be classified as primary injuries. |
| Blast injuries | Severe brain swelling, vasospasm and sub-arachnoid haemorrhage. |

These types of injury may be localised to only one part of the brain or diffuse.
(Maas *et al.* 2008)

**Table 16.2**  Effect on neurochemical mediators.

| Neurochemical mediator | Value | Effect |
| --- | --- | --- |
| Excitatory amino acids:<br>  Glutamate<br>  Aspartate | <br>↑<br>↑ | Cerebral swelling<br>Chloride shift<br>Calcium influx<br>Alteration in ATP<br>↑ Free radicals |
| Endogenous opioid peptides:<br>  Catecholamine<br>  Serotonergic system | <br>↑<br>↑ | ↑ Damage<br>↑ Metabolism<br>↓ Glucose utilisation |
| ECF $K^+$ | ↑ | Oedema |
| Cytokines | ↑ | Inflammation |
| ICF $Mg^+$ | ↓ | ↑ $Ca^+$ influx |
| Astrocyte damage | Hypertrophic and hyperplastic response to CNS injury | ↑ Neuronal survival:<br>  ↑ Protein kinase B/Akt<br>Activation of P2 purinergic receptors |

(Dawodu 2008)

**Table 16.3** Types of intracranial secondary brain injury.

| Type of injury | Explanation |
|---|---|
| ↑ICP | ICP >18 mm Hg, especially if > 40 mm Hg. |
| Cerebral oedema | Brain swelling as a result of interruption of cerebral structure and chemical alteration. |
| Epidural haematoma | Usually takes minutes but can be hours to show its clinical effect. |
| | Usually associated with a skull fracture of the temporal bone that disrupts the middle meningeal artery. Blood collects between the dura of the brain and the skull, creating a lens-like blood clot that compresses the underlying brain. |
| Subdural haematoma | Usually due to rupture of the veins that drain the brain into the dural sinuses. Blood collects underneath the dura, in a crescent-like shape, compressing the underlying brain and presenting with localised dysfunction. |
| Intracerebral haematoma | Bleeding and clot formation due to conversion of the intracerebral contusion from the primary injury. |
| Brain herniation: Supratentorial: Subfalcine | Midline shift where cingulate gyrus of frontal lobe is pushed under the falx cerebri. |
| | Cerebral hemispheres and basal ganglia pushed downwards and diencephalon and brain stem pass through the tentorium. |
| Transtentorial Uncal | Compression of midbrain when brain pushes through the tentorium cerebelli. |
| Infratentorial: Cerebellar | Cerebellar tonsils traverse foramen magnum. |
| CSF leak causing aerocele | Accumulation of air inside or on the surface of the brain, which as it enlarges, can cause pressure on the brain. |
| Meningitis | Due to access of microbes through a breach in the coverings of the brain. |

**Table 16.4** Types of extracranial secondary brain injury.

| Type of injury | Explanation |
|---|---|
| Hypoxia | Due to inadequate airway or aspiration, anaemia, hypovolaemic shock. |
| Raised intracranial pressure | Due to intervention, e.g. increased intrathoracic pressure from chest exercise therapy, incorrect positioning of patient, use of ventilator or positive end expiratory pressure, noxious stimulation, pain. |
| Hypotension | Due to blood loss from extracranial injuries. |
| Anaemia | Decreased haemoglobin carrying capacity due to extracranial bleeding. |
| Hyperthermia | Presence of infection. |
| | Malignant hyperthermia from brain injury. |

## OPEN AND CLOSED HEAD INJURY

It is important to differentiate between open and closed head injuries.

### Open head injury

In open injuries, the brain is exposed to air. There are three types of open injury:

- Penetrating injury, e.g. gunshot wound, stab wound.
- Compound depressed skull fracture with a tear of the dura mater.
- Basal skull fracture.

The risk with open injuries is infection (meningitis or brain abscess).

### Closed head injury

A closed head injury occurs when there is no disruption of the skull and no communication with the outside. The mechanism of injury relates to an acceleration/deceleration injury in which there is bruising, shearing and tearing of cerebral structures as they move against the rough internal base of the skull.

Closed head injuries may be classified as:

- Concussion.
- Contusion.
- Traumatic/Diffuse axonal injury.
- Intracranial haematoma.

### Severity of injury

Traumatic brain injury also varies in severity from the very severe to the very mild.

---

**Classification of head injuries (1)**

**Mild head injury:**
LOC <30 min
GCS >12/15
PTA 15–20 minutes - <24 hours

**Moderate head injury:**
LOC for ½–1 hours
GCS 9–12/15
PTA <24 hours

**Severe head injury:**
LOC >6 hours
GCS 3–8/15
PTA 1 week or longer

---

The classification of the severity of the injury includes the level of consciousness using the Glasgow Coma Scale score, as well as the period of PTA.

Other criteria such as the presence of neurological deficits, the need for operative intervention and the length of stay in hospital are also considered (Dawodu 2003: p. 2).

---

**Classification of head injuries (2)**

**Mild head injury:**
- Focal neurological deficit.
- No operative lesions.
- No CT scan abnormalities.
- Length of hospital stay <48 hours.

**Moderate head injury:**
- CT scan abnormalities.
- Operative lesions.
- Length of hospital stay >48 hours.

---

The boundaries between these categories are indistinct and it is important to understand that patients can move from one category to another (and back again).

### CONCLUSION

Early detection of secondary brain injury as well as appropriate patient management will ensure that the damage from secondary brain injury is limited or prevented. Knowledge of the classification of head injuries will aid in the appropriate management of neurotrauma patients.

---

### Activity 16.1

1. Compile a list of care aspects that could affect the secondary effects of brain injury.
2. In practice describe the methods used to decrease the risk of secondary effects of brain injury.
3. A patient has been admitted with an open head injury involving the left parietal region. Describe the management of this patient's open injury.
4. Differentiate between the clinical presentation of a patient with an open head injury and a closed head injury.

# Chapter 17
# Raised Intracranial Pressure

*Nadine Abelson-Mitchell*

School of Nursing and Midwifery, Faculty of Health, Education and Society, Plymouth University, Devon, UK

## INTRODUCTION

The management of intracranial pressure (ICP) is one of the most important aspects of neurotrauma practice. Small alterations in ICP can have severe consequences for the patient's morbidity and mortality.

## DEFINITION

Normal intracranial pressure is between 0–15 mm Hg. Raised ICP occurs when ICP is >15 mm Hg. Intracranial pressure is usually treated if ICP is >18 mm Hg.

## CAUSE OF INCREASED INTRACRANIAL PRESSURE

Causes of ↑ ICP related to brain injury can be classified as follows:

- Extradural, subdural, intraventricular, intracerebral haemorrhage.
- TBI.
- Meningitis, encephalitis and brain abscesses including subdural/extradural empyema.
- Hydrocephalus.
- Cerebral oedema, hypoxia and hypercarbia.
- Iatrogenic causes such as use of mechanical ventilation, incorrect positioning of the patient, e.g. in the head down position, obstructed airway, vigorous chest exercise therapy and medication such as Morphine, Fentanyl and Sufentanil (www.drugs.com).

## DIAGNOSIS

Diagnosis is based on the clinical features. Clinical features differ depending on whether the lesion is supratentorial, that is above the level of the tentorium cerebelli, or below the level of the tentorium cerebelli (Abelson 1982).

### Supratentorial lesions

Supratentorial lesions occur in the cerebral cortex, lateral ventricles, pituitary and any structures above the tentorium cerebelli. Raised intracranial pressure will result in tentorial herniation where the tips of the temporal lobes protrude through and are trapped in the tentorium cerebelli (see Chapters 18/22).

Supratentorial ↑ICP presents as follows:

- Nausea and vomiting due to pressure on the vomiting centre in the 4th ventricle. The type and frequency of vomiting must be recorded and reported.
- Headache due to stretching of the meninges. The nature, duration, severity and location of any headache must be

noted, as well as the relationship between headache, nausea and vomiting.

- ↓ Level of consciousness due to pressure, ischaemia, hypoxia to the RAS.
- Pupil changes due to pressure, ischaemia, hypoxia to the optic nerve (CN II) and occulomotor nerve (CN III) resulting in dilated pupils, initially, on the same side as the space occupying lesion and then on the other side. The patient may present with fixed dilated pupils. This is an indication of temporal herniation and is an ominous sign.
- One of the significant features of increasing intracranial pressure is an increase in systolic blood pressure more than in the diastolic pressure. This drastic increase in systolic pressure occurs in order to overcome the increased intracranial pressure by forcing oxygenated blood into the cerebral circulation. This is known as Cushing's law.
- Pulse changes due to pressure, ischaemia, hypoxia to the cardiac centre in the pons variola and medulla oblongata. This may result in an initial abrupt tachycardia leading to a bradycardia.
- Respiratory changes due to pressure, ischaemia, hypoxia to the respiratory centre in the pons variola and medulla oblongata.
- Changes to the pupils, pulse and respiration are referred to as Cushing's triad.

## Infratentorial lesions

Infratentorial lesions occur in the cerebellum, 4th ventricle, pons variola, medulla oblongata, midbrain, brain stem and cranial nerves. The space-occupying lesion develops below the level of the tentorium cerebelli and raised ICP will result in foramen magnum herniation with pressure on the pons variola and medulla oblongata causing respiratory arrest and cardiac arrest.

Infratentorial ↑ICP presents as follows:

- Respiratory arrest due to pressure, ischaemia, hypoxia to the pons variola and/or medulla oblongata.
- Cranial nerve deficits such as problems with swallowing, due to pressure, ischaemia, hypoxia to the cranial nerves.
- Signs of cerebellar disease due to pressure on the cerebellum (see Chapter 12 and Table 12.3).

When pressure is increased in the 4th ventricle this results in increased pressure above the tentorium and the patient then presents with signs and symptoms of supratentorial ↑ICP.

## INVESTIGATIONS

The investigations that will be undertaken depend on the suspected cause of the increase in pressure and the provisional diagnosis (see Chapter 13). This may include:

- A review of the clinical features (Teasdale and Jennett 1974).
- CT scan.
- MRI scan.
- Skull x-ray.

---

Implications for practice

**Do not perform a lumbar puncture** in the presence of ↑ICP and papilloedema as the patient will cone, i.e. the cerebellar peduncles will drop through the foramen magnum thus squeezing the brain stem and compressing the cardiac and respiratory centres. **This situation is irreversible and death will ensue**.

---

## TREATMENT

Numerous pharmaceutical agents are used to treat ↑ ICP (see Chapter 14 and Chapter 22). These include:

- Mannitol, an osmotic diuretic, that draws fluid from the cerebral structure and circulation away from the brain.
- Hypertonic saline.
- Barbiturates to decrease the brain's metabolic functioning.

## MANAGEMENT OF THE PATIENT

The unit may have a particular protocol for the management of patients with ↑ ICP (see Chapter 22 and Figure 22.5).

The following nursing diagnoses must be attended to within the nursing care plan: (see Chapter 23):

- Need for safe, therapeutic environment.
- Alteration in cerebral function.
- Potential increase in intracranial pressure.
- Increasing neurological deficit.
- Presence of behavioural disturbance.
- Alteration in respiratory function.
- Inability to maintain airway.
- Alteration in thermoregulation.
- Fluid volume deficit/overload.
- Alteration in nutritional status.
- Inability to attend to self-care needs.
- Altered psychological status.

## CONCLUSION

The nurse must be knowledgeable about ICP as increased ICP affects both the morbidity and mortality of patients with neurotrauma. Prevention, early detection and management of increased ICP are key elements of care. In-depth knowledge will enable the practitioner to understand physiological changes and explain these changes to the team and families when the need arises. Knowledge will also alert practitioners to the need to call for urgent medical assistance, investigation and intervention.

---

### Activity 17.1

#### Scenario

Trevor, 19 years old, has just been admitted to A&E (Casualty) after a motor vehicle accident. He was brought in by a paramedic ambulance crew. Trevor is unaccompanied. GCS 9/15.

The doctor is concerned that Trevor will develop raised intracranial pressure.

#### Exercises

1. Justify the observations you will undertake on Trevor, include the frequency and route of observation.

2. What manifestations will make you suspect Trevor is developing raised intracranial pressure?
3. Relate the clinical manifestations of brain injury to the anatomy and physiology of the brain.
4. Develop a care plan for a patient with raised intracranial pressure.
5. In practice, describe methods that will be used to maintain intracranial pressure within normal limits.

# Chapter 18
# Assessment of the Patient with Neurotrauma

*Nadine Abelson-Mitchell*

School of Nursing and Midwifery, Faculty of Health, Education and Society, Plymouth University, Devon, UK

## INTRODUCTION

As nurses accept responsibility and accountability for independent professional practice, improved assessment ability is mandatory to the delivery of optimum patient care. The nurses are the only members of the health team who attend to the patient for 24 hours out of every 24. Patient assessment requires intelligence, insight and an in-depth knowledge of general anatomy and physiology as well as neuroanatomy, neurophysiology and neuropathology. The nurse needs to be aware of the significance of the observations and, most importantly, when to summon medical assistance.

Patient assessment, both neurosurgical and general, is incorporated into, and is one of the most fundamental features of, neurosurgical nursing. Many of the patients who present with neurotrauma have other co-morbidity/ies. This may include respiratory or cardiac disease, previous trauma, dependence on substances such as recreational drugs or alcohol, diabetes mellitus, cancer as well as mental health issues. When conducting an assessment it is important to consider any co-morbidities.

Assessment can be presented in various ways. In this chapter assessment will be described as follows:

1. General principles.
2. Neurological observations.
3. Vital signs.
4. Recording the observations.
5. Undertaking a CNS examination
6. Recording the assessment.

## GENERAL PRINCIPLES

Assessment needs to occur at various stages throughout the patient's journey and takes place in various settings:

- At the scene: see Chapter 19.
- In the Emergency Department: see Chapter 21.
- In an acute setting: see Chapter 22.
- In a sub-acute setting.
- Rehabilitation (see Appendix 1).
- Community setting (see Appendix 2).
  - Home.
  - Residential setting.

### Purpose of an assessment

The purposes of undertaking an assessment can be summarised as follows:

- To establish a baseline of neurological function.
- To note any trend.
- To monitor for any changes in status or complications.
- To determine any associated risk.
- To treat alterations in status.
- To determine health needs.
- To decide on intervention.

- To prevent complications.
- To predict patient outcome.

An accurate initial assessment must be conducted and recorded to determine any deterioration in the patient's status (Maas *et al.* 2008). The findings must be assessed and recorded uniformly and accurately in order for them to be of diagnostic and prognostic value.

### Pre-requisites for effective assessment

To ensure an effective assessment you must provide the following:

- A safe, risk-free environment for the patient as well as the assessor:
  - Assessment of patients with neurotrauma is often difficult as the patient may have an altered level of consciousness. The patient may be agitated, confused or unconscious and therefore extra care must be taken to ensure an effective assessment with as little distress as possible. It is therefore important to be able to conduct a neurological assessment with all patients.
  - Patients who have suffered from neurotrauma may be admitted to the hospital unaccompanied. It may therefore be necessary to complete the assessment once a family member or friend has arrived.
- Effective communication:
  - It is important for the assessor to introduce themself and explain exactly what is to be done to the patient in a step-by-step fashion.
  - Establish whether the patient understands the language used by the assessor. If necessary seek out an interpreter to assist with the assessment.
  - Do not shout at the patient.
- Appropriate interpersonal relationships.
- Maintain confidentiality, dignity and respect.
- Equipment necessary to undertake a neurological examination:
  - A penlight torch.
  - A set of items to test sensory perception:
    - Clean cotton wool swab.
    - Sharp instrument such as a stylus.
  - Stethoscope.
  - Otoscope.
  - Reflex hammer.
  - Tuning fork.
  - Tongue depressor.

### Alcohol and assessment

Alcohol affects people in different ways and some patients who present with head injury will have consumed alcohol.

---

**Box 18.1** Tips for assessment

Ensure a conducive environment.
Determine the following:

- LOC.
- Is the patient accompanied by another person who could provide relevant information?
- Level of co-operation.
- Patient's level of understanding.

Maintain dignity and respect throughout assessment.

Document the findings and level of intervention required.

Reassure the patient throughout assessment.

---

In these circumstances be extra cautious in terms of the neurological examination and the need for regular monitoring. Focus on the patient's neurotrauma and not on the alcohol consumption as the alcohol could be masking the signs of serious neurological damage.

### The frequency of neurological assessment

It may be necessary to undertake a full neurological examination to establish a baseline for the patient, and thereafter prescribe the type and frequency of monitoring that is needed. The frequency of monitoring may be prescribed by a medical practitioner or by a registered nurse, based on their professional discretion. NICE guidelines (NICE 2007: p. 36) recommend that observations should be performed and recorded on a half-hourly basis until a GCS of 15/15 has been achieved. Once the patient's GCS is 15/15, the observations should be performed half-hourly for two hours, hourly for four hours and two hourly thereafter.

To avoid unnecessary repetition and disturbance to the patient it is possible for nurses and doctors to assess the patient simultaneously, to establish a baseline status that is essential for future management decisions. To ensure uniformity of assessment nurses should assess the patient together at the beginning and end of each shift. While testing the patient the nurse must read the previous observations and report variations.

### Performing the assessment

The neurological assessment is undertaken as part of a comprehensive assessment of the patient, using the Needs Approach Model (see Chapter 3 for details of needs assessment).

## NEUROLOGICAL OBSERVATIONS

### Assessing the level of consciousness

Consciousness, a person's level of awareness, may change after neurotrauma (Zeman 2001). The level of consciousness may deteriorate because of trauma, pressure, ischaemia and hypoxia to the RAS that is found in the midbrain and the brain stem – the part of the brain responsible for wakefulness.

### History

Is the patient conscious? Is the patient able to report the circumstances of the injury?

### Examination

#### *Glasgow Coma Scale (GCS)*

Used nationally and internationally, the Glasgow Coma Scale (see Table 18.1) (Teasdale and Jennett 1974) is a simple, sensitive, uniform, comprehensive and objective means of assessing and recording LOC that permits continuous evaluation with little inter-observer error (Kay and Teasdale 2001). The use of the GCS permits the assessor

to recognise degrees of altered consciousness while avoiding ill-defined terms such as semi-conscious or stupor.

The Glasgow Coma Scale (GCS) is scored out of 15 points. The scale consists of 3 components: eye opening, verbal response and motor response scoring between 1 and 4, 1 and 5, and 1 and 6 points respectively (Kay and Teasdale 2001).

*Eyes opening* (Table 18.2)

**Table 18.2** Eliciting a response to eye opening.

| Score | Category | Instruction |
|---|---|---|
| 4 | Spontaneously | When a person enters the room the patient opens his eyes spontaneously. |
| 3 | To speech | The patient opens his eyes to questions such as please open your eyes. |
| 2 | To pain | The patient only opens his eyes as a result of painful stimulation. |
| 1 | None | No response. |

*Verbal response* (Table 18.3)

**Table 18.3** Eliciting the verbal response.

| Score | Category | Instruction |
|---|---|---|
| 5 | Orientated | The patient is orientated to time, place and person. It is important to ask the patient questions applicable to his age and intelligence. |
| 4 | Confused | The patient is not orientated to time, place and person. It is important to ask the patient questions applicable to his age and intelligence. |
| 3 | Inappropriate | The patient gives an incorrect answer to a question asked, such as: Assessor: What is the time? Patient: I had egg and chips for lunch. |

**Table 18.1** Glasgow Coma Scale categories and scoring system.

| Eye opening | Score |
|---|---|
| Spontaneous | 4 |
| To voice | 3 |
| To pain | 2 |
| None | 1 |

| Verbal response | Score |
|---|---|
| Orientated (time, place, person) | 5 |
| Confused | 4 |
| Inappropriate words | 3 |
| Incomprehensible sounds | 2 |
| None | 1 |

| Motor response | Score |
|---|---|
| Obeys command | 6 |
| Localising to pain | 5 |
| Flexion to pain | 4 |
| Abnormal flexion to pain | 3 |
| Extension to pain | 2 |
| None | 1 |

**Table 18.3** *(Continued)*

| Score | Category | Instruction |
|---|---|---|
| 2 | Incomprehensible | One cannot understand the patient – he may be mumbling, groaning or swearing (remember that swearing might be appropriate if one is hurting the patient and this is his usual manner of behaviour). |
| 1 | None | No response. |

*Motor response* (Table 18.4)

**Table 18.4** Eliciting the motor response.

| Score | Category | Instruction |
|---|---|---|
| 6 | Obeys commands | When the patient is asked to lift his leg he follows instructions. |
| 5 | Localise pain | There is no response to verbal command therefore the patient's response to pain is tested using fingernail bed pressure or cranial nerve distribution. The patient tries to touch the area that has been tested. |
| 4 | Withdraws | When the nurse tests the patient's response to pain, the patient withdraws the limb being tested. |
| 3 | Flexion | On painful stimulation the patient adopts the decorticate position which involves flexion of the arms, wrists and fingers; adduction of the upper extremities; and extension, internal rotation and plantar flexion of the lower extremities.<br><br>This is a sign of damage in the hypothalamic area and cerebral peduncles. |

**Table 18.4** *(Continued)*

| Score | Category | Instruction |
|---|---|---|
| 2 | Extension | On painful stimulation, the patient adopts the decerebrate position. This involves extension and hyperpronation of the arms; extension and plantar flexion of the lower extremities.<br><br>This is a sign of pons variola and midbrain disruption. |
| 1 | None | There is no response to painful stimulation. |

The patient's eye opening, verbal and motor responses should be noted, as described in Table 18.1, 18.2, 18.3 and 18.4. The range of scores is therefore between 3 (lowest) and 15 (fully conscious). A patient with a GCS of 15 has spontaneous eye opening, is orientated in time, place and person and obeys commands (e.g. protrudes tongue to command). If a patient is dysphasic, they may not be able to answer or respond to questions appropriately. If this is the case, it is common practice to annotate 'dys' in the verbal section of the chart.

If the patient does not respond to voice, then test the patient's response to painful stimuli. Test for painful stimulation using nail-bed pressure (Maas *et al.* 2008) or pain should be stimulated in the distribution of a cranial nerve (i.e. central pain), such as pressure over the supraorbital area (oculomotor nerve, CN III) or squeezing the trapezius muscle (accessory nerve, CN XI). Normal flexion means bending of limb towards the painful origin (but not quite reaching it, which would be localising) whereas extension means straightening of limbs (i.e. withdrawal from pain). When using the Glasgow Coma Scale, once motor function in terms of the best motor response has been assessed, further observation of the patient's motor response is required (Abelson 1982).

It must be noted that when testing the patient's response to painful stimulation, it is essential for all assessors to use the same method of testing to ensure uniform assessment. The importance of the GCS is that if a patient is examined and on assessment scores 11 out of 15, and two hours later scores 7 out of 15, this is an indication that he is deteriorating. The nurse must summon the doctor as prompt intervention is imperative.

It has been reported that the motor part of the GCS is as good a prognostic indicator as the whole GCS (Jagger *et al.* 1983). In fact, a drop in the motor response is more significant than a drop in eye opening or verbal responses. Many neurosurgeons therefore advocate a deteriorating GCS to be a drop by one point in the motor domain or by two points in the other categories. Maas *et al.* (2008: p. 734) report that in 39–44% of patients there is a noted deterioration of the GCS motor score, and pupillary responses.

---

### Implications for practice

**Caution:**

- Remember that the patient must not be assaulted during testing.
- Test for painful response using fingernail bed pressure or distribution of cranial nerves.
- Do not use a sternal rub.
  A sternal rub does not stimulate pain along a cranial nerve distribution and should not be used to assess GCS. It is a technique that is unable to distinguish between localisation and flexion, and may give aberrant results in the presence of a spinal injury.
- Be consistent in method of testing selected.

---

### Pupils

Assess and record pupillary size, shape, equality and the reaction to light, the dilating pupil as well as any swelling or discolouration of the eye and eyelids. If concerned about the size, shape, reaction or inequality of the pupils, call for assistance.

Pupillary constriction is controlled by the parasympathetic fibres running in cranial nerve III. Any compressive lesions (e.g. haematoma, coning or cerebral herniation) may result in the malfunction of these fibres, leading to a dilated pupil with an absent reaction to light. Usually the pupil on the side of the lesion is affected first, and thereafter the pupil on the other side. Irreversible brain damage may have already occurred by this stage and without prompt treatment the patient is unlikely to survive.

When assessing pupils it is necessary to use a torch of 22 lumens. The recording of pupil size may be done in terms of:

- Millimetres measured against the actual size of the patient's pupil.

- A pre-measure set of pupil sizes.
- Coded numbers.

The important aspects of pupil observation are:

*Size*

Pupil size should always be interpreted by comparing with the previous sets of observations, in combination with the GCS, as a patient with a GCS of 15 and sitting up is unlikely to have cerebral herniation, even if the pupils are unequal in size. The interpretation of findings regarding pupil size and reaction can be difficult because pupil size and response are sensitive to a range of different influences such as light source in the room, medication such as Atropine and Morphine. Also, there may have been direct trauma to the globe of the eye, previous ophthalmic surgery, use of eye drops or there may be physiologically asymmetrical pupils. Alternatively, the constricted pupil may be the abnormal pupil, although in the context of severe brain injury, the dilated pupil should always be considered the abnormal pupil until proven otherwise.

The following must be observed:

- Is the pupil size changing?
- Is the pupil size normal (N)?
- Is the pupil size pinpoint (P)?
- Is the pupil size small (S)?
- Is the pupil size dilated (D)?

The above method of recording pupil size is simple and accurate.

Pupil size may also be assessed by measuring the actual pupil size against a pre-measured set of pupil sizes in millimetres (see Figure 18.1).

Whatever method of assessing pupil size is used, the important observation is to note any change and call assistance immediately.

*Reaction*

The following must be observed:

- Is the reaction normal (N)?
- Is the reaction sluggish (S)?
- Are the pupils fixed (F) with no reaction?

---

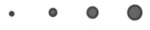

**Figure 18.1**   Picture of pupil sizes.

*Equality*

The following must be observed:

- Is the size and reaction of the left pupil equal to that of the right pupil?
- Is the left pupil larger than the right?
- Is the left pupil smaller than the right?

*Direct and consensual light reflex*

The direct and consensual light reflex must be assessed:

PROCEDURE

Using a penlight torch shine the light into the patient's left eye.

- The normal response is that the pupil on the left eye reacts by contracting in size to the bright light source. This is the direct light reflex.
- Now look at the right eye, in response to the bright light source in the left eye, the normal response is that the pupil on the right eye reacts by contracting in size. This is the consensual light reflex.

EXPLANATION

The light is shone on the retina in the left eye. The visual stimulation is detected by the optic nerve (CN II). The optic nerve (CN II) has two portions – a lateral portion that is found in the left eye and a medial portion that is located on the medial aspect of the retina in the right eye. The lateral portion of CN II travels back to the visual area in the occipital lobe via the optic chiasm (see Figure 18.2). It travels via the optic chiasm until it reaches the left side of the brain. The medial portion in the right eye travels to the optic chiasm and there it goes to the right side of the brain. Thus both the left side of the brain and the right side of the brain receive fibres from both eyes via the optic chiasm. The motor response to stimulation from the optic nerve is via the oculomotor nerve (CN III). The response is the consensual light reflex as there are fibres from both the left and the right eye on each side of the brain.

*Shape*

The shape of the pupil must be observed. Always bear in mind that the patient may have had a cataract operation, lens implant or an eye injury.

*Papilloedema*

Is papilloedema present?

To observe papilloedema an ophthalmoscope is required. Papilloedema occurs when there is engorgement of the retinal vessels and optic disc as a result of raised intracranial pressure and it is best seen in the area of the optic disc as retinal engorgement 'silver wiring' with nonpulsating vessels (see Chapter 17) (see Figure 18.3).

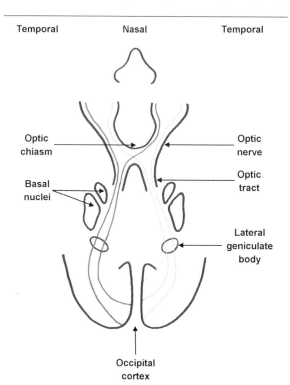

**Figure 18.2** Diagram of optic chiasm. For a colour version of this figure, please refer to the plate section.

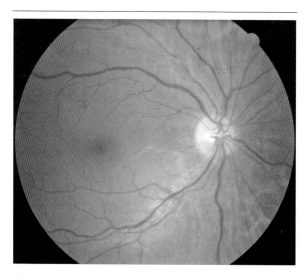

**Figure 18.3** Normal appearance of optic disc. For a colour version of this figure, please refer to the plate section.

## Eye movements

Eye movements may be affected in CNS disorders and must therefore be observed. Eye movements are controlled by the nerves as listed in Table 18.5.

**Table 18.5** Cranial nerves controlling eye movement.

| Number | Name of cranial nerve | Abnormal action |
|--------|-----------------------|-----------------|
| III | Occulomotor nerve | Pupil dilation, ptosis and outward movement of the eye. |
| IV | Trochlear nerve | Affected eye moving inwards. |
| VI | Abducens nerve | Loss of natural gaze and diplopia in the affected eye. |

In the unconscious patient it may not be possible to assess cranial nerve III, IV and VI. As an alternative, assess the patient's doll's eye movement, which is an occulo-cephalic response.

### Technique

If the head is moved upwards the eyes move downwards. This is a normal response and doll's eye movement is present. If, when moving the head to the left or right, up or down, the eyes remain centrally fixed, doll's eye movement is absent. This is pathological and must be reported.

### Motor assessment

Limb function should be assessed in order to identify the presence of cerebral space-occupying lesions or spinal injuries. Document any pre-existing weakness from previous illness as this will affect the interpretation of the assessment. The MRC (Medical Research Council 1981) grading system shown in Table 18.6 is used.

Each limb should be tested separately. If a patient is able to lift a limb off the bed (i.e. against gravity), then the power is at least 3/5. The presence of any resistance against the assessor will put the power at 4/5 whilst normal power is 5/5.

### Raised intracranial pressure

The patient must be assessed for any signs and symptoms of raised intracranial pressure (see Chapter 17).

**Table 18.6** MRC grading system.

| Muscle strength | Score |
|-----------------|-------|
| Normal strength | 5 |
| Reduced strength but can still move against resistance | 4 |
| Movement against gravity but not against resistance | 3 |
| Movement with gravity eliminated | 2 |
| Palpable contraction but no visible movement | 1 |
| No movement | 0 |

### Intracranial pressure monitoring

This is extremely important but is only done in specialised units where there are adequate resources. The intracranial monitoring device may be placed in the lateral ventricle, subdural space or extradural space. The following is noted:

- Systolic pressure.
- Diastolic pressure.
- Mean pressure.

The intracranial pressure should be kept below 25 mm Hg. The nurse must be aware of any patient intervention that will cause an increase in intracranial pressure, such as hurting the patient, suctioning the patient, taking arterial blood gases or causing interference with cerebral venous drainage by malpositioning the head and neck or nursing the patient in the head down position.

## Convulsions, seizures and fits

These are important and must be recorded. A seizure may be motor or sensory depending on the area involved. The following must be noted:

- Any predisposing factors.
- Type of seizure.
  - Generalised seizure.
  - Focal seizure.
- Duration.
- The progression of the seizure.
- Incontinence.
- Cyanosis.
- Pupil response.

## Cerebrospinal fluid leakage (CSF)

CSF leakage is an indication of neurotrauma. CSF may leak from the ears, nose and throat as well as from wounds, intraventricular drainage or monitoring circuits. The danger from CSF leakage is that of infection and air entry. A CSF leak can be recognised by the following.

- Patient signs and symptoms:
  - History of accident or a fight in which the nose was injured or broken.
  - There may be damage to the ethmoid and cribriform plate.
  - Recurrent attacks of meningitis after a fractured base of skull.
  - The nose runs when stooping, lifting anything heavy, or getting out of bed.
  - Salty taste in the mouth.
- Appearance of the CSF:
  - The CSF looks like an egg yolk and an egg white as the RBCs and CSF separate. This is noticed on the pillowcase or absorbent sheet on which the patient's head is resting (see Chapter 12, p. 97).
- Biochemistry of the CSF (see Chapter 12, p. 98).

---

Implications for practice

A CSF leakage is very dangerous and therefore must be reported immediately. It must not be plugged, but kept covered with a sterile pad and managed aseptically.

---

## VITAL SIGNS

The vital signs of blood pressure (BP), pulse (P), respiration (R) and temperature (T) reflect the patient's neurological status and general status and may profoundly affect the outcome (see Chapter 12).

### Respiration

The observation of the respiratory system is of paramount importance. Increasing $pCO_2$ causes vessel dilation and causes a further rise in intracranial pressure. The patient's respiration may change because of trauma to, pressure on, ischaemia, or hypoxia to, the respiratory centres which are found in the pons variola and medulla oblongata; raised intracranial pressure; fractured base of the skull and pontine lesions as well as chest trauma; aspiration, respiratory failure and respiratory embarrassment. The respiratory pattern may vary from midbrain-hyperventilation, irregular breathing, Cheyne–Stokes respiration, apnoeic attacks and respiratory arrest. If any abnormalities are present the

**Table 18.7** Observations of the respiratory system.

| Modality | Observations |
|---|---|
| Airway | Is the airway patent? |
| | Is there an obstruction (blood, teeth or vomitus) present? |
| Rate | What is the respiratory rate? |
| Rhythm | Is the respiration regular or irregular? |
| Volume | What is the depth of respiration? |
| Air entry | Is the air entry equal bilaterally? |
| | Presence of abnormal sounds? |
| Oxygen percentage | Is the patient receiving $O_2$? |
| | At what rate? |
| | According to blood gases? |
| Humidification | Is the air humidified? |
| Ventilator observations | When required. |
| Pulmonary oedema | Is there pulmonary oedema? |
| | With increased intracranial and arterial hypertension there is a redistribution of the blood into the pulmonary vasculature. This may cause pulmonary oedema. |

rate, rhythm and depth of respiration must be recorded for one minute.

Table 18.7 presents a list of the observations regarding respiration.

### Blood pressure

The systolic pressure, diastolic pressure and pulse pressure must be noted.

If the neurosurgical patient's blood pressure is dropping consider:

- Hypovolaemic shock from extracranial haemorrhage or diabetes insipidus.
- The patient is approaching the terminal stage.

### Pulse rate

Some authorities believe that the pulse rate increases and decreases with raised intracranial pressure, others believe that it decreases as a physiological response to an increased blood pressure. Changes in the pulse rate occur because the cardiac acceleratory centre is affected before the cardiac inhibitory centre – both of which are found in the medulla oblongata. Therefore the patient will develop a tachycardia which may be transient and then a bradycardia or just a bradycardia – both of which are significant.

Besides raised intracranial pressure, a change in pulse rate may be due to shock, hypovolaemia and an acid-base or electrolyte imbalance. The nurse must observe the pulse rate, rhythm, regularity and volume.

In the acute phase, the patient may be attached to a cardiac monitor. Arrhythmias that occur from CNS disturbances include sinus tachycardia, paroxysmal atrial tachycardia and bradyarrhythmias from supraventricular and ventricular foci. Lesions that affect the basilar skull, subarachnoid haemorrhage, lesions of the hypothalamus and strokes may present with an inverted T wave, a prolonged QT interval and prominent U wave (as an anterior myocardial infarction presents) but in this case the enzyme levels are normal.

## Haemodynamic status

The patient's haemodynamic status is also very important and must be monitored:

- Perfusion.
- Skin colour, temperature and moisture.
- Fluid intake – oral, nasogastric and intravenous.
- Fluid output – urine, faeces, nasogastric and any other drainage.

## Temperature

Damage to the hypothalamus may affect the patient's temperature causing hyper- or hypothermia. Blood in the CSF from a subarachnoid haemorrhage or post-operatively will cause a pyrexia, as will a urinary tract infection or chest infection.

The temperature of an unconscious patient must be taken per axilla. Variance between the core body temperature and the temperature per axilla is <2.2 °F (1.2 °C). Rectal temperature assessment using a thermocouple is preferable.

## RECORDING THE OBSERVATIONS

There is no universally accepted method of assessing and reporting neurosurgical observations but, in an endeavour to improve the standard of neurosurgical patient observation and management, a concise patient management plan has been produced. The recorded observations should include RR, oxygen saturation ($O_2$Sats), fraction of inspired oxygen ($FiO_2$), P, BP and T, GCS, pupillary size and reac-

tion to light and the presence of any limb weakness (see Figure 18.4).

## Patient deterioration

When concerned about a patient, summons assistance. The importance of accurate and prompt reporting of any variations that occur, as well as summoning medical assistance, must be stressed (Abelson 1982). When there is a change in the patient's neurological status, this should be confirmed by a second member of staff immediately. If this is not possible, then a doctor should be informed. Once the change is confirmed, further action will need to be taken. This usually comprises stabilisation of the patient and then obtaining an urgent CT scan of the brain.

## UNDERTAKING A COMPREHENSIVE CNS EXAMINATION

Although the stress is on neurological examinations it is important to remember that the neurological examination is a component of a thorough systematic examination of the neurotrauma patient.

## General assessment

A general assessment of all body systems must be completed to ensure any other disorders/injuries/conditions are determined as these could affect the patient's current management, morbidity and mortality. The general assessment includes:

- Obtaining a general history about the patient.
- Obtaining a history of the incident/progress since the time of the incident.
- Current medication/reaction to medication.
- Previous/presenting problems.
- Examination of the body systems:
  - The condition of the eyes, nose and mouth regarding ulceration, infection or any other feature.
  - The skin – abrasions, bruising, decubitus ulcers and allergies.
  - State of hydration – a change in output may indicate one of the following:
    - Diabetes insipidus after head injury or with pituitary lesion or operation.
    - Decreased fluid intake – due to nausea and vomiting, lethargy or unconsciousness.
    - Inappropriate ADH secretion after head injury.
    - Haemodynamic disturbances or renal complications.
    - Nutritional state.

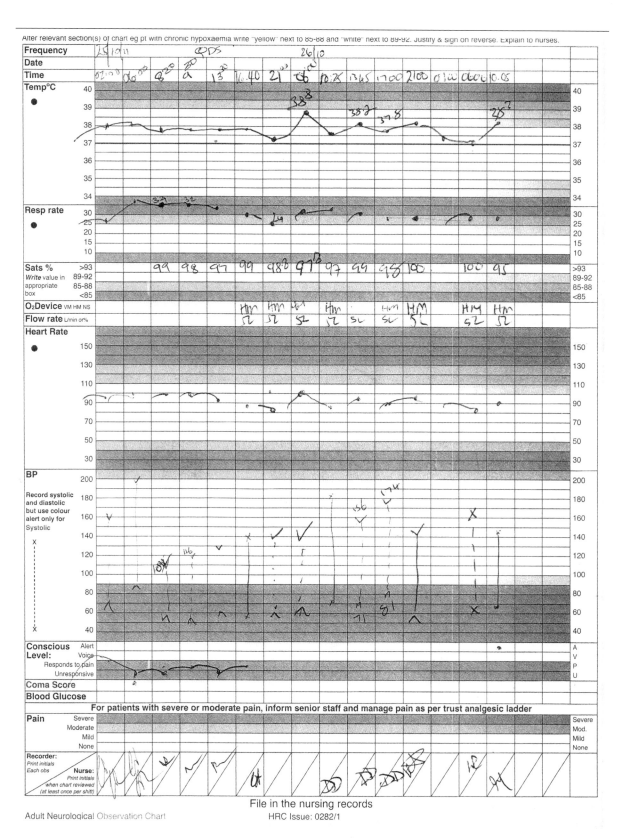

**Figure 18.4** A copy of a neuro-observations chart used at Derriford Hospital, Plymouth.

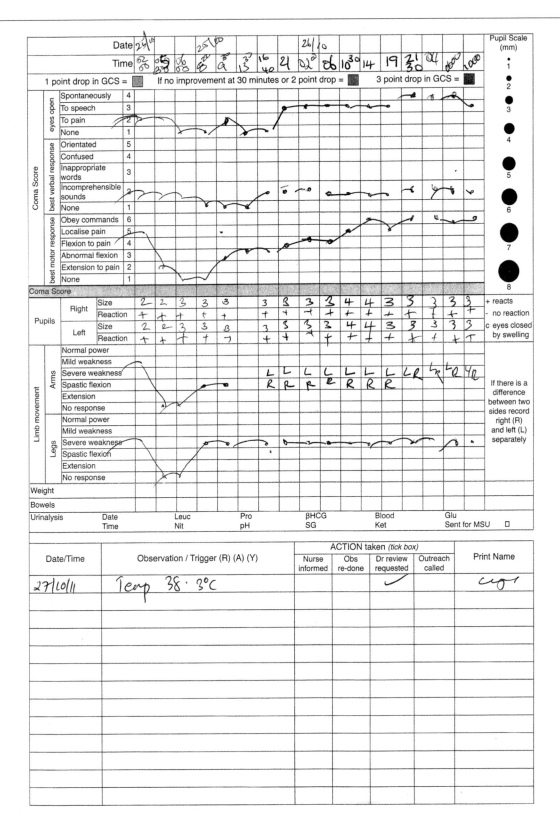

**Figure 18.4** *(Continued)*

- The results of investigations. It is essential to know the normal values to be able to report when a result is abnormal.

The neurological examination includes history taking, physical examination and requesting further investigations.

The neurological assessment includes the assessment of:

- Skull integrity.
- General cerebral function.
  - General behaviour.
  - Intellectual performance.
- Specific cerebral function.
  - Assessment of speech.
  - Sensory system.
  - Specific sensory systems.
  - Examination of the cerebellum:
    - Motor function.
    - Reflexes.
    - Cranial nerves.

### Skull integrity

Is there any obvious sign of scalp or skull injury? Any bleeding from the scalp/skull? Palpate the skull for any lesions.

### General cerebral function

#### General behaviour

Behaviour patterns may be an indication of cerebral pathology and must therefore be observed (see Table 18.8). There are often personality, mood and behaviour changes in frontal lobe pathology.

#### Intellectual performance

Talking to the patient will elicit some indication of the patient's intellectual performance (see Table 18.9).

### Specific cerebral functions

#### Assessment of speech

##### History

Ask the patient whether they had any abnormalities of vision or speech prior to this incident.

##### Examination

Test for signs of agnosia, apraxia and aphasia (Tables 18.10, 18.11 and 18.12).

#### Sensory function

A neurological deficit may involve sensory pathways, and therefore the patient's sensory function must be assessed.

**Table 18.8** Enquiry regarding behaviour patterns.

| Presentation | Enquiry |
|---|---|
| Mood | Does the patient have frequent alterations in mood? |
| | Check the patient's emotional status, for example agitated, angry, depressed, tearful or euphoric? |
| Personality | Has there been a personality change? |
| Intellect | Does the patient understand the conversation? Has there been a change in intellectual ability? What about powers of concentration? |
| Activities and socialisation patterns | In general, is the patient displaying normal behaviour? Is the behaviour acceptable? Is the behaviour appropriate for the cultural setting? |

**Table 18.9** Enquiry regarding memory.

| Activity | Enquiry |
|---|---|
| Short term memory | Can the patient remember recent events? Ask the patient to repeat a series of number such as one to 10 and then ask the patient to repeat the series backwards. Check the patient's arithmetic ability by asking them to multiply or divide some numbers. |
| Establish whether the patient has any PTA | Questions could be asked relating to the time of day, what the patient did this morning or what they had for dinner last night. |
| Long term memory | Can the patient remember past events? Questions could be asked relating to their youth or activities undertaken in the previous year. |

**Table 18.10** Test for signs of agnosia, apraxia and aphasia.

| Test for | How performed |
|---|---|
| Sound recognition | With patient's eyes closed ask him to identify familiar sounds. |
| Auditory-verbal comprehension | Does patient answer questions and carry out instructions? |
| Recognition of body parts and sidedness | Does he recognise body parts? Does patient know left from right? |
| Performance of skilled motor acts | Can he complete motor acts such as drinking from a cup, closing a safety pin or using common tools. |
| Visual object recognition | Ask patients to identify familiar objects such as a pencil or mobile phone. |
| Visual-verbal comprehension | Ask patient to read a sentence from a book or a newspaper and explain its meaning. |
| Motor speech | Ask patients to imitate different sounding phrases such as A, E, I, O, U. |
| Automatic speech | Ask patient to repeat days of the week or months of the year. |
| Volitional speech | Does the patient answer questions relevantly? |
| Writing | Can the patient write his name and address? |

(Reproduced with permission from Vazuka 1962)

**Table 18.11** Types of agnosia.

| Type of agnosia | Affected cerebral area |
|---|---|
| Visual | Occipital lobe |
| Auditory | Lateral and superior portion of the temporal lobe |
| Tactile | Parietal lobe |
| Body parts and relationships | Posterior-inferior region of parietal lobe |

(Reproduced with permission from Vazuka 1962)

**Table 18.12** Types of aphasia.

| Type of aphasia | Brain area involved |
|---|---|
| Auditory-receptive | Temporal lobe |
| Expressive speaking | Inferior posterior frontal areas |
| Visual-receptive | Parieto-occipital area |
| Expressive writing | Posterior frontal area |

(Reproduced with permission from Vazuka 1962)

Sensory function is represented in the sensory homunculus (see Chapter 12, p. 87).

The sensory system consists of two systems:

*The generic sensory system:*

• Pain.
• Temperature.
• Coarse touch.
• Fine touch.
• Pressure.
• Proprioception.

*Specific sensory systems:*

• Taste.
• Smell.
• Touch.
• Vision.
• Hearing.

---

**Implications for practice**

**Caution:**

• Ensure hands washed before undertaking examination.
• Wash hands when necessary during examination.
• Do not injure patient.
• Maintain surgically clean procedures at all times.
• Discard items used for testing after use.
• Disinfect reusable implements.

---

*The generic sensory system*

PAIN/COARSE TOUCH/FINE TOUCH/PRESSURE

*History*   Ask the patient:

• About the site of the pain.
• Rate the pain from 1–10 where 1 is minimal pain and 10 is maximum pain.
• What increases or relieves the pain?
• Is patient taking medication for the pain?

*Examination*   Examine the area of pain:
- Is there any discolouration, bruising or evidence of trauma?
- Check for any abnormal movements in the area.
- Is it superficial pain or deep pain, i.e. organ pain?
- Test for superficial tactile sensation using a wisp of cotton wool. Test hands, forearms, upper arms, trunk, thighs, lower limbs and feet as well as perineal and perianal areas. Ask the patient if they can feel fine touch or pressure.
- Test for superficial pain using a pin or sharp object. Test hands, forearms, upper arms, trunk, thighs, lower limbs and feet as well as perineal and perianal areas. Ask the patient if they can feel pain in the area that is being tested.

TEMPERATURE
*History*   Ask the patient:
- Whether they can determine changes in temperature.

*Examination*   Examine the area:
- Test for temperature sensation by using test tubes filled with hot and cold water. Apply the test tubes to the various parts of the body. Test hands, forearms, upper arms, trunk, thighs, lower limbs and feet. Ask the patient if they can feel hot and cold. Do not burn the patient.

PROPRIOCEPTION
Proprioception is joint position sense. The way in which, when walking or running or in an emergency situation, a person automatically knows where their feet are, for example in order to stop falling in a hole in the pavement.

*History*   Ask the patient:
- If they are able to walk in the dark.
- When walking, do they watch the position of their feet?

*Examination*
- Test the joint position sense in the fingers and toes by asking the patient to close their eyes and let the assessor know if the digit is being moved upwards or downwards. Be careful not to place pressure on the skin as this will give the patient a clue as to the movement of the digit.
- Use a tuning fork on bony prominence such as the wrist, elbow, shoulder, hip, knee, shin and ankle. Note the patient's ability to feel the vibration and determine when the vibration has stopped.

*Specific sensory systems*
TASTE
*History*   Ask the patient:
- If they are able to taste various substances, such as salt, sweet, sour or bitter substances.

*Examination*
- Test taste sensation on both sides of the tongue using a few grains of sugar or lemon juice.
- Can the patient differentiate the tastes on both sides of the tongue? When testing taste or smell it is important to use items with which the patient is familiar otherwise they will not be able to determine the substance.

SMELL
*History*   Ask the patient:
- If they suffer from nasal congestion or sinusitis as this could affect their sense of smell.
- If their appetite is good and if they can smell food and other items such as flowers, perfume or if something is burning.
- If they are able to smell various substances such as coffee, cinnamon or curry.

*Examination*
- Look into nostrils to check that there is no obstruction or discharge.
- Test smell in both nostrils using a few grains of coffee, cinnamon or curry.
- Can the patient differentiate the smell in both nostrils?

TOUCH
*History*   Ask the patient:
- If they can feel different sensations applied to various parts of their body.
- Sensations of light pressure and deep pressure being applied.

*Examination*
- Patient to close their eyes.
- Apply touch to all four limbs to check if they can feel sensation (see Chapter 12).

VISION
*History*   Ask the patient:
- Are they are able to see clearly?
- Can they determine colours?
- Are they experiencing any problems with their eyes or their vision?

*Examination*
- Test the patient's visual acuity using a Snellen's chart.
- Test the patient's visual fields. Use a white and red tipped applicator to check visual fields. The assessor brings the white or red applicator into the peripheral field of vision at 180°. The applicator is then brought in an arc to the midline until such time as the patient notices the indicator. This is repeated with the other eye.
- Check the eyes for any redness, discharge, etc.
- Refer the patient to an ophthalmologist or optometrist if necessary.

HEARING
*History*  Ask the patient:
- Are they are able to hear clearly?
- Can they determine sounds/frequencies?
- Are they experiencing any problems with their ears or hearing?

*Examination*
- Check the ears for any obstruction, discharge, etc.
- Test patient's hearing.
- Use tuning fork to test for air and bone conduction in both ears.
- Refer the patient to an audiologist, ENT specialist, if necessary.

*Examination of the cerebellum*
The cerebellum is responsible for fine motor movement, balance and coordination.

HISTORY
Check whether the patient presents with any history of imbalance, falling over and tremors, perhaps an inability to do up and undo their buttons, pick up objects or do fine work such as needlework.

EXAMINATION
Stand in front of the patient, the assessor raises the index finger about 12–15 cm from the patient's nose. The assessor asks the patient to use their index finger to touch his finger and touch their nose. The assessor may alter the position of his finger and increase the speed of this activity. The patient must do this test with both hands.

In a sitting position ask the patient to pat their knees by alternating the supine and prone area of their hand.

Ask the patient to use his thumb and forefinger and allow them to touch in rapid succession.

Ask the patient to walk normally and thereafter in a heel to toe fashion.

*Motor function*
Motor function may be affected because of trauma, ischaemia, pressure and oedema or hypoxia to the pyramidal motor tract.

The neurological examination includes the examination of muscles for muscle size, muscle strength and muscle tone as well as any involuntary movements.

When assessing motor function it is essential to assess all four limbs individually and comparatively for position, power, tone and reflexes. To simplify the recording of motor function the various aspects of motor function can be coded, as shown below.

POSITION
See Table 18.13.

**Table 18.13**  Position of limbs.

| Score | Category | Explanation |
|-------|----------|-------------|
| 3 | Normal | When one examines the patient the limbs are in a normal position. |
| 2 | Decorticate | The arms are flexed, the legs are extended. |
| 1 | Decerebrate | The arms and legs are extended. |

POWER
This is coded according to the internationally accepted method of assessing power (see Table 18.6).

MUSCLE TONE
Muscle tone is the resistance to passive movement and is tested in all four limbs by asking the patient to push against some form of resistance. This could be the assessor's hand.

Muscle tone is coded as shown in Table 18.14.

**Table 18.14**  Muscle tone.

| Tone | Explanation |
|------|-------------|
| Normal tone | The response in terms of tone is normal. |
| Increased tone | The muscles show increased resistance to pressure. |
| Decreased tone | The muscles show no resistance to pressure and may be flaccid. |

MUSCLE SIZE

Muscle size is determined in the following way.

The muscle bulk is assessed by palpating the muscle as well as measuring the muscle on each side using a tape measure. The size of the muscle and any difference between the two muscles is reported.

INVOLUNTARY MOVEMENTS

Any involuntary movement must be noted (see Table 18.15). The involuntary movements may include:

**Table 18.15**  Types of involuntary movement.

| Name | Movement |
|------|----------|
| Athetosis | Snakelike movements of the limbs. |
| Chorea | Thrashing arm movements, known as St Vitus dance. |
| Tremor | Tremor may occur at rest or on activity and may involve a hand, limb or more than one limb or the entire body. |

REFLEXES

When undertaking a full examination of the CNS the patient's reflexes must be assessed.

There are two types of reflexes that are assessed:

- Deep reflexes.
- Superficial reflexes.

When examining reflexes it is important for the patient to be relaxed. The reflex is tested by tapping briskly on a tendon or bony prominence using a patella hammer. It is important to check each reflex and be able to compare left- and right-sided reflexes.

DEEP REFLEXES   See Table 18.16.

In addition, it is important to check for ankle clonus (see Chapter 12).

SUPERFICIAL REFLEXES   Superficial reflexes (Table 18.17) are tested by stroking the skin with an object that will not break the skin, for example, cotton wool, a spatula or the end of the patella hammer.

PATHOLOGICAL REFLEXES   The Babinski response is elicited by stroking the lateral aspect of the soul of the foot. In pyramidal tract disease extension or dorsiflexion of the big toe occurs.

CRANIAL NERVE FUNCTION

There are 12 cranial nerves that need to be examined to detect any deficit, such as bulbar palsy (absence of coughing and swallowing) or facial palsy.

*History*   Ask patient whether they have had any problem with their vision, visual acuity, swallowing, eating, facial pain or hearing.

**Table 18.16**  Deep reflexes.

| Reflex | Site of stimulus | Normal response | Related CNS area |
|--------|------------------|-----------------|------------------|
| Biceps | Biceps tendon | Contraction of biceps | Cervical 5/6 |
| Brachoradialis | Styloid process of radius | Flexion of the elbow and pronation of the forearm | Cervical 5/6 |
| Triceps | Triceps tendon above the olecranon | Extension of the elbow | Cervical 6/7/8 |
| Patellar | Patellar tendon | Extension of the leg at the knee | Lumbar 2/3/4 |
| Achilles | Achilles tendon | Plantar flexion of the foot | Sacral 1/2 |

**Table 18.17**  Superficial reflexes.

| Reflex | Normal response | Related CNS area |
|--------|-----------------|------------------|
| Upper abdominal | Umbilicus moves up and towards area being stroked | Thoracic 7/8/9 |
| Lower abdominal | Umbilicus moves down | Thoracic 11/12 |
| Cremasteric | Scrotum elevates | Thoracic 12/Lumbar 1 |
| Plantar | Flexion of the toes | Sacral 1/2 |
| Gluteal | Skin tenses at gluteal area | Lumber 4 through Sacral 3 |

*Examination* See Table 12.4 Cranial nerves p. 92.

## RECORDING THE ASSESSMENT

All findings of the CNS examination MUST be recorded in detail in the patient's notes. It is also imperative that if abnormalities are found these are reported to the medical practitioner in charge of the patient. All records are medico-legal documents, and according to law if is not recorded it was not undertaken. This could have serious implications if there is a medico-legal enquiry regarding the neurotrauma.

## CONCLUSION

A fundamental aspect of neurotrauma care is patient assessment. Registered Nurses must be able to assess neurotrauma patients in all settings, in order to plan relevant management and determine when it is necessary to summon medical assistance. Patient morbidity and mortality is affected by the nurse's ability to assess patient needs effectively.

### Activity 18.1

**Note**

Before undertaking independent neurological examinations please ensure that these are included in your scope of practice.

**Exercises**

1. Ask a senior colleague or physician to demonstrate how to conduct a comprehensive neurological examination.
2. Depending on your professional status perform a full neurological examination under supervision. Record your findings.

### Activity 18.2

**Scenario**

Mrs Jones, 28 years old, has been admitted to the Emergency Department after being involved in a pedestrian vehicle accident. The Glasgow Coma Scale score is 7/15. She is restless and is unaccompanied.

**Exercises**

1. Undertake a comprehensive neurological assessment of Mrs Jones.
 Document your findings.

### Activity 18.3

**Scenario**

Charles Smith, 65 years old, has been admitted to the ward after falling on the pavement this morning. It was reported that after he fell:

- They could not wake him but now he seems to be waking up.
- His GCS is 10/15.
- His breath smells quite strongly of alcohol.
- He is accompanied by his wife.

**Exercises**

1. Undertake a comprehensive neurological assessment of Charles.
2. Document your findings.
3. You are concerned that it is still morning and he smells strongly of alcohol. Describe how you will discuss this situation with his wife.

### Activity 18.4

**Scenario**

The direct and consensual light reflex.

**Procedure**

Using a penlight torch shine light into the patient's right eye.

**Exercises**

1. What do you expect to happen?
2. Why does this occur?
3. What happens if the patient is blind?
4. What is hemianopia and physiologically why does it occur?
5. What is homonymous hemianopia and why does it occur?

# Section 4
# MANAGEMENT OF NEUROTRAUMA

## INTRODUCTION

This section includes chapters to enable the reader to understand the management of neurotrauma at the scene, in the Emergency Department and in the hospital. Nursing management is described in detail. Prognosis, outcome, dying and death are also included to enable health professionals to manage these situations and prepare for palliative care or rehabilitation.

As not all hospitals have dedicated neurosurgical centres, it is possible that head injured patients may be admitted to and managed on general wards (Das-Gupta and Turner-Stokes 2002). It is therefore essential for health professionals to have a working knowledge of head injury management from a holistic, interdisciplinary perspective. The availability of neurosurgical centres and neurosurgical beds is limited. There are 36 neurosurgical units in the UK, with 43 neurosurgical ICU beds available for a population of 63.3 million (Crimmins and Palmer 2000: p. 8). As beds are limited there may be delays in admissions due to bed blocking, transfers and management that may affect patient outcome (Bradley *et al.* 2006; Crimmins and Palmer 2000).

---

## Key objectives

On completion of this section you should be able to achieve the following:

- Describe the management of the patient at the scene.
- Describe the transport of a patient to the Emergency Department.
- Describe the key elements of patient handover.
- Describe the management of the patient in the Emergency Department.
- Describe the details required when transferring a patient to a regional neurosurgical centre.
- State which investigations will need to be undertaken in the following patients:
  - Patient with GCS 13/15.
  - Patient with GCS 9–12/15.
  - Patient with GCS ≤8/15.

- Describe the principles of management of the patient:
  - At the scene.
  - In the Emergency Department.
  - In the ICU/HDU/ward.
- Describe multidisciplinary management of the patient in hospital.
- Compile a nursing care plan for a patient with a:
  - GCS 14/15.
  - GCS 10/15.
  - GCS 6/15.
- List the drugs that could be used to control the patients intracranial pressure (see Chapter 17).
- Discuss prognosis/outcome following head injury.
- Understand dying and death in relation to neurotrauma patients.
- Prepare a session for colleagues about delivering bad news to families.

## Ethical/legal considerations

Debate the ethical issues related to this section.

Debate the role of the multidisciplinary team using the following statement:

Whose patient is it? (see Chapter 5)

Consider and apply the legal and ethical issues highlighted in these chapters to neurotrauma practice:

- Quality assurance.
- Clinical governance.
- Patient dignity and respect.
- Confidentiality.
- Advocacy.

- Lasting power of attorney.
- Living wills.

Discuss views related to euthanasia and assisted suicide:

- Collect newspaper articles for debate regarding assisted suicide.

Relevant acts, e.g.

- Data Protection Act 1998.
- Freedom of Information Act 2000.
- Human Tissue Act 2004.

# Chapter 19
# Management of Neurotrauma at the Scene

*Henry Guly*

Accident and Emergency Services, Plymouth NHS Trust (Retired), Devon, UK

## INTRODUCTION

The first priority in managing a patient at the scene of an incident is to ensure safety. This includes:

- Safety of yourself and other rescuers.
- Safety of the scene and other people.
- Safety of the casualty.

Examples of dangers following a road traffic collision could include:

- Danger from other traffic.
- Sharp metal and broken glass from the damaged vehicles.
- Spilt diesel leading to a risk of slipping.
- Fire.
- Risk of infection from blood (e.g. hepatitis, HIV).

This list is not exclusive and other incidents will have other risks.

It is also important to get help, so contact the emergency services early.

The pre-hospital management of head injury can be divided into:

- Severe and moderate head injury (GCS <14/15).
- Minor head injury (GCS 14–15/15).

## SEVERE AND MODERATE HEAD INJURY

The theory of managing head injury is the same whether the patient is in an emergency department or at the roadside and can be summarised as ABCDE:

- *Airway with cervical spine control.*
- *Breathing.*
- *Circulation.*
- *Disability.*
- *Exposure and environment.*

However, the practicalities are different. For example, an injured car driver may be trapped in a sitting position or an injured motorcyclist may be dressed in leathers and a full face helmet and be found lying prone in a ditch. Circumstances will dictate how one should, e.g. manage the airway in such cases and how one can move the casualty from the position in which they are found, to lying supine with full cervical spine protection. Darkness and bad weather cause additional problems in assessing the patient.

*Neurotrauma: Managing Patients with Head Injuries*, First Edition. Edited by Nadine Abelson-Mitchell.
© 2013 Blackwell Publishing Ltd. Published 2013 by Blackwell Publishing Ltd.

## AIRWAY WITH CERVICAL SPINE PROTECTION

Airway care is vital and a patent airway must be obtained. The initial steps are:

- Basic airway manoeuvres – chin lift, jaw thrust.
- Simple adjuncts – suction, oropharyngeal airway, nasopharyngeal airway.

Problems arise when the airway cannot be maintained by these simple measures. In hospital, the patient would be intubated with the use of drugs in a rapid sequence induction (RSI) of anaesthesia, as would any patient with GCS ≤8/15, but most paramedics are not trained to perform this skill.

Advanced airway management in head injured patients is a major controversy in pre-hospital care. Possible alternatives are:

- Paramedics could be taught this skill. However, teaching all paramedics would be difficult and costly and even more difficult would be ensuring that they maintained the skill. An alternative would be for some paramedics to have this skill (e.g. those on helicopters) with these advanced paramedics being preferentially tasked to serious trauma. Unfortunately there is little evidence of benefit from pre-hospital intubation (Lecky *et al.* 2008).
- Intubation without drugs. If a patient is so deeply unconscious that they can be intubated without drugs, the prognosis is very poor. In addition, this will cause a rise in intracranial pressure.
- Use of doctors in pre-hospital care. Doctors in anaesthesia, intensive care and (increasingly) emergency medicine already have the skills of RSI and practice them in hospital. Training and skill retention is therefore not a problem.
- Laryngeal mask airway (LMA) and similar supraglottic devices. These are very effective at maintaining an airway but they do not fully protect the airway from aspiration.
- Cricothyroidotomy. This is a valuable technique for securing an airway if it is not possible in other ways but it does require training.

Head injuries are commonly associated with cervical spine injury and, in a patient with a decreased level of consciousness, it is impossible to clear the cervical spine clinically and so, at the same time as maintaining an airway, it is important to protect the cervical spine. This is initially done with in-line manual immobilisation and, as soon as it is possible to do so, with a firm cervical collar, sand bags and tape or head restraints.

The patient will also, usually, be immobilised on a spinal board. However, if a patient is very restless and combative, attempting to restrain their head movement may be counter-productive, and it may be better to apply a cervical collar only.

In summary, the maintenance of a clear airway with cervical spine protection is the top priority in head injured patients and must be achieved at the scene. If it is not possible to maintain the airway by simple manoeuvres and adjuncts, there are a variety of techniques that can be used, or more experienced assistance can be called on, depending on local arrangements and the paramedic's training, equipment and skills. However, the mainstay of management is likely to be the use of an LMA. If all else fails, the patient should be put into the recovery position. Clearly this MAY be injurious if a patient has a cervical spine injury but a head injured patient with an obstructed airway will die.

## BREATHING

It is important to maintain a high $PaO_2$ and so all seriously-injured patients should receive high concentrations of oxygen and oxygenation should be monitored by pulse oximetry (see Chapter 12). Immediate life-threatening chest injuries (e.g. open and tension pneumothorax) should be treated as a means of maintaining the $PaO_2$ and thus treating the head injury. If an appropriately trained doctor attends the scene, they may elect to treat associated chest injuries more aggressively with chest drains and intubation/ventilation.

## CIRCULATION

It is important to maintain the systolic blood pressure in a head injured patient, in order to maintain the cerebral perfusion pressure (see Chapter 12). Major bleeding must be stopped, initially by applying direct pressure to stem any external bleeding and tourniquets may occasionally be useful to prevent catastrophic bleeding from limbs. If a pelvic fracture is suspected, a pelvic binder should be applied.

Pre-hospital fluid replacement in trauma patients is controversial with increasing evidence to support permissive hypotension, especially in penetrating trauma. However, this is probably inappropriate for head injured patients. Fluid replacement should be considered in the hypotensive patient and it has been recommended that this should be done if the systolic BP is below 90 mm Hg. If IV cannulation is performed, this should usually be done in the ambulance so as not to delay the patient on scene.

## DISABILITY

This refers to a basic neurological assessment consisting of:

- Consciousness level (Glasgow Coma Scale).
- Pupils and their reaction to light.
- Gross motor movements.

This is important information as a baseline. A patient arriving at hospital with a GCS of 10 has a moderate head injury. However, if at the scene the GCS was 6, they are clearly getting better, whereas if at scene the GCS was 14, the patient is deteriorating (see Chapter 18).

## EXPOSURE AND ENVIRONMENT

In hospital, a patient will be completely stripped to ensure that no injury is overlooked. This is usually inappropriate at the scene. However, it may be necessary to fully expose part of the body to assess and treat any injury. If this is done, it is important that the patient is covered up again to prevent heat loss.

It is important that seriously injured patients are transported to hospital as soon as possible but paramedics attending the scene are often able to obtain information that will be of help to the hospital in assessing and treating the patient which they would otherwise be unable to obtain. Important information to obtain is:

- Mechanism of injury – speak to witnesses. In some cases a digital photograph may be better at describing the mechanism of injury than any number of words.
- Identity of the patient.
- Any details of the past medical history and medication – speak to relatives and, in the event of an injury occurring in the home, pick up the patient's medications.

There are two major decisions to be made in the pre-hospital management of the head injured patient.

### 'Stop and stabilise' versus 'load and go'

In the past there has been much argument about whether it is better to 'stop and stabilise' the patient before transfer or whether just to 'load and go' to hospital. These are two extremes, both of which are wrong and the decision to be made is: How much treatment should be undertaken at the scene?

Obviously, if a patient is trapped, there is no possibility of loading and going and much stabilisation can be done while waiting for the patient to be freed. In these circum-stances, it will usually be appropriate to call for additional help. Otherwise, the aim should be:

- Airway care with cervical spine protection.
- High concentration of inspired oxygen and treatment of any life-threatening chest injury.
- Stop significant bleeding.
- Straighten any obviously bent limbs.
- Obtain brief history if available.
- Load into ambulance.
- Baseline observations (heart rate, blood pressure, respiratory rate, oxygen saturation, GCS, pupils).
- Leave for hospital.
- IV cannulation and IV fluids if necessary (in the ambulance).

### Where to take the patient?

The next decision is which hospital to take the patient to. Patients with significant head injuries do better when managed in neurosurgical units, even if they do not require any surgical procedure. A patient taken to a hospital without a neurosurgical unit may well need a secondary transfer later. If they are taken straight to the hospital with neurosurgery, not only will they have surgery (if required) earlier but it will avoid the extra work and risks of a secondary transfer. Each area should have protocols for where to take patients but a few general guidelines would be:

- If the incident occurs equidistant between hospitals with and without a trauma centre or neurosurgical unit, take the patient to the hospital with a neurosurgical unit.
- If the patient is stable, it is worth going to the hospital with a neurosurgical unit, even if that is further away.
- As management of airways, breathing and circulation is the priority in managing a head injury, if the patient is unstable they should be taken to the nearest hospital.

### Advanced warning for the hospital

Hospitals should operate a trauma team for the management of severely injured patients. For this to be standing by when the patient arrives, the hospital requires advance warning of a seriously injured patient. Hospitals with different levels of staffing may have different requirements for which patients they want to be notified about – follow local guidelines. However, what they will want is objective information: the words 'serious head injury' mean nothing whereas 'head injury GCS 6' is objective information that will have the trauma team standing by, with equipment ready for an RSI. A useful mnemonic for passing information is ATMIST:

- *Age.*
- *Times* – time of injury, expected time of arrival.
- *Mechanism of injury.*
- *Injuries.*
- *Signs* – vital signs including GCS.
- *Treatment given.*

Other information may also be useful, e.g. if the patient is pregnant knowing this in advance will allow a gynaecologist to be part of the trauma team. This information is always best passed by the paramedic treating the patient, directly to the nurse-in-charge of the emergency department as passing information via a third party (e.g. ambulance control) allows distortion. The same can also occur when a patient is attended by a paramedic in a land ambulance who assesses, treats and 'packages' a patient who is then brought to hospital by a helicopter crew who may not know full details. In these circumstances, it is useful for the initial paramedic to speak to the ED so that the hospital gets first hand, rather than second hand, information.

### The handover

The handover can also use the ATMIST format. The ambulance crew need to be aware of the information that the hospital will require as detailed in Chapter 21. If the ambulance crew is re-tasked, they should ensure that the hospital personnel know how to contact them if further information is needed later.

### MINOR HEAD INJURY

A small proportion of patients with a seemingly minor head injury turn out to have a more serious (potentially fatal) injury. It is important therefore to have a low threshold for transporting a patient to hospital where they can be evaluated more thoroughly than can be done at the scene of the incident. NICE (2007) recommends that the following patients are taken to hospital:

- GCS less than 15 on initial assessment.
- Any loss of consciousness as a result of the injury.
- Any neurological deficit since the injury (including problems understanding, speaking, reading or writing, decreased sensation, loss of balance, general weakness, visual changes, abnormal reflexes and problems walking).
- Any suspicion of a skull fracture or penetrating head injury (see Chapter 16/Chapter 18).
- Amnesia for events before or after the injury.
- Persistent headache since the injury.

- Any vomiting episodes since the injury.
- Any seizure since the injury.
- Any previous cranial neurosurgical intervention.
- A high-energy head injury (e.g. pedestrian struck by motor vehicle, occupant ejected from motor vehicle, fall from a height of greater than one metre or more than five stairs, diving accident, high-speed motor vehicle collision, rollover motor accident, accident involving motorised recreational vehicles, bicycle collision or any other potentially high-energy mechanism).
- History of bleeding or clotting disorder or anti-coagulant therapy such as Warfarin.
- Current drug or alcohol intoxication.
- Age 65 years or older.
- Suspicion of non-accidental injury.
- Continuing concern by the professional about the diagnosis.

In addition, consider referral to an Emergency Department if any of the following factors are present depending on their own judgement of severity:

- Irritability or altered behaviour.
- Visible trauma to the head not covered above but still of concern to the professional.
- Adverse social factors (e.g. no-one able to supervise the injured person at home).
- Continuing concern of the injured person or their carer about the diagnosis.

---

### Activity 19.1

#### Scenario

You are walking along the street when you witness a car pull out in front of a motorcyclist travelling at about 30 miles per hour. The motorcyclist hits the car and flies over it, landing in the road about 5 metres from the car and apparently striking the ground with his helmet. He is lying on his front, making no movements.

#### Exercises

1. What is your first priority?
2. You approach the casualty. What are your priorities?
3. How can you quickly assess ABCDE?
4. What are the signs of airway obstruction?
5. He is making snoring noises, how do you relieve his airway obstruction?
6. The ambulance arrives: What are their priorities?

## Activity 19.2

**Scenario**

A 65 year old lady phoned for an ambulance after falling down a flight of stairs and injuring her head. She did not lose consciousness. When the ambulance got to the house, she was up and walking around. She lives on her own. She did not know why she had fallen but assumed that she had slipped. She said that her only injury was to her head where she had a large bruise over the right temporal region. She denied any neck pain. Initially she had had a headache but said that she had taken Paracetamol and this was now easing. She apologised for calling the ambulance but said that she had panicked when she found herself at the bottom of the stairs. She thanked them for coming but no longer required their services.

**Exercise**

1.  What should the ambulance crew do?

# Chapter 20
# Management of Neurotrauma on Transfer

*Henry Guly*

Accident and Emergency Services, Plymouth NHS Trust (Retired), Devon, UK

## INTRODUCTION

Patients in the Emergency Department with a head injury will eventually need to be transferred for a CT scan, may need admission to a ward or operating theatre or may need to be transferred to a regional neurosurgical unit, which may be 50, or more, miles away. Similar principles apply whether a patient is moved 50 metres to a CT scanner or 50 miles to another hospital.

Arrangements will, of course, depend on the patient's current state as a patient who is intubated and ventilated and who has other injuries will need much more equipment than a patient with an isolated head injury and a GCS of 15. However there is one principle that must operate whatever the transfer: *Anticipate all possible problems and act to prevent them, if possible, and to ensure that you have the personnel and equipment to deal with them if they occur.*

Rather than searching to find bits of equipment prior to transferring a patient, a transfer bag containing all equipment likely to be necessary for the majority of transfers should be available. However, this should be checked to ensure that all equipment is available before moving a patient. It is unlikely to contain all that is needed (e.g. controlled drugs and drugs that are normally kept refrigerated) and so these should be added.

It must first be decided whether the patient is safe to be transferred. A head-injured patient bleeding to death from a ruptured spleen needs to be moved to the operating theatre for this to be dealt with, rather than moved to CT or transferred to a neurosurgical centre.

## AIRWAY WITH CERVICAL SPINE PROTECTION

As has been seen, a patent airway is paramount in the care of the head injured patient. If the patient is intubated, the tube may become dislodged during movement. This should be prevented by securing the tube well. In addition, full intubation equipment and anaesthetic drugs should be taken in case this happens. Cervical spine immobilisation should be maintained during transfer (unless the spine has been cleared). This is particularly important while moving a patient (e.g. into the CT scanner).

If the patient is not intubated, one needs to anticipate the possibility of the patient developing airway problems during the transfer. Endotracheal intubation in the back of an ambulance or helicopter or in the CT scanner may be very difficult and so if there is a possibility of intubation being required, it should be done electively before the patient is moved. Even if it is considered that airway problems are unlikely, a transfer bag containing airway equip-

*Neurotrauma: Managing Patients with Head Injuries*, First Edition. Edited by Nadine Abelson-Mitchell.
© 2013 Blackwell Publishing Ltd. Published 2013 by Blackwell Publishing Ltd.

ment, including suction, intubation equipment and drugs, should be available.

## BREATHING

Just as intubation is easier in the ED than in the CT scan venue or during transfer, so are all other procedures. A pneumothorax may increase in size and while sometimes one may wait to decide whether or not to insert a chest drain, if required, if a patient needs transfer, it should be inserted before the patient is transferred.

A severely injured patient will be on oxygen – ensure that any cylinder taken is full and, for a long transfer, take a spare cylinder. Ventilators may stop working so a bag-valve-mask should be taken as a back-up.

## CIRCULATION

It is not uncommon for IV lines to become dislodged when the patient is moved so ensure they are secured well and that there are at least two IV cannulae in situ so if one is dislodged, IV access is still possible.

Beware of continued blood loss. Fractures and wounds will continue to bleed. Fractures should be splinted and wounds should be dressed. Adequate volumes of suitable IV fluids (including blood, if appropriate) need to be taken. Scalp wounds, in particular, tend to be overlooked and the patient may lose a lot of blood without it being realised. The best way to prevent scalp wounds bleeding is to suture them (the sutures can always be taken out and the wound re-sutured, more neatly, later).

Patients should have the same monitoring available during transfer as they did in the ED. If monitors are battery-operated, take spare batteries. Records of vital signs should be maintained during transfer.

All equipment will need to be secured in the ambulance: the ambulance crew will advise.

## DISABILITY

If the patient is judged as likely to have a seizure the patient should have prophylactic anticonvulsants (e.g. Phenytoin) before transfer and Benzodiazepines should accompany the patient.

If the patient's condition is deteriorating, Mannitol or hypertonic saline may be required (according to local protocol).

## EXPOSURE

Ensure the patient is kept warm during the transfer.

## OTHER

Urinary catheters and gastric tubes, if required, should be inserted before transfer. Ensure good pain relief. If a patient has other injuries, they may need top-ups of opiate analgesia.

## WHO SHOULD ACCOMPANY THE PATIENT?

The person (or persons) who should accompany the patient will be those who are best able to manage any problems that might be expected to occur. Inter-hospital transfers will usually be done by a doctor and nurse though critical-care-trained paramedics may replace hospital staff on the transfer team. The person escorting a patient to a ward or to another hospital must know the patient's history to be able to give a hand-over.

The patient with multiple injuries, who is intubated and ventilated, will usually be accompanied to CT by an ITU doctor, an ED doctor and at least one ED nurse. At the other extreme, a patient with a relatively minor head injury who meets one of the criteria for a CT scan but whose scan is expected to be normal, may walk to the scanner with a porter.

### If a patient is being transferred to another hospital such as the regional neurosurgical unit

Find out exactly where the patient needs to go. Notify the next-of-kin of the transfer. Decide how the patient should get there and how quickly they need to get there. Helicopters fly much faster than ambulances can drive, and so may be quicker if the helicopter can fly directly from one hospital to the other. However, if the helicopter takes half an hour to arrive and there needs to be ambulance transfers at either end, it may not prove to be faster overall. It will also involve more movement of a severely ill patient and will certainly be more expensive. Helicopter transfer is also riskier than ambulance transfer. Some helicopters are not able to fly at night.

Take adequate quantities of all drugs including oxygen. If the ambulance breaks down or the helicopter needs to divert to another landing site for whatever reason, the journey may take longer than expected. Take copies of all the notes, observation sheets, x-rays, scans and pathology results. If blood has been cross-matched, take that. If results from blood tests are awaited, someone should phone or fax them through to the receiving unit when they are ready. Some units will have a specific transfer document that will contain the information required by the receiving unit and a checklist of things to be done before transfer. The receiving hospital needs to be told not only what has been done to the patient but what has not yet been done, e.g. 'we have not yet done a secondary survey'.

Personnel accompanying the patient, if time is available, should fill their stomach (unless suffering from motion sickness) and empty their bladder. Hopefully the ambulance taking the patient to the neurosurgical unit will be able to bring any accompanying people back. However, it may be re-tasked to an emergency and may not be able to

do so, so the accompanying people need to be prepared to return independently and so should take:

- Warm clothes.
- Mobile phone.
- Money and/or credit card for food, drink and fares.
- An overnight bag (if appropriate).

The Association of Anaesthetists of Great Britain and Ireland (AAGBI 2009) have produced guidelines on the safe transfer of patients.

---

## Activity 20.1

### Scenario

John Smith is a 19 year old, previously fit, man who was accidentally hit on the head with a golf club. There was no loss of consciousness and he walked into the ED. On examination his GCS was 15 and he had no neurological deficit. On examination he had a stellate laceration of his forehead. A CT showed a depressed fracture underlying this laceration but no other intracranial injury. He needs to be transferred to the neurosurgical unit 30 miles away

for this to be debrided and for the fracture to be elevated.

### Exercises

1. How will you organise this?
2. Who should accompany the patient?
3. A paramedic ambulance has been booked and will arrive in 10 minutes: what else do you need to consider?

---

## Activity 20.2

### Scenario

Judith Brown is a 54 year old woman who has been involved in a road traffic crash. Her main injury is a head injury. On arrival she had a GCS of 12 (E3, M5, V4) with no localising signs. A CT has shown multiple contusions. When she returned from CT, her GCS had fallen to 10 (E2, M5, V3). She still has no localising signs. The CT of her neck, chest, abdomen and pelvis showed no injuries. She does, however, have an obvious open fracture of her left tibia and a swollen right foot but neither of these has been x-rayed yet. Her cardiovascular system is stable.

It has been decided that she needs to be transferred to the neurosurgical unit 60 miles away and she has been

accepted by the neurosurgeons there who have asked that she be transferred as soon as possible.

### Exercises

1. What needs to be done before she is transferred?
2. Should this patient be transferred by ambulance or helicopter?
3. It is decided to transfer the patient by ambulance. Who should accompany the patient?
4. What equipment will be needed?
5. The nurse accompanying the anaesthetist has never done a hospital transfer before and asks what else they should take? How do you respond?

# Chapter 21
# Management of Neurotrauma in the Emergency Department

*Henry Guly*

Accident and Emergency Services, Plymouth NHS Trust (Retired), Devon, UK

## INTRODUCTION

The words 'head injury' are often used very loosely and it is better to refer to 'traumatic brain injury' as it is the brain that is important rather than the scalp or skull.

## PREPARING FOR THE ARRIVAL OF A SERIOUSLY INJURED PATIENT

To allow the management of a severely injured patient to start as soon as the patient arrives in the Emergency Department requires advance warning to be given by the ambulance service. This advance warning should result in a trauma team being present in the resuscitation room as the patient arrives. The constitution of a trauma team will vary from hospital to hospital but ideally will consist of:

- A team leader who should be a consultant, probably in emergency medicine or intensive care.
- An anaesthetist to maintain the airway as well as anaesthetist assistant.
- A general surgeon.
- An orthopaedic surgeon.
- Two nurses.
- A radiographer.
- A scribe.

The team should put on personal protective equipment (gloves, apron, eye protection) and should also wear lead aprons so that essential x-rays can be done at the same time as resuscitation is performed.

## SEVERE AND MODERATE HEAD INJURY

The aim of the treatment of head injuries is to get oxygen to the brain. This involves getting oxygen into the blood (airway and breathing) and getting blood to the brain (circulation). It is therefore useful to consider the management of a brain injury in the ED using the ATLS (American College of Surgeons Trauma Committee 2008) format of:

- Primary survey, consisting of:
  - *A*irway with cervical spine control
  - *B*reathing
  - *C*irculation
  - *D*isability
  - *E*xposure and Environment.
- Secondary survey.
- Definitive treatment.

The ATLS course teaches that these are done sequentially. However, much information can be obtained very quickly

*Neurotrauma: Managing Patients with Head Injuries*, First Edition. Edited by Nadine Abelson-Mitchell.

by looking at the patient and asking: 'what happened'? If the patient is not distressed and responds clearly this confirms the mechanism of injury and that the airway is intact, the breathing is not too bad, the circulation is sufficient to allow adequate brain perfusion and the GCS is probably 15/15.

In hospital, when the patient is treated by an experienced trauma team, these stages can often be done simultaneously.

## Primary survey

### Airway

Airway problems in head injury are common due to:

- Decreased level of consciousness causing loss of muscle tone and airway obstruction from the tongue falling back and obstructing the pharynx.
- Aspiration of blood or vomit due to lack of a gag reflex.
- Associated facial or laryngeal injury.
- Blood in the airway from head, facial or chest injury.

Even one episode of hypoxia will significantly worsen the prognosis of a head injury and so a patent airway is essential. If a patient is not maintaining their airway, initial immediate actions should be:

- Simple airway manoeuvres (chin lift and jaw thrust), while avoiding movement of the cervical spine.
- Removal of any obvious obstructing foreign body, for example broken dentures.
- Suction.

If the patient is unconscious and will tolerate it, an oropharyngeal (Guedel) airway can be used. If it is not possible to insert an oropharyngeal airway (e.g. the teeth are tightly clamped) or if the patient will not tolerate it, a nasopharyngeal airway is better tolerated. It is best avoided in patients with basal skull fracture but a patent airway is the first priority and so a basal skull fracture should not be regarded as an absolute contra-indication to its use.

These manoeuvres and adjuncts may open an obstructed airway but do not protect the airway from aspiration, so the patient who is at risk of this needs a cuffed endotracheal tube (ETT) inserted. This should be done routinely in any patient with a GCS of 8 or below (a GCS >8/15 does not mean that the patient does not need intubation as there may be other indications for intubation.) Intubation normally requires a rapid sequence induction of anaesthesia. This may not be easy, especially if there is facial

trauma, and so alternative methods of securing an airway such as a laryngeal mask airway or a cricothyroidotomy should be available if intubation fails.

The position of the tube needs to be confirmed clinically by listening to the chest and by the detection of carbon dioxide using capnography. Although a cuffed ETT should prevent aspiration of vomit or blood from facial injuries from entering the trachea, a patient bleeding from a lung contusion or other chest injury may still have an obstructed airway. Such patients need suction of their ETT.

Head injuries are commonly associated with cervical spine injuries. If a patient has a decreased level of consciousness they will not complain of pain and neurological abnormalities may not be detected. For this reason ALL patients with a decreased level of consciousness due to a head injury must be assumed to have a cervical spine injury until it can be proved otherwise. Thus the cervical spine needs to be immobilized. This can be achieved by either:

- Inline manual immobilisation, i.e. by holding the head in a neutral position compared to the rest of the body; or
- Firm cervical collar (to prevent flexion and extension of the neck) AND head blocks (to prevent lateral movement).

### Breathing

Hypoxia worsens the prognosis of a head injury. So, too, does hypercarbia which causes the intracranial pressure to rise. All severely injured patients should initially receive high concentrations of oxygen. This chapter discusses the management of head injury rather than the multiply injured patient but in order to achieve good oxygenation, any associated chest injury (e.g. pneumothorax, haemothorax) must be treated. Breathing may also be compromised by injuries of the cervical spinal cord causing weakness of respiratory muscles. Adequate treatment of the head injury thus requires treatment of the patient's other injuries. A severe head injury may, itself, cause hypoventilation. If there is any evidence of respiratory insufficiency, the patient must be intubated and ventilated even if this was not required for the protection of the airway.

Patients should have the adequacy of their breathing monitored by continuous measurement of the oxygen saturation by pulse oximetry and by regular blood gas estimations. The inspired oxygen concentration will be adjusted depending on the arterial oxygen concentration. All ventilated patients should have their end-tidal $CO_2$ monitored by capnography and the ventilation should be adjusted to maintain this within normal limits.

A chest x-ray should be taken early to diagnose treatable chest injuries.

### Circulation

It is vital to get oxygen to the brain and this demands not just oxygenated blood, but a good blood flow to the brain. The cerebral blood flow depends on the cerebral perfusion pressure (CPP) (see Chapter 12).

It is not possible to measure the intracranial pressure (ICP) pre-hospital and it is rare for it to be measured in the ED but the normal ICP is less than 10 mm Hg. The aim is to maintain the CPP above 70 mm Hg. The ICP is frequently raised after a head injury so if we assume it to be 20 mm Hg, it is important to maintain a MAP of 90 mm Hg which equates to a systolic BP of approximately 120 mm Hg.

Maintenance of blood pressure is vital in brain injured patients and this is done by stopping bleeding and giving adequate fluid replacement. Occasionally drugs may be given to increase the blood pressure in such patients. Invasive blood pressure monitoring should be used in severely injured patients. This also allows easy monitoring of arterial blood gases.

All severely injured patients should have two large-bore IV cannulae inserted. A patient with an isolated, closed head injury and a normal blood pressure may not require any fluids. However, a patient with blood loss will need warmed IV fluids to maintain their blood pressure as above. Initial fluids will be crystalloids (normal saline or Hartman's solution up to two litres in adults), but if further fluids are required these should be given as blood and blood products.

Bloods should be taken for full blood count, urea and electrolytes, blood sugar, clotting studies, blood grouping and saving serum for possible cross-matching later (or for immediate cross-matching if there has been significant blood loss). Arterial blood gases should be measured and females of child-bearing age should have a blood or urine pregnancy test. ECG monitoring should be applied and a 12 lead ECG performed (see Chapter 13). If the mechanism of injury suggests any possibility of a pelvic fracture, a pelvic x-ray should be taken early as unstable pelvic fractures may be associated with significant blood loss and yet may not be clinically obvious.

### Disability

Disability refers to an assessment of the central nervous system. If the patient is to be intubated, this assessment should be done before the patient is anaesthetised as it cannot be done afterwards. This assessment should consist of:

- Level of consciousness (Glasgow Coma Score see Chapter 18). This is vital as not only is this a measure of the severity of the brain injury but the initial GCS acts as a baseline against which improvement or deterioration can be judged.
- Pupils (size, reaction to light, presence or absence of a squint).
- Gross muscle power. Compare left with right and upper limb with lower limb. Weakness of one side (assuming it is not caused by a limb injury) usually indicates a hemiplegia caused by a local brain injury and gross weakness of the legs, compared to the arms, indicates a probable spinal cord injury.

Under the heading of disability, it is also important to exclude other causes of a decreased level of consciousness. In particular, it is important to exclude hypoglycaemia by measuring the blood glucose. Alcohol intoxication may cause a decreased level of consciousness but finding a raised blood alcohol level does not exclude a head injury, so a decreased level of consciousness in a head-injured patient must never be attributed to alcohol (except in retrospect).

Brain injuries may be complicated by seizures. If hypoglycaemia has been excluded, a seizure may be stopped with IV Lorazepam or Diazepam. A patient who has had one seizure is at risk of further seizures and so should be given a loading dose of Phenytoin IV (this should be given slowly and the patient needs ECG monitoring). Seizures are also predisposed to by intracranial haematomas and depressed skull fractures associated with a dural tear. These patients may also be given Phenytoin.

### Exposure and environment

A full examination requires that the patient is stripped fully as otherwise important injuries may be missed. The patient must then be covered up and efforts made to prevent heat loss as hypothermia will worsen the prognosis.

### Secondary survey

The aim of the primary survey is to detect and treat life-threatening injuries. Once this has been done and the patient is stable, the secondary survey is performed which aims to detect ALL injuries. This will start with a history and examination.

### History

It is important to get a clear idea of exactly what happened. Depending on the circumstances this information might be available from the patient, a witness, the police or the ambulance crew. Questions to ask are:

- Events.
  - What happened and how did it happen? In other words the mechanism of injury. As an example, if the injury was from a fall, determine the following:
    - Did the patient have a medical cause for the fall? For example, become unconscious and then fall, hitting their head, or did they trip and hit their head and become unconscious as a result of their fall?
  - When did it happen?
  - Where did it happen?
  - Why did it happen?
  - Who is the patient? Who was involved? Who witnessed it?
  - What has happened since: e.g. what was the consciousness level when they were found? If the GCS is 11 now but was 6 when the ambulance arrived, this may indicate an improvement in the patient's condition, but if it is now 11 but was 15 when first seen, this indicates a deterioration in the patient's condition and may be an emergency situation.
  - Has the patient had any other symptoms, e.g. headache, vomiting, convulsion?
- Past medical history (are there any medical problems that might affect the management of the patient, e.g. insulin dependent diabetes).
- Medication. Of particular importance in head-injured patients are anti-coagulants (e.g. Warfarin) and antiplatelet agents (e.g. Aspirin, Clopidogrel) as these may predispose to intracranial bleeding.
- Allergies.
- When did they last eat or drink? An anaesthetist may want to know this but in reality, it will rarely alter the patient's management.

A frequently-taught mnemonic is that one should take an AMPLE history:

*Allergies*
*Medication*
*Past history*
*Last ate or drank*
*Events*

This contains all the information one needs to collect but the order is not sequential!

## Examination

The patient should be fully examined from head to toe. For the head, particular attention should be paid to:

- Wounds: size, depth, location (i.e. what underlying structures may be damaged). Scalp wounds sometimes bleed profusely and cause significant blood loss. This can most easily by stemmed by suturing the wound. Before a scalp wound is sutured, a finger should be put into the wound by a suitably trained professional to feel the underlying skull as this may reveal a depressed fracture. If brain tissue is seen in a wound, this indicates that there must be an underlying depressed fracture with a tear in the dura mater. These patients will need neurosurgery.
- Bruises and swellings.
- Facial injuries.
- Eyes. The pupils and the presence of a squint. Eye injury is common in association with head and facial injury.
- Signs of basal skull fracture. Fractures of the base of the skull usually involve fractures into the nose, the sinuses and the ear. These are important because of the risk of infection. Signs of a basal fracture are:
  - Bleeding from the ear. Blood in the ear may have trickled in from the outside or it may have come from the ear. This may be from a local injury but it is more likely to be caused by a basal skull fracture.
  - Blood in the middle ear. If the tympanic membrane is intact, then bleeding into the middle ear will show itself as dark discolouration of the tympanic membrane.
  - Cerebrospinal fluid (CSF) from the ear or the nose. This is a common sign of a basal skull fracture but is not often seen in the ED as the clear CSF is obscured by blood. It is more commonly detected the following day when the bleeding has ceased.
  - Bruising over the mastoid (Battle's sign).
  - Bilateral black eyes (panda eyes). Most black eyes are caused by facial injury but if a patient has bilateral black eyes following an injury to the back of the head, this is highly suggestive of a basal skull fracture.

The rest of the body, including the back (examined during a log-roll), will also need to be examined.

At this stage management of the severely injured patients will include:

- A urethral catheter inserted to check for haematuria and to monitor urine output. In an adult, aim for a urine output of at least 0.5 ml/kg/hr. A full bladder may cause agitation and restlessness which can be cured by catheterisation. Urethral catheterisation is contra-indicated if there is suspicion of a ruptured urethra.

- A gastric tube inserted. This is done to decompress the stomach. This helps to protect the airway against aspiration and will also allow better ventilation. If a patient is to have an abdominal CT scan, a gastric tube will allow oral contrast to be given (if required). The usual route for a gastric tube is via the nose (naso-gastric tube) but this is contra-indicated in a patient with a basal skull fracture when an oro-gastric tube should be inserted by the most appropriate person.
- Analgesia. It used to be taught that opioid analgesia should not be given to head-injured patients because of the risk of respiratory depression and the effects of opioids on the pupils. However, quite apart from humanitarian concerns, pain will raise the intracranial pressure and so should be treated. The best way of treating pain is with small doses of intravenous opioids (e.g. morphine 10 mg, diluted to 10 ml) titrated against clinical response and baseline cardiorespiratory measurements. Do not forget other techniques to reduce pain, for example, nerve blocks and splintage of fractures.

Procedures such as x-rays, catheterization, gastric tubes, splintage, etc. require that the conscious patient does not resist. If the patient is combative, they should be anaesthetised to allow adequate investigation and treatment.

## *Investigations*

All patients should have an early chest x-ray and those where the mechanism of injury suggests the possibility of a pelvic fracture should have a pelvic x-ray. In the seriously injured patient, these should be done during the primary survey.

All patients with a severe or moderate head injury should have a head CT scan. It is important to exclude a cervical spine injury in all patients with a severe head injury. If a patient is having a head CT scan, the easiest way to exclude a bony neck injury is to do a cervical spine CT scan at the same time. If, for any reason, a CT head scan is not being performed, a series of cervical spine x-rays should be performed, ensuring that the C7/T1 junction is seen.

If a patient is unconscious or anaesthetised, it is impossible to exclude an abdominal injury clinically. If the mechanism of injury (e.g. fall from a height, RTC) suggests the possibility of such an injury, it should be excluded by further investigations. An abdominal ultrasound or FAST scan (Focused Abdominal Sonography for Trauma) can diagnose free intraperitoneal blood but a normal FAST scan does not exclude an abdominal injury. Patients with high velocity injuries will also need imaging of the thoracic and lumbar spine. Most patients, therefore, with a severe head injury from a high velocity mechanism, should have a CT of the head, neck, chest, abdomen and pelvis with reformats to show the thoracic and lumbar spine. This is commonly called a pan-CT (see Chapter 13).

Other investigations will be done based on the clinical picture.

### Further monitoring

If the patient is not anaesthetised, they can be monitored by regular observation of the GCS, pupils and vital signs. A falling GCS, especially if associated with dilatation of one or both pupils, will require a further CT to be performed.

If the patient is anaesthetised, they will be admitted to an intensive care unit (ICU). Monitoring of the GCS is impossible and an intracranial pressure monitor will usually be inserted to monitor the ICP.

Arranging a transfer may take some time and this time can be used for suturing scalp wounds (administering tetanus prophylaxis) and treating other injuries.

### Definitive management of the severe head injury

If there is an intracranial haematoma (extradural, subdural or intracerebral), a neurosurgical opinion should be obtained as soon as possible as to its suitability for surgery. If the patient is taking anti-coagulants, these should be reversed with vitamin K and either prothrombin complex concentrate or fresh frozen plasma.

If surgery cannot be performed immediately (e.g. the patient needs to be transferred to a neurosurgical unit) and the patient is deteriorating, it may be possible to 'buy time' by using Mannitol or hypertonic saline to lower the ICP – ask advice from the neurosurgeon.

If there is no surgically-treatable problem, the patient should, ideally, still be transferred to a neurological centre but will be managed conservatively. Unfortunately, patients frequently spend many hours in the ED waiting for transfer so their active management must start in the ED. The management can be divided into monitoring and treatment.

### Non-surgical management of severe head injury

The non-surgical management of a head injured patient comprises:

- Maintaining blood oxygenation.
- Maintaining cerebral perfusion pressure:
  - Maintaining blood pressure.
    - Stop blood loss.
    - IV fluids.
    - Inotropes (possibly).

- Reducing ICP (requires the ICP to be monitored):
  - Sedation.
  - Ventilation to maintain normal $pCO_2$.
  - Head-up position (once it is known that there is no cervical spine injury).
  - Removing collar (cervical collars can raise the ICP by pressure on the jugular vein).
  - The ETT should be secured by tape rather than a tie that goes round the neck as that, too, can raise the ICP by pressure on the jugular vein.
  - Consider Mannitol for cerebral oedema.
  - Consider barbiturates.

It is important to avoid the causes of secondary brain injury. These are:

- Hypoxia.
- Hypercarbia.
- Hypotension.
- Hypoglycaemia.
- Hyponatraemia.
- Hyperpyrexia.
- Convulsions.
- Infection: this occurs late and not in the ED, prophylactic antibiotics are of no value.

In addition, do not forget the normal nursing care of the unconscious patient especially the prevention of pressure sores (see Chapter 23).

## MINOR HEAD INJURY

Minor head injuries are very common but a small proportion of patients with apparently minor injuries turn out to have a more serious injury, which may be rapidly fatal if it is not recognised and treated. The two major problems in this group of patients are intracranial haematoma and compound depressed skull fracture. It is, of course, also important not to miss any associated cervical spine (or other) injury.

### Intracranial haematoma

The most common intracranial haematoma to complicate an apparently minor head injury is an extradural haematoma. This is usually caused by an injury to the middle meningeal artery, which causes bleeding between the skull and the dura (in the extradural space) (see Chapter 12 p. 75). In adults it is usually associated with a skull fracture.

The patient may have had a brief loss of consciousness before regaining a normal conscious level or they may have suffered no loss of consciousness. This would indicate that there is either no primary brain injury or that it is very minor and so if the haematoma is evacuated early, the prognosis is excellent.

The typical picture is that following a short period when the patient feels well, they develop a severe headache and may vomit. As the haematoma expands, the ICP increases and the level of consciousness falls. As the pressure increases, 'coning' occurs with dilation of the pupil on the side of the haematoma followed by dilatation of the other pupil. This may be associated with a rise in blood pressure, a fall in the heart rate and respiratory depression. This is a neurosurgical emergency and the haematoma must be evacuated rapidly (see Chapter 12 p. 94 and Chapter 17).

Subdural and intracerebral haematomas also occur but these are usually associated with a significant primary brain injury so they usually come into the ED with a reduced level of consciousness and there are often localising neurological signs, e.g. weakness of one arm and leg. As the haematoma expands, the level of consciousness decreases further and coning occurs.

Chronic subdural haematomas usually occur in the elderly; they may present months after a minor injury and the patient may give no history of injury. The usual symptom is a fluctuating level of consciousness.

Predisposing factors to intracranial haematomas are:

- Bleeding disorders, especially anti-coagulant treatment.
- If there is brain shrinkage, this leaves a potential space for a haematoma to form. Causes of this include:
  - Alzheimer's disease and similar causes of dementia.
  - Chronic alcohol abuse (these patients have the added problem that they frequently fall and injure their heads).
  - Patients with hydrocephalus treated with a shunt.

Basal skull fractures may also present as minor injuries. The other problem that must not be missed is a compound depressed skull fracture with a dural tear because, untreated, this may be complicated by infection (meningitis or brain abscess). This is normally caused by an injury with a small, hard object, for example a golf club or a hammer in which the force is localised and drives a small piece of bone through the dura into the brain. As the brain injury is a local laceration there may be no loss of consciousness and so the severity of the injury may be under-estimated.

It is vital to have a low threshold for doing a CT of the head to detect complications early while accepting that it is important to reduce exposure to ionising radiation. There are many studies looking at the clinical features that predict an intracranial injury so that unnecessary scans can be reduced while abnormalities are not missed. Two recent reviews (NICE 2007; SIGN 2009), both from the UK, have made very similar recommendations regarding the indications for scanning. Both divide the indications into scans that should be done immediately and those that should be done within 8 hours of injury. The indications are shown in Tables 21.1 and 21.2.

Where CT is not available, it is important that local guidelines are drawn up on how head-injured patients will be investigated and managed.

A significant proportion of head injuries occur to those who have been drinking alcohol, and if a patient has altered behaviour or a reduced level of consciousness it may be difficult to know whether this is due to the alcohol or to

**Table 21.1** Indications for immediate CT scan. Head injury: Triage, assessment, investigation and early management of head injury in infants, children and adults. NICE Clinical Guideline 4. Copyright © 2003 NICE.

| NICE Guidelines 2007 (NICE 2007) | SIGN Guidelines 2009 (SIGN 2009) |
|---|---|
| GCS <13 on initial assessment in the ED | GCS 13 or 14 with failure to improve within 1 hr of observation or 2 hr of injury |
| GCS <15 at 2 hr post injury | |
| Suspected open or depressed skull fracture | Suspected penetrating injury |
| Any sign of basal skull fracture | Severe and persistent headache |
| More than one episode of vomiting | Coagulopathy and loss of consciousness*, amnesia or any neurological feature |
| Focal neurological deficit | |
| Amnesia for events more than 30 minutes before impact | |
| Post-traumatic seizure | |

NICE expresses concern about Clopidogrel use but advises clinical judgement.
*Coagulopathy includes Warfarin use.

**Table 21.2** Indications for CT scan within 8 hours. Head injury: Triage, assessment, investigation and early management of head injury in infants, children and adults. NICE Clinical Guideline 4. Copyright © 2003 NICE.

| NICE guidelines (2007) | SIGN Guidelines (2009) |
|---|---|
| Dangerous mechanism of injury (pedestrian struck by motor vehicle, occupant ejected from motor vehicle, fall from height) | Dangerous mechanism of injury (pedestrian struck by motor vehicle, occupant ejected from motor vehicle, fall from height) |
| GCS 15 but history of loss of consciousness or amnesia and age >65 | Significant assault, for example blunt trauma with a weapon |
| History of loss of consciousness or amnesia AND dangerous mechanism of injury (pedestrian struck by motor vehicle, occupant ejected from motor vehicle, fall >1 metre or 5 stairs) | Amnesia for events more than 30 minutes before impact |
| | Any seizure activity |
| History of loss of consciousness or amnesia AND coagulopathy* | Clinical evidence of a skull fracture, for example boggy haematoma |

*NICE expresses concern about Clopidogrel use but advises clinical judgement.

the head injury. However, even if a patient is known to be intoxicated and has a greatly raised blood alcohol level, this does not exclude a significant head injury and, as has been noted above, patients with chronic alcoholism are more at risk of intracranial haematoma. The only safe way to manage head-injured patients is to ignore the fact that they have been drinking and to apply the same criteria for CT scanning.

## ADMISSION

The NICE guidelines (2007) recommend that the following patients should be admitted to hospital following a head injury:

- Patients with new, clinically significant abnormalities on imaging.
- Patients who have not returned to GCS 15 after imaging, regardless of the imaging results.
- When a patient fulfils the criteria for CT scanning but this cannot be done within the appropriate period, either because CT is not available or because the patient is not sufficiently co-operative to allow scanning.
- Continuing worrying signs (e.g. persistent vomiting and severe headaches) of concern to the clinician.
- Other sources of concern to the clinician (e.g., drug or alcohol intoxication, other injuries, shock, suspected non-accidental injury, meningism and cerebrospinal fluid leak).

## DISCHARGE FROM THE ED

The following groups of patients are likely to be able to be discharged from the ED:

- Patients in whom a CT is not indicated on the basis of history and examination.
- Patients with normal imaging of the head as long as no other factors that would warrant a hospital admission are present and there are appropriate support structures for safe discharge and for subsequent care (e.g. competent supervision at home).

Patients who presented to the emergency department with drug or alcohol intoxication should receive information and advice on alcohol or drug misuse before being discharged.

All patients with any degree of head injury who are discharged from an ED or observation ward should receive a written head injury advice card (see Box 21.1). This should be explained to the patient and any carers.

If a patient returns unexpectedly after being discharged, this may indicate that there has been a problem at the initial consultation; either an under-estimation of the severity of an injury or a misunderstanding between patient and doctor. When a head-injured patient returns, there is a high incidence of abnormalities found on CT scanning. Patients with a head injury who return unexpectedly should, ideally, be seen by or at least discussed with, a senior doctor. A significant number of patients who are discharged after a head injury may continue to complain of symptoms such as headache, dizziness, difficulty in concentration, etc. Arrangements should be made for all of them to be followed up, either by their general practitioner or by a specialist nurse, so that they can be reassured and so that those with severe symptoms can be detected and referred for neuropsychological review.

## MANAGEMENT OF PATIENTS WHO ARE ADMITTED FOR OBSERVATION

Patients with significant problems will usually be admitted to a neurosurgical or intensive care unit. The management of these patients is discussed in Chapter 22).

Many other patients will be admitted for a short period of observation only. This is frequently done in a short-stay observation ward. These patients should be actively observed and not just left to 'sleep it off'. The observations required are:

- GCS, pupil size and reactivity, limb movements;
- RR, HR, BP, T, blood oxygen saturation.

The NICE guidelines (NICE 2007: p. 36) recommend that observations should be performed and recorded on a half-hourly basis until a GCS of 15/15 has been achieved. Once the patient has a GCS 15/15, they recommend that observations should be performed:

- Half-hourly for 2 hours.
- Then 1-hourly for 4 hours.
- Then 2-hourly thereafter.

These observations should be started once the patient arrives in the ED and should not be delayed until the patient arrives on the observation ward. Should a patient with GCS of 15 deteriorate at any time after the initial 2-hour period, observations should revert to half-hourly and follow the original frequency schedule.

Any of the following examples of neurological deterioration should prompt urgent reappraisal by the supervising doctor:

---

**Box 21.1** Suggested written discharge advice card for patients > 12 years who have sustained a head injury (NICE 2003: p. 23). Head injury: Triage, assessment, investigation and early management of head injury in infants, children and adults. NICE Clinical Guideline 4. NICE copyright © 2003 NICE.

It is alright to leave hospital now. Your symptoms have been checked and you seem to be well on the road to recovery. At home it is very unlikely that you will have any further problems. But, if any of the following symptoms do occur, come back, or get someone to take you to your nearest hospital emergency department as soon as possible:

- Unconsciousness, or lack of full consciousness (for example, problems keeping eyes open).
- Any confusion (not knowing where you are, getting things muddled up).
- Any drowsiness (feeling sleepy) that goes on for longer than one hour when you would normally be wide awake.
- Any problems understanding or speaking.
- Any loss of balance or problems walking.
- Any weakness in one or more arms or legs.
- Any problems with your eyesight.
- Very painful headache that won't go away.
- Any vomiting – getting sick.
- Any fits (collapsing or passing out suddenly).
- Clear fluid coming out of your ear or nose.
- Bleeding from one or both ears.
- New deafness in one or both ears.

*Things you shouldn't worry about:*
Other symptoms over the next few days which should disappear in the next 2 weeks such as a mild headache, feeling sick (without vomiting), dizziness, irritability or bad temper, problems concentrating or problems with your memory, tiredness, lack of appetite or problems sleeping. If you feel very concerned about any of these symptoms in the first few days after discharge or if these problems do not go away after 2 weeks see your own doctor. Seek a doctor's opinion about your ability to drive a car or motorbike.

*Things that will help you get better:*
If you follow this advice you should get better more quickly and it may help any symptoms you have to go away:

- DO make sure you stay within easy reach of a telephone and medical help.
- DO have plenty of rest and avoid stressful situations.

DO NOT:
- Stay at home alone for the first 48 hours after leaving hospital.
- Take any alcohol or drugs.
- Take sleeping pills, sedatives or tranquilisers unless they are given by a doctor.
- Play any contact sport (e.g. rugby or football) for at least 3 weeks without talking to your doctor first.
- Return to your normal school, college or work activity until you feel you have completely recovered.
- Drive a car, motorbike or bicycle or operate machinery unless you feel you have completely recovered.

Hospital contact details: Telephone number.

---

- Development of agitation or abnormal behaviour.
- A sustained (that is, for at least 30 minutes) drop of one point in GCS (greater weight should be given to a drop of one point in the motor response score of the GCS).
- Any drop of three or more points in the eye-opening or verbal response scores of the GCS, or two or more points in the motor response score.
- Development of severe or increasing headache or persistent vomiting.
- New or evolving neurological symptoms or signs such as pupil inequality or asymmetry of limbs or facial movement.

To reduce inter-observer variability and unnecessary referrals, a second member of staff competent to perform observation should confirm deterioration before involving the supervising doctor, but if it is not possible to do this immediately the doctor should be called.

## SOCIAL ASPECTS

It is not uncommon for severely injured people to be unidentified when they arrive in the ED. It is important to try to identify the patient, and the police are usually very helpful in this respect. The police are also helpful when trying to identify and trace the next-of-kin. The police will also ask for a prognosis as the death of a patient following trauma will require investigation and decisions, e.g. when to re-open a road may depend on the anticipated outcome. However, prognosis may be difficult.

Relatives will also need to be talked to and this should be done jointly by the trauma team leader and a nurse. It is important to be honest about the extent of the injuries and the prognosis but unless the severity of injury is such that death is inevitable, always hold out some hope.

Where the prognosis seems hopeless and the patient has severe pre-existing disease or disability, it may, on occasion, be appropriate not to treat the injury. In these circumstances it is important to speak to the relatives to find out whether the patient had ever expressed an opinion on what they would like to happen in such circumstances (see Chapter 24/Chapter 26).

## Activity 21.1

### Scenario

You are working in an emergency department when, with no prior warning, an ambulance arrives with a young man who has been involved in a motorcycle crash. His name is unknown.

You receive the following ATMIST handover:

- Age: unknown but looks in his late teens.
- Time of accident: about 40 minutes ago.
- Mechanism: the patient was riding his motorcycle very fast when a car pulled out of a side road. The motorcycle hit the car and the rider was thrown over the car, landing in the road at least 10 metres away. He then slid along the road. His helmet was cracked.
- Injuries: he has clearly had a head injury and also appears to have a fractured right femur.
- Vital signs: at scene his GCS was 7 (E2V2M3), pulse 80, BP 120 systolic.
- Treatment: his neck has been immobilised on a spinal board with a cervical collar and head blocks. He is tolerating an oropharyngeal airway and has been given oxygen.

### Exercises

1. What are you going to do?
2. Three ED doctors and three ED nurses respond immediately to your call for help. How will they be used?

**Further information is then provided**. The primary survey reveals:

- Airway: the patient is tolerating an oropharyngeal airway. With this in place, the airway is patent.
- Breathing: RR 12, there is bruising over the left lower chest but there is good air entry on both sides of the chest. Oxygen saturation 97% on oxygen at 15 litres per minute via a mask with a reservoir bag.
- Circulation: Heart rate 70 beats per minute, BP 160/80 mm Hg. There is no evidence of external blood loss.

Disability:
- Conscious level. Eyes: no response to painful stimulus (PS). Verbal: no sound to PS. Motor: left side has abnormal flexion to PS and right side extends to PS.
- Pupils equal and react to light.
- Blood sugar 7 mmol/L.
- Exposure: the patient has been fully stripped. The only obvious injury is a deformity of the right thigh suggestive of a fractured femur. Pulses in the right foot are present.

3. What is the GCS?
4. What do these observations tell you?
5. For things to run smoothly, it is necessary to plan ahead: what will need to be done over the next 15 minutes (or shorter time if possible)?
6. The patient is now in CT with a team of ED and ITU doctors and nurses. You are still in the ED. What else is likely to be needed when he returns from CT?

## Activity 21.2

### Scenario 2

It is 10am and you are working in an Emergency Department when you get a phone call from an ambulance crew to warn you that they are bringing you a 72 year old woman who has fallen down stairs and who has a severe head injury. They will be with you in 10 minutes.

1. What further information do you need?

#### *Further history*:

When the ambulance crew arrives they give some further history. Her name is Mrs. Mary Jones and she was found at the bottom of the stairs by a carer. She was in her night clothes and it is uncertain how long she has been there but could have been there all night.

#### *Initial assessment* **reveals**:

- **A**irway: patent and breathing normally.
- **B**reathing: RR 16, good air entry on both sides of the chest and no evidence of chest injury. Oxygen saturation 96% on air.

- **C**irculation: she has clearly lost some blood from her scalp laceration but it is no longer bleeding. Her heart rate is still 60 beats per minute and her BP is still 160/100 mm Hg.
- **D**isability: her GCS is E4M6V4. She is confused and does not know where she is or what day it is. She is unable to give a history. Her pupils are equal and react to light and she will move all four limbs to command.

There is no other obvious injury. She is log-rolled off the spinal board onto the ED trolley while maintaining in-line manual immobilisation of her cervical spine and the cervical collar and head blocks are replaced.

2. What thoughts are going through your mind about this patient's injury?
3. How could you get further information?
4. What investigations will be needed?
5. When doing head injury observations, what signs would indicate that she was developing an intracranial haematoma?

# Chapter 22
# Hospital Management of Neurotrauma

*Kevin Tsang[1] and Peter Whitfield[2]*

[1]Frenchay Hospital, North Bristol NHS Trust, UK
[2]South West Neurosurgery Centre, Plymouth NHS Trust / Peninsula College of Medicine and Dentistry, Plymouth, Devon, UK

## INTRODUCTION

Those with moderate or severe head injuries need care under neurotrauma specialists, consisting of neurosurgeons, intensive care physicians and neurorehabilitation professionals.

Hospital management of these patients depends on the underlying pathology. Space-occupying haematomas may require urgent surgical evacuation and decompression (Royal College of Surgeons of England 2005; Seelig *et al.* 1981; Wilberger *et al.* 1991). Management, whether ward-based or set in the intensive treatment unit (ITU), aims to prevent secondary brain injury by avoiding hypoxia, hypotension, hypoperfusion, raised intracranial pressure (ICP), hyper/hypothermia, hyper/hypoglycaemia and electrolyte imbalance. Utilisation of ITU treatment protocols has been shown to improve patient outcome (Clayton *et al.* 2004; Patel *et al.* 2002). This chapter provides an overview of the various treatment modalities used in the management of these patients to enable health professionals to prepare for the admission of such patients and the delivery of quality care.

## INITIAL ASSESSMENT OF TRAUMA PATIENTS

Neurological examination involves documenting the patient's Glasgow Coma Scale (GCS), pupillary size and reaction to light and the presence of focal neurological deficits (see Chapter 18) as well as deciding which patients require CT scanning (see Figure 22.1).

### Patient stabilisation

The patient may need to be intubated to protect the airway. The criteria for intubation are listed in Table 22.1.

**Table 22.1** Criteria for intubation and ventilation (NICE 2007). Head injury: triage, assessment, investigation and early management of head injury in infants, children and adults. NICE Clinical Guideline 56, NICE copyright © 2007 NICE.

| Assessment | Action |
|---|---|
| GCS ≤8 | Intubate immediately |
| Absence of laryngeal reflexes | |
| Hypoxia (PaO$_2$ <13 kPa whilst on O$_2$) | |
| Hyper- or hypocarbia (PaCO$_2$ >6 kPa or <4 kPa) | |
| Irregular breathing patterns | |
| Drop in GCS motor score of ≥1 | Intubate prior to transfer |
| Facial fractures or copious bleeding into mouth | |
| Seizures | |

(NICE 2007)

# Investigation for clinically important brain injury

**CT imaging of the head is the primary investigation of choice.**

## Selection of adults for CT scanning of head

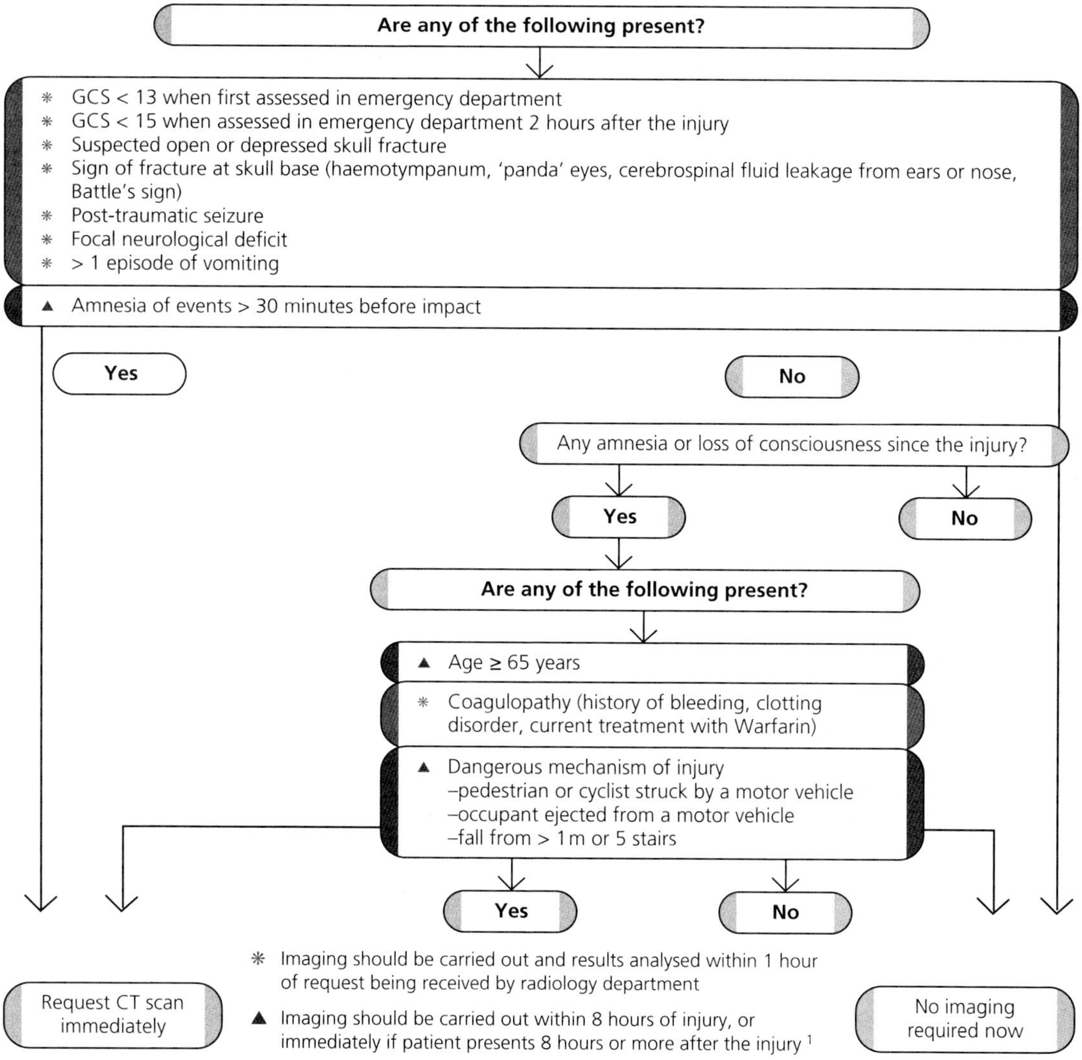

**Are any of the following present?**

* GCS < 13 when first assessed in emergency department
* GCS < 15 when assessed in emergency department 2 hours after the injury
* Suspected open or depressed skull fracture
* Sign of fracture at skull base (haemotympanum, 'panda' eyes, cerebrospinal fluid leakage from ears or nose, Battle's sign)
* Post-traumatic seizure
* Focal neurological deficit
* > 1 episode of vomiting

▲ Amnesia of events > 30 minutes before impact

**Yes** / **No**

Any amnesia or loss of consciousness since the injury?

**Yes** / **No**

**Are any of the following present?**

▲ Age ≥ 65 years

* Coagulopathy (history of bleeding, clotting disorder, current treatment with Warfarin)

▲ Dangerous mechanism of injury
  –pedestrian or cyclist struck by a motor vehicle
  –occupant ejected from a motor vehicle
  –fall from > 1 m or 5 stairs

**Yes** / **No**

* Imaging should be carried out and results analysed within 1 hour of request being received by radiology department

▲ Imaging should be carried out within 8 hours of injury, or immediately if patient presents 8 hours or more after the injury [1]

Request CT scan immediately

No imaging required now

[1] If patient presents out of hours and is ≥ 65, has amnesia for events more than 30 minutes before impact or there was a dangerous mechanism of injury, it is acceptable to admit for overnight observation, with CT imaging the next morning, **unless CT result is required within 1 hour because of the presence of additional clinical findings listed above**

**Figure 22.1** Indications in NICE guidelines for CT scanning in head injury (NICE 2007). Head injury: triage, assessment, investigation and early management of head injury in infants, children and adults. NICE Clinical Guideline 56. Copyright © 2007 NICE.

The aim is to allow optimal oxygenation ($PaO_2$ >13 kPa) and ventilation ($PaCO_2$ 4.5–5 kPa) and to prevent aspiration. Arterial blood gases should be repeated before and after intubation to ensure achievement of the above.

The patient should also be sedated (e.g. Propofol), given analgesia (e.g. Fentanyl) and paralysed (e.g. Atracurium) to allow, firstly, safe intubation and secondly, reduction of cerebral metabolism and energy requirement. Beware that anaesthetic agents often cause hypotension and the patient will therefore require intravenous crystalloids (e.g. 0.9% $NaCl^2$) and often other medications (e.g. Metaraminol) to help maintain the blood pressure (aiming for a mean arterial pressure, MAP, $\geq$60–80 mm Hg). Therefore, the patient should have at least one, if not two large-bore cannulae in place and should also have a urinary catheter inserted for accurate fluid balance monitoring.

Once the patient is sedated and paralysed, it is no longer possible to assess the GCS. Pupil examination therefore becomes the most important neurological assessment and this must be repeated and documented clearly.

The transfer should not commence until adequate resuscitation and stabilisation are completed.

## MANAGEMENT IN THE NEUROSCIENCE UNIT

When a patient reaches the neurosurgical unit, a repeat primary survey (ATLS protocol) is performed to ensure that there has been no change during transfer. Any deterioration in the patient's status would warrant immediate attention and this would include a new scan if the deterioration were neurological. Subsequent treatment would depend on the findings.

### Surgical treatment

#### *Indications*

Once a trauma patient obtains a CT scan of the head, a decision is required with regard to the definitive management plan. The options include watch and wait, surgical intervention or intensive care management.

The process of decision-making is not simple. In principle, a space-occupying haematoma should be evacuated. However, many factors may affect this decision (Bullock *et al.* 2006), including the patient's age, pre-morbid status, CT finding and current neurological status (including changes since the event). It has been shown that age over 60 years is an independent poor prognostic indicator in patients with severe head injuries (Brain Trauma Foundation 2008), especially if their initial GCS is 8 or less (Wilberger *et al.* 1991). In fact, it has been demonstrated

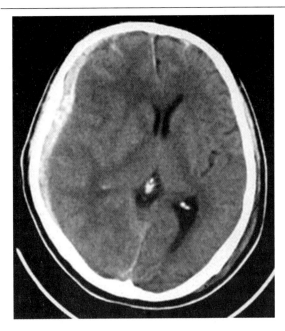

**Figure 22.2** CT scan showing a right-sided acute subdural haematoma (ASDH) with significant midline shift. With kind permission from Derriford Hospital, Plymouth Hospitals NHS Trust.

that GCS itself is a good predictor of outcome, regardless of the patient's age (Murray *et al.* 2007).

Many authors have attempted to use CT findings to calculate the probability of a good or bad outcome and hence utilise this data to decide on a management plan (Bullock *et al.* 2006). The volume of haematoma, the amount of midline shift (transfalcine herniation, see Figure 22.2) and the absence of CSF in the basal cisterns have all been studied.

Although these are all poor prognosticators, no actual criteria have been concluded. Most surgeons operate if the patient has an operable haematoma or contusion causing significant mass effect, provided some patient factors are favourable (e.g. age, neurological status on presentation, pre-morbid factors).

In the case of traumatic axonal injury (TAI, also known as diffuse axonal injury, DAI) (see Figure 22.3), where there is no space-occupying haematoma but global cerebral swelling resulting in high pressures, the decision-making is more difficult (Smith *et al.* 2003).

TAI tends to carry a worse prognosis and although many treatment modalities are available, none has been shown to be superior. In general, these patients are treated in the intensive care unit with maximal medical therapy and

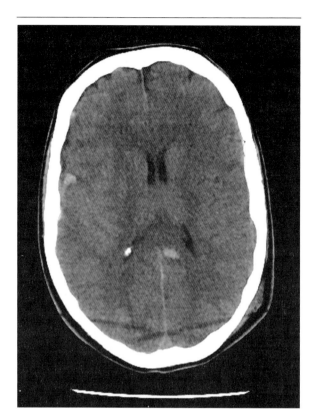

**Figure 22.3** CT scan showing petechial haemorrhages at the grey-white margin and in the corpus callosum, in keeping with traumatic axonal injury (TAI). With kind permission from Derriford Hospital, Plymouth Hospitals NHS Trust.

surgery is only considered if there is still difficulty in controlling the raised intracranial pressure (ICP).

### Timing of surgery

Once the decision is made that a patient requires an operation, this should occur as soon as possible. The Brain Trauma Foundation and the Royal College of Surgeons of England recommend that all patients with severe head injury requiring neurosurgical intervention should receive this within four hours of the injury (Royal College of Surgeons of England 2005). Although one group has shown that operating beyond four hours significantly worsens the prognosis, another group has actually demonstrated that there is a difference in patient outcome between patients operated within or beyond two hours of the injury (Bullock *et al.* 2006).

In reality, a multitude of factors may affect the timing of surgery, such as the need to stabilise the patient, the timing of obtaining a CT scan, the timing of transferring the patient to the neurosurgical unit, and so on (Bulters and Belli 2009).

### Surgical procedures

In the trauma setting, three main operations may be performed: burr-hole evacuation of haematoma, craniotomy and evacuation of haematoma or decompressive craniectomy, or a combination of these.

A burr-hole is created with either a hand-held twist-drill or an electric drill. The size of the burr-hole is normally 11 mm; therefore only liquid blood can be evacuated through this. A burr-hole may be used in chronic subdural haematoma or in an emergency where the patient cannot wait for a craniotomy to be performed. In these circumstances, a burr-hole may be used to temporarily relieve the pressure; usually with the adjunct of nibbling adjacent bone away to enable a decompression.

A craniotomy is the standard operation in most head injuries. This involves creation of a large bone flap to allow access to the extradural and subdural spaces. Acute extradural, subdural and intracerebral haematomas can be evacuated through this. It gives very good exposure and allows easier access and control of bleeding. At the end of the procedure, the bone flap is often replaced prior to suturing of the scalp. This operation may also be performed in those with depressed skull fractures. These patients have a high risk of bleeding, contusion, subsequent infections and seizures. A craniotomy can be performed to allow elevation of the depressed fragments, repair of the dura and reconstruction of the skull.

If the patient has very high ICP and there are signs of cerebral herniation, or the brain is contused and has the potential to cause raised ICP, the bone flap can be left out such that there will be a defect in the skull to allow for a degree of brain swelling. This is called a decompressive craniectomy (see Figure 22.4).

This is performed when a medically-treated patient continues to have refractory high ICP or, at the time of the initial surgery for evacuation of a haematoma, if the surgeon considers that there is a high chance of future brain swelling. This remains an issue with differing opinions (Woertgen *et al.* 2006).

## INTENSIVE CARE MANAGEMENT

The aim of treatment in the intensive care unit is to prevent secondary assault to the brain. This is achieved via tight control of breathing and ventilation, haemodynamic status, ICP, temperature, nutrition and glucose (Maas *et al.* 2008). Most units have a set protocol which the nurses and doctors

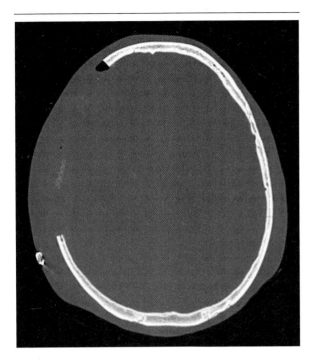

**Figure 22.4** A post-operative CT scan showing the extent of a decompressive craniectomy. With kind permission from Derriford Hospital, Plymouth Hospitals NHS Trust.

follow on admitting such a patient, as this seems to reduce confusion amongst healthcare professionals and allows for a better outcome (Clayton *et al.* 2004; Patel *et al.* 2002). The protocol for the South-West Neurosciences Unit, Plymouth, is shown in Figure 22.5.

**Airway and breathing**

In patients with severe head injury (GCS ≤8), airway and ventilatory support is mandatory. The criteria for intubation have been listed in Table 22.1. This allows the physician to tightly control the patient's oxygen and carbon dioxide levels. Regular blood gases are taken from an arterial line to look at the partial pressures of oxygen ($PaO_2$) and carbon dioxide ($PaCO_2$), and to assess the patient's acid-base balance (see Chapter 12/Chapter 14).

Ideally, the patient should be well oxygenated with $PaO_2$ of 10–13 kPa (Meyer *et al.* 2010). This is achieved by delivery of a fixed amount of oxygen ($FiO_2$) and adjustment of the Positive End-Expiratory Pressure (PEEP). PEEP allows splinting of the alveoli at the end of expiration and therefore recruits more alveoli for the next breath. Beware that in a patient with normal lung compliance, this increase in intrathoracic pressure may transmit up the jugular veins and result in raised ICP.

Carbon dioxide is a potent vasodilator. This means that a high $PaCO_2$ can result in cerebral vasodilation, an increase in cerebral blood volume (CBV) and thus raised ICP. The optimum $PaCO_2$ is estimated to be between 4.5–5 kPa, as a lower $PaCO_2$ can be harmful (via its effects of vasoconstriction and subsequent reduction in CBF (Coles *et al.* 2007; Curley *et al.* 2010).

Every treatment has potential side-effects and endotracheal intubation is no exception. The endotracheal tube can cause laryngeal damage, it makes mouth hygiene difficult and patients are at higher risk of lower respiratory tract infection (LRTI), DVT, pressure sores and so on. In those requiring long-term mechanical ventilation, a tracheostomy reduces some of these side-effects. The decision on timing of tracheostomy insertion is a contentious issue but is usually deferred for about a week after the injury to provide an adequate opportunity to avoid this intervention (Barquist *et al.* 2006; Bouderka *et al.* 2004).

**Circulation**

As in all trauma scenarios, it is very important to maintain a stable cardiovascular system to allow adequate perfusion of all major organs. In patients with severe head injury, cerebral perfusion is of utmost importance to prevent ischaemic events. In order to allow adequate oxygen extraction in the brain, the CPP, should be at least 60 mm Hg (Trivedi and Coles, 2009). In the normal brain, autoregulation maintains a constant CBF within a wide range of MAP (see Figure 22.6).

This mechanism can be impaired in head injury patients such that even minor fluctuations in MAP can result in large rises or falls in CBF (Fortune *et al.* 1994).

In order to maintain tight BP and CPP control, all severely head-injured patients should have invasive BP monitoring via an arterial line. If the patient is sedated, then an ICP monitor should be inserted to allow its measurement and hence deduction of CPP.

Several options are available to maintain an adequate BP. The initial management should be fluid resuscitation. In fact, regardless of BP, ICP and CPP control, negative fluid balance is associated with a poorer outcome (Clifton *et al.* 2002). The type of fluid used is dependent on the patient's electrolyte balance, but hypotonic fluid (e.g. dextrose) should be avoided as this may exacerbate cerebral oedema. Isotonic saline use (0.9% $NaCl_2$) has been studied extensively and the conclusion is that it is the best option for fluid replacement (The SAFE study investigators 2007).

# ICP Treatment Guidelines

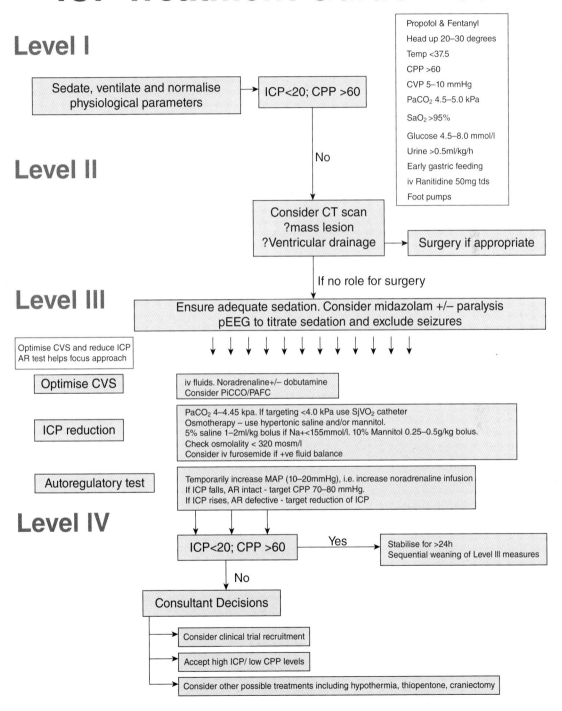

*Peter Whiffield and Elfyn Thomas 2009*

**Figure 22.5** Protocol for control of ↑ICP, South-West, Neurosciences Unit, Plymouth. With kind permission from Derriford Hospital, Plymouth Hospitals NHS Trust.

If the patient remains hypotensive despite adequate fluid resuscitation (confirmed by either urine output or direct measurement of central venous pressure using a central line), one must suspect on-going blood loss from a body cavity such as abdominal or pelvic or from fractured bones. If no other sources of bleeding are found, then the blood pressure needs to be elevated using medications such as

inotropes. These include Noradrenaline, Dopamine and Dobutamine. The use of these drugs is supervised by the intensive care physicians and the choice is dependent on the patient's renal and cardiac functions. Remember that these drugs all cause splanchnic vasoconstriction and prolonged use of high doses can result in gut ischaemia and infarction causing peritonitis and death.

### Intracranial pressure control

ICP is determined by the Monro–Kellie doctrine, which states that the skull is a closed box with three contents: brain, blood and CSF (see Figure 22.7). Since it is a closed box, expansion of volume of one content will need to be compensated by reduction in volume of another to prevent a rise in the ICP. This forms the basis of its control during management of severe head injury (Tsang and Whitfield 2011).

ICP is measured in sedated patients using a monitor (see Figure 22.8), which is a small probe inserted into the brain which can transduce pressure in mmHg.

Normal ICP should be between 5–10 mmHg and in head injury patients, up to 20 mmHg is often accepted.

### Control of blood flow

As there are three components within the cranium, ICP can be reduced by removing one of the three components. Adequate blood flow is obviously required for cerebral perfusion, but excess cerebral blood volume (CBV) can increase ICP. The simplest method of reducing CBV is by

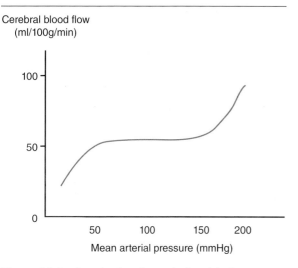

**Figure 22.6** Graph showing relationship between cerebral blood flow (CBF), arterial pressure (MAP), and autoregulation between 50–150 mm Hg. With kind permission from Derriford Hospital, Plymouth Hospitals NHS Trust.

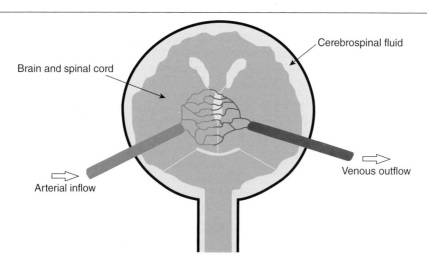

**Figure 22.7** Schematic diagram showing the contents of the cranium according to the Monro–Kellie doctrine. With kind permission from Derriford Hospital, Plymouth Hospitals NHS Trust. For a colour version of this figure, please refer to the plate section.

(a)

(b)

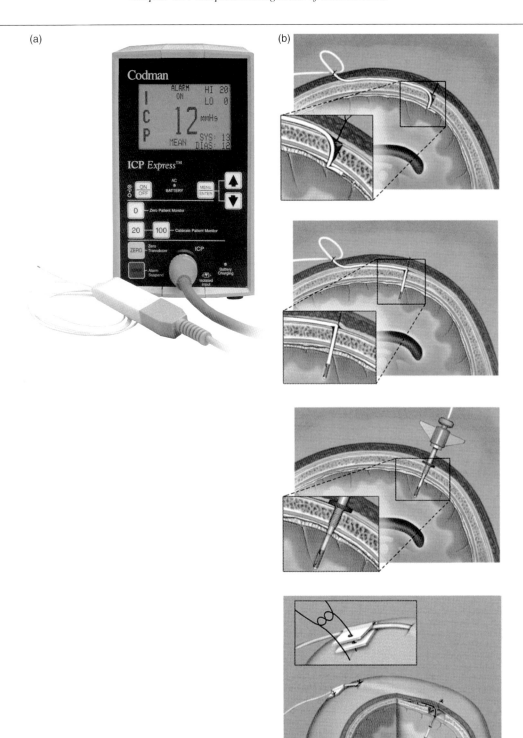

**Figure 22.8** ICP monitor and probe insertion. With kind permission from Codman.

encouraging venous return to the heart. This can be achieved by elevating the patient's head up to 30° and loosening anything around the neck which may be obstructing the jugular veins (e.g. tie around endotracheal tube, collars).

The next step would be to control the carbon dioxide level. $CO_2$ is a potent vasodilator and this can increase the CBV, resulting in higher ICP. Controlling the $PaCO_2$ level to 4.5–5 kPa will readily reduce the ICP. In refractory cases, the $PaCO_2$ can be reduced to 4–4.5 kPa but this also increases the risk of cerebral ischaemia (from vasoconstriction due to low levels of $CO_2$). Lower parameters are therefore no longer recommended (Curley *et al.* 2010).

### Control of CSF

The body is able to reduce the amount of CSF within the cranium by encouraging its flow down the spinal cord within the subarachnoid space into the lumbar theca. If excess CSF is still present within the cranium (e.g. hydrocephalus), this can be removed via an external ventricular drain (see Figure 22.9).

This drain is inserted via a burr-hole into the frontal horn of the lateral ventricle. The zero reference point is then set at the level of the Foramen of Monro (connection between lateral and third ventricles, surface landmark being the tragus of the ear). The amount of CSF drainage can be adjusted by setting the chamber at a height relative to the zero reference point. The higher the setting, the less CSF will be drained.

### Control of brain swelling

The final content of the cranium is the brain. In severe head injury, especially in diffuse injury, there can be widespread swelling of the brain resulting in high ICP despite control of the other contents. The initial management should

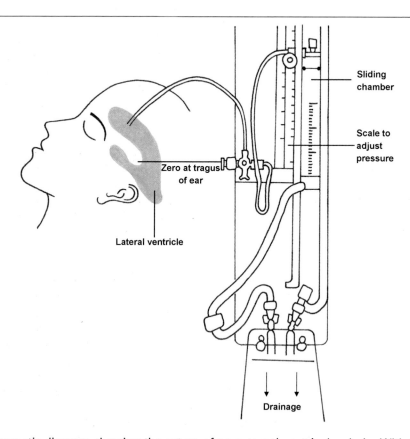

**Figure 22.9**  Schematic diagram showing the set-up of an external ventricular drain. With kind permission from Codman.

involve sedation (e.g. Propofol) and analgesia (e.g. Fentanyl), as this will reduce stimulation to the brain and also reduce its metabolic requirements. The use of benzodiazepines (e.g. Midazolam) and paralytic agents (e.g. Atracurium) can be added to optimise sedation.

If ICP continues to be high despite all of the above, osmotherapy can be used: 5% $NaCl_2$ solution attracts fluid into the vasculature via its hypertonic properties. This readily reduces cerebral oedema and is very useful as a temporising measure. Mannitol is another fluid used for the same effect, but its mechanism of action is dependent upon its osmotic diuretic properties, encouraging the fluid to be removed by the kidneys. It has been shown that hypertonic saline is superior to Mannitol and should be used in the first instance (Oddo *et al.* 2009).

In extreme circumstance where none of the above manages to control the raised ICP, a decompressive craniectomy can be performed (hence opening the 'closed box' to relieve pressure). This is a controversial topic and is under intense research. A recent study in Australia showed that decompressive craniectomy was superior in terms of mortality rate, but the outcome of those alive was worse (Cooper *et al.* 2011). Finally, in refractory situations, the patient may be treated with intravenous barbiturates to induce a metabolic coma. This reduces the oxygen demands of the brain but is fraught with adverse effects.

### Other aspects

It is very easy to focus on the acute issues listed above and forget about the long-term, ongoing risks of a ventilated patient at bed rest. These include nutrition, pressure areas, chest infections, muscle wasting and thrombo-embolic prophylaxis.

Adequate nutrition is necessary for all critically ill patients as these patients require even more energy than usual for recovery. A nutritionist should be consulted to help create the best regime for each individual patient, and this would involve looking at the patient's electrolytes (e.g. $Na^+$, $K^+$, $Mg^{2+}$, $PO_4^-$), protein and albumin levels, fluid balance and overall metabolism. Gastric feeding is the preferred method, and this can be achieved either via an orogastric or a nasogastric tube (the latter is contraindicated in patients with base of skull fractures). Failing these, parenteral feeding can be used but this should only be for the short term, and a definitive gastric feeding tube should be established as soon as possible. A percutaneous endoscopic gastrostomy (PEG) tube can be placed if it is clear that recovery of the swallowing reflexes is likely to be protracted.

Patients lying in the same position can develop pressure sores over bony prominences and these can become infected with varying degrees of soft tissue loss and be very difficult to treat. This can be very easily prevented by using a specially made mattress and good nursing care. These patients should be turned from one position to another every 3–4 hours. Any signs of skin irritation should be attended to immediately and may require the help of tissue viability nurses.

Patients on bed rest have an increased risk of infections and muscle wasting, resulting in prolonged periods of mechanical ventilation and subsequent rehabilitation. These risks can be minimised with good nursing care and liaison with physiotherapists. Regular chest physiotherapy along with suctioning and oral hygiene is of utmost importance. The patient's joints should also be regularly exercised to prevent muscle wasting and increased tone. Occasionally, splinting may be required for increased tone and contractures, and medications such as Baclofen or Botox injections may be necessary in some cases.

Thrombo-embolism is extremely common in trauma patients, with up to 58% of patients being diagnosed with DVT and 2% with pulmonary embolism; carrying a mortality rate of up to 43% (Reiff *et al.* 2009). Many of these patients have some form of bleeding in the brain and therefore many physicians would not advocate the use of chemical prophylaxis (e.g. Enoxaparin) initially. However, a few studies suggest that early use of Enoxaparin does not significantly increase the risk of further bleeding (Norwood *et al.* 2008). On the other hand, it has also been shown that mechanical prophylaxis (pneumatic compression devices) alone is at least as efficient as chemical prophylaxis without any risk of bleeding (Kurtoglu *et al.* 2004). A cautious approach is therefore normally taken.

### FURTHER MANAGEMENT AND PROGNOSIS

The management strategies outlined in this chapter relate to the patient's acute condition and aim to reduce mortality and morbidity. However, the treatments that will allow the patient to return to normal activities do not stop here. In fact, this is the beginning of the road to rehabilitation, involving a large multidisciplinary team of experts aiming at improving the patient's quality of life. They include physiotherapists, occupational therapists (OT), speech and language therapists (SALT), clinical psychologists and social workers. Most patients are transferred from the tertiary centre to their local rehabilitation unit to continue with these therapies.

## Case Study

### History

A 46 year old lady was found collapsed by the road-side at 3am and an ambulance was called to the scene. When paramedics arrived at the scene, she was found to be protecting her own airway, breathing spontaneously with no signs of external haemorrhage. Her GCS was 11 (E2V3M6) with equal pupils which reacted to light. She was therefore immediately taken to the local emergency department.

### Emergency department assessment

On arrival at the hospital, her GCS deteriorated to 8 (E2V1M5) but her pupils were still equal and reactive to light. The rest of her observations were within normal limits. She was sedated, intubated and ventilated and transferred to the CT scanner. The CT scan of the head (see Figure 22.10) showed the presence of large temporal

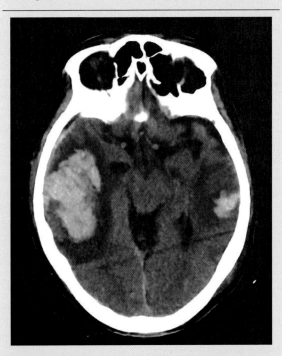

**Figure 22.10** CT scan showing a patient with bitemporal contusions, worse on the right than the left, associated with a thin right-sided acute subdural haematoma. With kind permission from Derriford Hospital, Plymouth Hospitals NHS Trust.

contusions, worse on the right, associated with a very thin acute subdural haematoma.

She was transferred back to the emergency department where an anaesthetist was called and the patient was referred for neurosurgical advice.

In the emergency department, the anaesthetist ensured the airway was secured, checked for bilateral air entry and inserted an arterial line for invasive blood pressure monitoring. An arterial blood gas was obtained and this was used to aid control of the patient's ventilation (in terms of $CO_2$ levels). The patient was connected to a continuous infusion of Propofol and Alfentanyl. A urinary catheter was inserted. The patient was then transferred to the local neurosurgical unit.

### Neurosurgical treatment

Due to the presence of a large temporal contusion in the non-dominant hemisphere, along with the patient's rapid deterioration, a decision was made to operate on the patient urgently. She was transferred directly to the operating theatre on arrival at the tertiary hospital.

A thorough hand-over was obtained from the transfer team and the patient was re-assessed. Apart from the patient being sedated and hence a GCS could not be obtained, there were no other changes to her assessment. She did, however, require several boluses of Metaraminol to maintain an adequate blood pressure during transfer.

The patient underwent a right-sided temporal craniotomy and evacuation of contusion. Haemostasis was obtained and an ICP monitor was inserted at the end of the operation. She was then transferred to the intensive care unit.

### Intensive care treatment

During her stay in the intensive care unit, her ICP remained below 20 mm Hg with a CPP of between 60–70 mm Hg. Therefore, after 24 hours of stable observations, she was weaned off the sedation for a neurological assessment. She was initially very slow to wake initiating a repeat CT scan (see Figure 22.11).

This showed adequate evacuation of the contusion and subdural haematoma. Eventually the patient recovered to a GCS of 10+T (E4V$_T$M6) and was moving both sides of

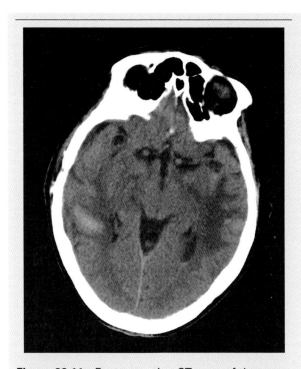

**Figure 22.11** Post-operative CT scan of the same patient as in Figure 22.10 showing satisfactory resolution of the contusions. With kind permission from Derriford Hospital, Plymouth Hospitals NHS Trust.

her body equally. She was extubated successfully. Following another 24 hours of monitoring, she was transferred back to the neurosurgical ward.

**Rehabilitation**

Whilst she was on the neurosurgical ward, her GCS remained stable at 14 (E4V4M6) and she gradually started to mobilise with the physiotherapists. She had some expressive dysphasia and had multiple assessments by the SALT team. Due to the persistence of cognitive impairment, word-finding difficulties and the need for assistance whilst mobilising, she was transferred back to her local hospital to continue with rehabilitation.

She was seen back in the neurosurgery clinic three months after the injury, and she walked into the clinic without any aids and her GCS was back to 15. However, on direct questioning, she still had memory problems and would find it difficult to perform certain daily tasks, therefore she was still living with her elderly parents and not yet back at work.

# Chapter 23
# Nursing the Patient with Neurotrauma

*Nadine Abelson-Mitchell*

School of Nursing and Midwifery, Faculty of Health, Education and Society, Plymouth University, Devon, UK

## INTRODUCTION

Nursing the patient with neurotrauma is a challenge but also an opportunity to provide holistic, individualised, needs-based, patient-centred care along the patient's journey.

The nurse is in a unique position as she provides 24-hour care to the patient and is therefore able to monitor the patient's status and report the findings to the appropriate health professional. The nurse needs to be mindful of her scope of practice as set out by the regulating body (e.g. ARN 2008; NMC 2008). Training and competence, responsibility and accountability for actions underpin nursing practice (Hoeman 2008; ARN 2008). The nurse must be knowledgeable, have the correct aptitude and attitude as well as clinical competence in order to provide quality care to patients and families.

The role of the nurse must not be under-estimated; it extends from primary prevention, through acute management in a secondary care setting to tertiary care in a rehabilitation centre, residential facility or within the home environment (ARN 2008; Audit Commission 2000; Pryor 2002; RCN 2007a, 2007b).

Nurses have practiced rehabilitation for many years as part of nursing intervention, e.g. prevention of complications, prevention of decubitus ulcers, prevention of foot-drop, halitosis and dental caries as well as the prevention of deep vein thrombosis.

The role of the nurse (Figure 23.1) includes, but is not limited to, the following:

## ADVOCATE

The nurse needs to be knowledgeable to protect the interests of the patient, ensure the patient is provided with reasonable care and enable the patient and family to make informed choices (Griffith and Tengnah 2008). The patient, their family and carers have to make important decisions that may be life changing. Patients who have had neurotrauma are often unconscious, unable to talk for themselves or lack capacity (Joyce 2009; Leatherman and Goethe 2009; Nicholson *et al.* 2008). They may also have difficulty understanding or interpreting what has been said. The nurse acts as the patient's 'advocate' (ARN 2008, www.rehabnurse.org/advocacy/content/pethical.html). It is important to establish whether the patient has a nominated lasting power of attorney for personal care and financial matters (Chatfield and Menon 2011; DH 2007b; Nicholson *et al.* 2008). Whilst the nurse acts informally as the patients advocate, at times it may be necessary to involve a social worker, solicitor or lawyer in the patient's management and affairs (see Chapter 32).

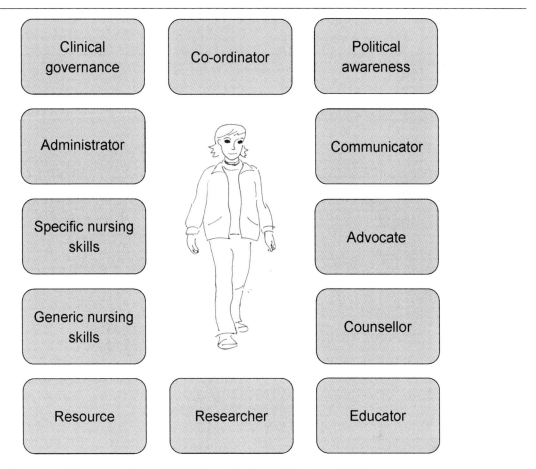

**Figure 23.1** The role of the nurse (Pryor 2002; Royal College of Nursing 2007a).

## ESSENTIAL NURSING SKILLS

Essential nursing skills include direct patient care and involve techniques, skills and risk management. It is imperative that nurses are competent practitioners, responsible and accountable for their practice that involves identification of patient's needs, appropriate use of the nursing team to meet the needs of the patient, patient evaluation and effective documentation.

Generic nursing skills include all nursing skills utilised for all patients. With regard to neurotrauma, the nurse may need to adapt the technique to the patient's circumstances, e.g. the unconscious or restless patient (DH 2004b).

## THERAPEUTIC PRACTICE

Nurses must be competent in numerous techniques in order to enhance the patient's journey and experience.

For example in rehabilitation this will include:

- Patient monitoring.
- Early stimulation programmes.
- Behaviour modification programmes.
- Feeding and nutrition.
- Continence.

Specific nursing skills are those skills for which nurses have been especially trained and for which they are competent to complete.

*Such skills may include:*

- Assessment of the central nervous system.
- Neurological observations.
- Cranial nerve assessment.

- Intracranial pressure monitoring.
- Pain control.
- Head dressings.
- Management of seizures.
- Behaviour modification.
- Preparation for neurosurgery.
- Preparation for neurological investigations.
- Nutrition.
- Specific rehabilitation techniques.

*Generic skills may include:*
- Maintaining a conducive environment.
- Care of the unconscious patient.
- Maintaining patient hygiene.
- Temperature control.
- Insertion of urinary catheter.
- Feeding patients.
- Intravenous therapy.
- Patient mobilisation.

A Nursing Care Plan has been developed to cover the needs of the neurotrauma patient (Table 23.1).

## CO-ORDINATION

Working as an equal partner in a multidisciplinary team is an integral part of nursing. The nurse participates in decision-making regarding the patient's care and anticipated outcomes. Team responsibilities include co-ordinating health team activities and services, collaboration with team members, networking, liaison and consultation.

## CLINICAL GOVERNANCE

Quality assurance in neurotrauma management is essential. The nurse is responsible for maintaining the quality of care (DH 2006b, 2007b, 2007c).

## ADVICE/COUNSELLING

The nurse provides support to patients and families.

## POLITICAL AWARENESS

Nurses need to be aware of government initiatives and policies of importance to neurotrauma management, e.g. the National Service Framework for Long Term Conditions (DH 2005a), NICE guidelines for head injury management (NICE 2003, 2007) as well as policies related to staffing, and so on.

## EDUCATION

One of the foundations of nursing is learning and teaching staff, patients, families, carers, friends and communities. Education is essential to enable health professionals to provide effective, efficient and competent care throughout the patient's journey (Baker 2011; DH 2007a, 2007c, 2007f, 2010c).

## RESEARCH

Professionals working within neurotrauma practice are in a research rich milieu. It is essential to ensure that valid and reliable research is undertaken and published to support effective, evidence-based nursing practice related to neurotrauma (DH 2007a).

## ETHICAL CONSIDERATIONS

Ethical issues, related to health practice and the patient journey, present many challenges within neurotrauma practice as personnel are often working with vulnerable patients or patients who lack capacity (DH 2007a). The fundamental principles of autonomy, beneficence, justice and non-maleficence apply at all times (American Association of Rehabilitation Nurses: www.rehabnurse.org/advocacy/content/pethical.html).

The ethical issues that prevail include decisions regarding patients' rights such as patient choice and 'Do Not Resuscitate' orders, issues of informed consent, confidentiality, substance abuse, the use of restraints in practice, abuse of patients and professional/patient relationships. Other issues relate to healthcare reform such as access to healthcare, cost containment, quality of care, length of stay, criteria for admission to rehabilitation services and patient non-compliance (American Association of Rehabilitation Nurses www.rehabnurse.org/advocacy/content/pethical.html).

## REHABILITATION NURSING

Rehabilitation nursing is defined as the process of facilitating or enabling clients to achieve maximum functional capacity with minimum disruption to their daily lives. In acute care, due to the patient's condition, the nurse often undertakes activities for the patient, the nurse is the 'doer'. In rehabilitation the nurse encourages and facilitates the patient to undertake the activity for themselves.

Additional information related to nursing the patient with neurotrauma can be found in the various chapters of this book.

**Table 23.1** Nursing care plan.

| Nursing diagnosis | Potential problems | Possible cause/s | Planned intervention | Expected outcome (linked to timeframe) |
|---|---|---|---|---|
| **Safety & environment** | | | | |
| Provision of therapeutic patient environment. | Noisy environment. Agitated patient. Family distress. | Admission of patient to unit. Performance of numerous therapeutic activities. GCS<12/15. | Assess environmental needs of patient. Maintain adequate: Lighting. Ventilation. Environmental temperature (21 °C). Clean room daily and when necessary. Keep neat and uncluttered. Have equipment readily accessible. Maintain patient privacy. Maintain safe environment. Protect patient from injury. Control extraneous noise and activity. Maintain quiet atmosphere. Minimise untherapeutic noise. Place clock/calendar strategically. Ensure adequate staffing. | Therapeutic environment. Safety of patient. Early reality orientation. |
| Potential for injury/trauma. | Falling out of bed. Seizure activity. Self-inflicted injury from friction and side-rails. Aggression. Depression. Frustration. Lack of insight. Restlessness. | Altered level of consciousness related to CNS dysfunction. | Assess risk of injury/trauma. Maintain safe environment. Close observation of patient. Seek cause of agitation/restlessness. Ensure well protected side-rails in situ. Reassure patient. Avoid restraints if possible. Apply restraints if necessary as ordered by physician. Explain reason for applying restraints. Administer medication as prescribed. Sedatives to be used with caution. May require 1:1 supervision. | Provision of safe environment. Absence of injury complications. Minimise agitation. No masking of cerebral signs. |

*(Continued)*

**Table 23.1** (*Continued*)

| Nursing diagnosis | Potential problems | Possible cause/s | Planned intervention | Expected outcome (linked to timeframe) |
|---|---|---|---|---|
| Alteration in level of consciousness. | GCS<12/15. | Head injury. Raised intracranial pressure. | Ensure safe environment. Monitor 15 minutes – daily depending on condition: Neurological status, using GCS. Vital signs. Fluid and electrolyte balance. Notify physician if alteration occurs. Re-orientate patient to time, place and person. Reassure patient. Do not undertake activities that will increase intracranial pressure beyond reasonable limits, for example playing music. | Neurological examination within normal limits. Absence or resolution of increased intracranial pressure. Patient orientated to place, time and person. Introduce early stimulation programme. |
| | Noxious stimulation. | Environmental noise. Inappropriate stimulation programme. | Provide therapeutic environment by avoiding or minimising factors that may precipitate an increase in intracranial pressure: Extensor spasms. Head down/prone or flat position. Hypercarbia. Hypertension. Hyperthermia. Hypoxia. Increased intrathoracic pressure. Isometric muscle contractions. Pain. Exercise therapy. Suctioning. Taking of blood samples. Tension of the neck. Tight endotracheal/tracheostomy tape. Turning. Valsalva manoeuvre. Ventilator resistance. Decrease extraneous noise. Avoid emotionally disturbing dialogue. Talk to and reassure patient. Notify physician of any change in patient status. | Neutral therapeutic environment. Minimise the effect of noxious stimulation. |

| Patient problem | Cause | | Nursing action | Expected outcome |
|---|---|---|---|---|
| Restlessness/agitation. | Head injury. Raised intracranial pressure. Alteration in patient comfort, e.g. pain, full bladder, constipation. | | Ensure safe environment. Ensure side-rails in situ at all times. Monitor patient status. Seek cause: Ensure bed clean and dry. Ensure bladder empty. Reduce extraneous stimulation to a minimum. Apply restraints as ordered by the physician if this is the only way of protecting patient. Notify physician of change in patient's status. | Safe patient environment. |
| **Mentation** Alteration in cerebral perfusion and intracranial pressure. | Decreased cerebral perfusion. Cerebral ischaemia CPP < 60 mm Hg. Increased intracranial pressure >15 mm Hg. | Head injury. Intracranial hypertension. Systemic hypertension. Loss of cerebral autoregulation. Space occupying lesion. Cerebral oedema. Concussion/Contusion. Fluid overload. Haemorrhage. Haematoma. Skull fracture. Vasospasm. Raised intracranial pressure. ↑ $pCO_2$ ↓ $pO_2$ | Monitor for clinical manifestations of raised intracranial pressure: Nausea and vomiting. Headache. Deteriorating level of consciousness. Pupil changes. Increased systolic blood pressure. Bradycardia. Widened pulse pressure. Altered respiration. Establish neurological baseline and vital signs on admission. Perform on-going assessments every 15–60 minutes. Note any skull wound. Note any CSF leakage/drainage. Assist with insertion of intracranial pressure monitoring device. Monitor values and waveforms of intracranial pressure recordings. Raise head of bed to 15–30° provided airway maintained. Maintain bedrest as ordered. Maintain body in neutral position. Maintain controlled ventilation according to doctor's orders. Administer medication as ordered. | Maintain intracranial pressure within normal limits. Control or resolution of increased intracranial pressure. Maximum neurological functioning. Absence of complications. MICP ≤10 mm Hg. Maintain normal cerebral perfusion. CPP = ±80 mm Hg. Maintain cerebral perfusion: >60 mm Hg. |

*(Continued)*

**Table 23.1** (*Continued*)

| Nursing diagnosis | Potential problems | Possible cause/s | Planned intervention | Expected outcome (linked to timeframe) |
|---|---|---|---|---|
| | | | Administer fluid as ordered – 1500–2000 ml/ 24 hours according to doctor's orders. Administer treatment as ordered. Notify physician of alteration in patient status. Monitor and record intracranial pressure and vital signs. Maintain blood pressure within patient's normal limits. Ensure adequate oxygenation. Minimise noxious stimulation. | |
| Presence of/potential for intracranial bleed. | Intracranial bleed: Extradural haematoma. Subdural haematoma. Subarachnoid bleed. Intraventricular bleed. Intracerebral bleed. | Disruption of cerebral blood flow. Skull fracture. | Monitor and record neurological status and vital signs every 15–60 minutes. Note classic sign of extradural haematoma: Change and restlessness. Clinical manifestations of raised intracranial pressure. Dilating ipsilateral pupil. Administer emergency medications such as osmotic diuretic agents and treatment as ordered. Prepare patient for operative procedure. Ensure informed consent. Notify physician immediately of any change in neurological status/vital signs. | Early detection of intracranial haemorrhage. Absence of uncal herniation. Maximum neurological functioning. |
| Presence of or potential for seizure activity | Seizure activity. Status epilepticus. Hypoxia. | Cerebral oedema. Cerebral ischaemia. Irritative effect of blood. Neuronal alteration. | Implement seizure precautions: Oxygen and suction apparatus at bedside. Airway, emergency equipment and medication available. Bed height at lowest level. Padded side-rails up at all times when patient alone. Prevent precipitating factors (fever, hypoxia, electrolyte disturbance, lack of sleep, noxious stimulation). | Absence of seizures. Control of seizure activity. Education and counselling of patient and family. |

| | | | |
|---|---|---|---|
| | | Monitor and record seizure activity:<br>　Type of seizure.<br>　Duration.<br>　March.<br>　Presence of:<br>　　Cyanosis.<br>　　Incontinence.<br>　　Eye deviation.<br>Seek cause of seizure activity.<br>Administer anti-convulsant medication as prescribed.<br>Record effects and side-effects of medication given.<br>Control and prevent status epilepticus.<br>Record and notify physician of any precipitating factors that exist and of seizure activity.<br>Reassure and support patient and family.<br>Discharge planning regarding seizure activity. | |
| Alteration in skull integrity. | CSF leak<br>Base of skull fracture.<br>Penetrating/open head wounds.<br>Skull fracture. | Assess for CSF leak.<br>Monitor and record 1–2 hourly:<br>　Neurological status.<br>　Presence of skull fracture/wound.<br>　Signs of CSF leak:<br>　　Rhinorrhea (anterior fossa fracture).<br>　　Ottorrhea (posterior fossa fracture).<br>　Signs of meningitis/meningism:<br>　　Pyrexia.<br>　　Stiff neck.<br>　　Photophobia.<br>　　Positive Kernig's sign.<br>　　Positive Brudzinski's sign.<br>　Vital signs.<br>If CSF leak occurs:<br>　Nasogastric tube to be inserted by appropriately trained person.<br>　Avoid nasotracheal suction.<br>　Manage CSF leak aseptically.<br>　Make use of aseptic technique for oropharyngeal care. | Absence/Resolution of CSF leak.<br>Minimum neurological deficit.<br><br>Prevent intubation of the cranial cavity via the oropharynx or nose. |

*(Continued)*

**Table 23.1**  (*Continued*)

| Nursing diagnosis | Potential problems | Possible cause/s | Planned intervention | Expected outcome (linked to timeframe) |
|---|---|---|---|---|
| | | | Cover with sterile pad and change pad when necessary. Allow free drainage of leak – DO NOT PLUG. Monitor site, amount and quality of drainage. Collect and test a specimen for the presence of glucose. Administer medication (prophylactic antibiotics/treatment) as ordered. | |
| | Recurrent meningitis. | Persistent CSF leak. | Reverse barrier nurse. Monitor patient status. Prepare patient for investigative and operative procedure/s. Notify physician. | Absence of CSF leak. |
| | Skull fracture. Base of skull fracture. | | Monitor and record: Neurological status. Sense of taste/smell. Vital signs. Aseptic wound/ear management. | Stabilisation of fracture. No neurological deficit. |
| Cerebral dysfunction. | Presence of neurological deficit. | Motor deficit: Hemiplegia. Paralysis. Paresis. Spasticity. Sensory deficit: Anosmia. Speech. Vision. | Monitor and record neurological status and vital signs. On admission, establish and implement nursing care plan, including preventive rehabilitation, based on individual needs and specific deficits present. Institute measures to promote optimal skin integrity, muscle tone, functioning, maintenance and circulation. Ensure patient carries out exercise programme 2–4 hourly. Involve clinical nurse specialist in patient/family counselling and support. Ensure adequate comprehensive rehabilitation available throughout recovery of patient. Involve health team personnel as soon after admission as possible. When necessary obtain health team referrals, in particular speech therapist and neuropsychologist. Help patient to accept/adjust to neurological deficit. | Absence of complications. Maximal neurological functioning. |

| | | |
|---|---|---|
| | Work through process of adjustment with patient.<br>Encourage patient.<br>Mobilise patient as soon as possible.<br>Ensure patient undertakes occupational therapy instituted.<br>Through preventive and curative rehabilitation programme avoid complications:<br>  Decubitus ulcers.<br>  Foot drop/wrist drop.<br>Notify physician of worsening neurological deficit.<br>Refer patient to rehabilitation liaison officer/psychiatrist and team personnel for further care.<br>Commence discharge planning. | |
| Continued presence of neurological deficit. | Collaborate with physician and health team re: prognosis and expected level of recovery.<br>Ensure patient adheres to rehabilitation programme.<br>Ensure correct referral to other health services.<br>Assess specific needs of patient according to neurological deficit.<br>Assess level of independence for self-care and ADL.<br>Interagency/Intersectoral assessment to be arranged.<br>Monitor level of achievement toward maximum and potential independence; means to promote as 'normal' a lifestyle as possible.<br>Re-inforce any gains of independence patient achieves.<br>Encourage and reassure patient.<br>Assess families need for information.<br>Appropriate discharge planning.<br>Refer to hospital and community services. | Maximal independence:<br>  Self-care activities.<br>  Activities of living.<br>  Use of therapeutic devices.<br>Absence/minimise complications of neurological deficit.<br>Acceptance of neurological deficit. |

(Continued)

**Table 23.1** (*Continued*)

| Nursing diagnosis | Potential problems | Possible cause/s | Planned intervention | Expected outcome (linked to timeframe) |
|---|---|---|---|---|
| Inadequate therapeutic stimulation. | Boredom. Depression. Lack of independence. Lack of reality orientation. Slowed psychosocial and emotional recovery. | ↓LOC | Ensure appropriate attitude of staff. Implement an early stimulation programme in a conducive environment. Switch the light off at night. Avoid sedation unless absolutely necessary. Employ reality orientation: Begin re-orientation and re-association as soon as possible. Talk about familiar topics. Re-orientate to time, place and person. Orientate to body signals. Interaction with others. Mobilise the patient as soon as possible. Sensory stimulation. Introduce therapeutic activities to aid learning; such as games. Improve patient's level of motivation: Frequent encouragement and praise. Positive re-inforcement. Feedback of progress. Incorporate health team personnel in stimulation programme. Institute co-ordinated comprehensive programme of physical and mental stimulation. Maintain/re-inforce motivation of staff, patient and family. Assess stage and progress of patient: Co-ordination. Insight. Memory. Speech. Understanding. Incorporate family/patient in planning/implementing stimulation programme. Utilise all 5 senses progressively. | Intentional therapeutic stimulation. Adequate reality orientation. Stimulation of desire to resume self-care activities and independence. Maximum cognitive, psychosocial and emotional independence. Means of stimulation does not affect intracranial pressure adversely. |

(Continued)

| Problem | Cause | Nursing action | Goal |
|---|---|---|---|
| | | Auditory stimulation:<br>  Voice.<br>  Talking.<br>  Radio.<br>  Tape recorder.<br>Tactile:<br>  Intentional touch.<br>  Ice.<br>Visual:<br>  Bright posters.<br>  Calendar.<br>  Clock.<br>  Magazines.<br>  Photographs.<br>Smell.<br>Taste.<br>Introduce activities gradually.<br>Recognise personal preferences – music, games.<br>Remember the importance of physical contact:<br>  Hold patient's hand.<br>  Touch limbs/trunk.<br>Encourage, teach the family means of stimulating patient:<br>  Talking.<br>  Reading.<br>  Playing games.<br>Offer positive re-inforcement and encouragement.<br>Record methods used to stimulate patient and responses. | |
| **Respiratory**<br>Potential for suffocating.<br>Inability to maintain own airway. | Accompanying facial injury:<br>  Le Fort's fracture.<br>Unconscious state. | Assess respiratory function.<br>Position patient correctly to prevent obstruction and aspiration.<br>Position pillow/s correctly.<br>Remove dentures.<br>Utilize oral airway when necessary | Patent airway. |

**Table 23.1** (*Continued*)

| Nursing diagnosis | Potential problems | Possible cause/s | Planned intervention | Expected outcome (linked to timeframe) |
|---|---|---|---|---|
| | Inability to cough, swallow or gag. | Unconscious state. | Nil per os.<br>Insert nasogastric tube.<br>Oropharyngeal suction when necessary.<br>Pulmonary toilet.<br>Test for cough, swallow and gag reflex. | Return of cough, swallow and gag reflex.<br>Prevention of aspiration. |
| | Aspiration of gastric contents. | Unconscious state. | Monitor:<br>  Respiratory function.<br>  Nausea, vomiting.<br>  Manifestation of paralytic ileus.<br>Avoid supine position unless intubated/tracheostomy tube in situ.<br>Test for cough, swallow and gag reflex prior to feeding.<br>Insert nasogastric tube for gastric decompression.<br>When patient starts feeding, remain with patient.<br>Allow patient to rest after feeds.<br>Raise head of bed to 30° after feeding.<br>Chest physiotherapy. | Avoidance of gastric aspiration. |
| Respiratory dysfunction. | Hypoxia.<br>Hypercarbia.<br>Respiratory insufficiency/failure. | Anaemia.<br>Atelectasis.<br>CNS dysfunction.<br>Chest trauma.<br>CN dysfunction.<br>Haemorrhage.<br>Pneumonia.<br>Pulmonary embolism.<br>Pulmonary oedema. | Monitor patient status hourly:<br>  Respiratory rate, rhythm, volume.<br>  Skin colour, perfusion, temperature.<br>  Signs of respiratory failure.<br>  Presence of cyanosis.<br>  Clinical features of deep vein thrombosis and pulmonary embolus.<br>  Auscultate chest bilaterally to detect aeration or obstruction.<br>Check results of investigations:<br>  Arterial blood gases.<br>  Chest x-ray.<br>Explain procedures, equipment and need for respiratory assistance to patient and family.<br>Administer drugs as ordered. | Normal respiratory rate and pattern.<br>Adequate alveolar ventilation and perfusion.<br>Arterial blood gas levels within patient's normal limits.<br>Normal arterial blood gas values:<br>  pH      7.36–7.44<br>  $pO_2$    10.0–13.0kPa<br>  $pCO_2$  4.5–6.0kPa<br>  SB      21–23 mEq/L<br>  BE      −1–+1 |

| Problem | | Intervention | Rationale |
|---|---|---|---|
| Problems related to endotracheal intubation/ tracheostomy. | Airway obstruction. Aspiration. Atelectasis. Haemorrhage. Pneumonia. | Assess respiratory function. Monitor: Signs and symptoms of respiratory distress. Vital signs. Document size of tube in situ. Keep tracheal dilator at bedside. Tape spare tubes (same size, one larger and one smaller) to head of bed. Keep suction equipment and resuscitator bag with appropriate connection at bedside. Suction tracheostomy frequently then less often as mucous decreases and according to chest sounds. Insert catheter – less deeply for tracheostomy than for intubation. Maintain aseptic technique during intervention. | Patent airway. Prevent increase in intracranial pressure, hypoxia and hypercarbia. No irritation of carina. Decrease coughing spasms and risk of mucosal damage. Absence of infection. |
| Crusting/thick secretions. | | Humidify inspired air. Irrigate tube with sterile saline solution (0. 5–1 ml) if secretions are thick. Remove and clean inner cannula (if present) 2–4 hourly using sterile technique. | Easily removable secretions. $\uparrow$ ICP |
| Dislodgement of tube. Tube not secured effectively. Restless patient. | | Secure tube with adhesive plaster, twill or umbilical tape. Use square knots, allow only 1 small finger's space between tape and patient's neck. Two people are needed to change tapes, especially with combative patient. Do not remove old ties until new ties are securely in place. Restrain patient as needed to prevent removal of tube. | Tube secured in situ. No $\uparrow$ICP from venous obstruction. |

*(Continued)*

**Table 23.1** (*Continued*)

| Nursing diagnosis | Potential problems | Possible cause/s | Planned intervention | Expected outcome (linked to timeframe) |
|---|---|---|---|---|
| | Stomal infection or peristomal skin breakdown. | Poor aseptic technique. | Observe stoma for erythema, exudate, odour and crusting lesions. Use sterile technique to suction and care for stoma. Cleanse stoma with hydrogen peroxide and sterile water 2–4 hourly and when necessary. Keep skin/stoma as dry as possible. Protect stoma edges. Change tapes as needed. Culture discharge/stoma. Notify physician. Apply antibiotic ointment as ordered. | Absence of stomal infection. |
| | Possible tracheal erosion | Tube movement. High pressure cuff. | Monitor tube shape and position. Prevent tube dislodgement. Avoid movement or tension on tube when suctioning, cleaning stoma or changing tapes. Keep cuff deflated when possible. Change tube weekly or according to hospital policy. | Absence of tracheal damage. Ability to resume upper airway ventilation following closure of tracheostomy. Prevention of tracheal stenosis. |
| | Respiratory distress | Atelectasis. Consolidation. Hyperventilation. Hypoventilation. Peri-operative sedation. Pneumonia. Pneumothorax. Tracheostomy leakage. | Check for airway obstruction. Keep resuscitator bag at bedside. Assess respiratory status. Assess patient for lower airway problems. Provide humidity with or without oxygen. Administer chest exercise therapy including percussion, vibration and postural drainage (if tolerated). | Adequate ventilation as measured by equal and adequate lung aeration. Absence of pulmonary congestion and increased respiratory effort. |

| | | | |
|---|---|---|---|
| Pneumonia. Pulmonary infection. | Bypass of normal filtering system. Repeated traumatic suctioning procedure. Breach of aseptic suctioning procedure. | Monitor vital signs 2–4 hourly for manifestations of pulmonary infection. Change humidification system and ventilator tubing daily and manual breathing bag every 3 days. Use sterile distilled water to fill nebuliser. Ensure suction apparatus at bedside. Employ aseptic suctioning technique. Perform frequent oral hygiene. Send tracheal aspirates if infection suspected. Change position of patient 2 hourly. Control hyperthermia. Prevent aspiration by: Careful attention during feeding. Inflating cuff prior to feeding. Checking position of nasogastric tube prior to feeding. Administer chest physiotherapy. Notify physician of abnormality. Administer medications as ordered. | Absence of clinical or radiological evidence of pneumonia or pulmonary infection. Afebrile patient. Chest clear. |
| Hypoxia. | Altered blood gas picture. | Monitor blood gas results 15–20 minutes after ventilation settings changed. Monitor for signs and symptoms of hypoxia. Check arterial PO$_2$ level. Notify physician. | Effective mechanical ventilation. Maintenance of ventilation perfusion ratio. Adequate oxygenation. |
| Hypoventilation. | Pneumothorax. Haemothorax. Atelectasis. Pneumonia. | Monitor: Respiratory rate ½–1 hourly. Blood gases. Ventilator settings. Breath sounds. Augment chest physiotherapy. Notify physician. | PCO$_2$ and PO$_2$ within normal limits. Full lung expansion. Prevention of atelectasis. |
| Hyperventilation. | Settings for mechanical ventilation. | Continue assisted or controlled ventilation. Monitor PCO$_2$ levels. Ensure adequate dead space. Administer carbogen as ordered. Administer medications (sedation) as ordered. | Maintain normal blood gases. |

*(Continued)*

**Table 23.1** (*Continued*)

| Nursing diagnosis | Potential problems | Possible cause/s | Planned intervention | Expected outcome (linked to timeframe) |
|---|---|---|---|---|
| | Oxygen toxicity. | Use of 100% $O_2$ for extended periods. | Monitor arterial blood gases. Progressively decrease $FO_2$ to below 0.5 within 24–48 hours of initiating mechanical ventilation. Institute other remedial measures (as ordered). | Maintain: pO₂ 10.0–13.0kPa pCO₂ 4.5–6.0kPa Absence of oxygen toxicity. Achieve adequate oxygenation. |
| | Transient hypertension | Increased intracranial pressure. PEEP. | Monitor BP, P, CVP and urine output. Notify physician. | Haemodynamic stability. |
| | Airway obstruction | Accidental extubation. Bronchospasm. Excessive accumulation of secretions. Improper position of endotracheal tube. Thick secretions. | Keep spare inhalation bag at bedside. Ensure proper positioning of tube. Insert oral airway if patient is biting or gumming the tube. Provide for patency of ventilator tubing. Auscultate lungs. Oropharyngeal and bronchial toilet 1–2 hourly and when necessary. Administer chest physiotherapy 2 hourly unless contra-indicated. Administer drugs as ordered. | Patency of airway. |
| | Tension pneumothorax. | Hyperventilation. | Monitor: Signs and symptoms of tension pneumothorax. Arterial blood gases. Chest x-ray results. Controlled use of mechanical ventilation. Assist with insertion of underwater chest drain if pneumothorax present. | Bi-lateral full lung expansion. |
| | Ventilator malfunction. | | Monitor ventilator 1–2 hourly: Functioning panel light indicators: Setting of alarm system. Correct ventilator settings. Delivery of correct oxygen concentration. Humidity, temperature. Tube attachments secure. Patency of tubes. Presence of air leaks. | Maximum ventilator function. Ventilator delivers required volume of humidified oxygen. Emergency electricity supply. |

**Haemodynamic**

| Problem | Nursing action | Goal |
|---|---|---|
| Alteration in cardiac function. | Spare ventilator available<br>Manual ventilation in case of emergency<br>Adequate training of personnel in case of ventilator malfunction. | |
| Decreased cardiac output:<br>Shock.<br>Hypotension<br>Cardiac contusion. | Seek cause.<br>Emergency apparatus on hand.<br>Monitor:<br>Vital signs 1–4 hourly.<br>Blood pressure.<br>Pulse.<br>Respiration.<br>Temperature.<br>Urine output.<br>Hgb and Hct values.<br>Monitor cardiac function:<br>PCWP, CVP, radial line.<br>Note ECG pattern.<br>Monitor clotting profile.<br>Note extracranial injuries.<br>Arrest bleeding.<br>Administer fluid as ordered.<br>Administer medications as ordered. | Adequate cardiac output.<br>Haemodynamic stability.<br>Maintain:<br>CPP > 50 mm Hg.<br>Mean arterial blood pressure<br>>50 mm Hg.<br>(N = 70–80 mm Hg)<br>CVP = 5–15 cm H2O.<br>PCWP = 6 mm Hg<br>Sinus rhythm on ECG.<br>Absence of shock. |
| Haemorrhage.<br>Associated extracranial injury.<br>Polytrauma. | Comprehensive assessment of all body systems.<br>Resuscitate patient.<br>Monitor patient initially every 15–60 minutes for signs and symptoms of multiple trauma/haemorrhage:<br>Haematuria, limb swelling, fracture, abdominal distension, changes in vital signs, urine output.<br>Notify physician of signs and symptoms of haemorrhage.<br>Cross match blood type, check Hb, PCV, Hct.<br>Monitor and record fluid balance.<br>Administer blood, blood products as ordered by physician. | Absence/early detection of haemorrhage/extracranial injury.<br>Normal urine output.<br>Prevention of acute renal failure. |

*(Continued)*

**Table 23.1** (*Continued*)

| Nursing diagnosis | Potential problems | Possible cause/s | Planned intervention | Expected outcome (linked to timeframe) |
|---|---|---|---|---|
| | | | Administer medications and treatment as ordered by physician. | |
| | | | Check acid-base and electrolyte balance. | |
| | | | Assist physician to insert central venous pressure line, radial artery cannula. | |
| | | | Prepare patient for investigation/operative procedure. | |
| | | | Reassure patient and family. | |
| | Gastro-intestinal bleeding related to: Curling's ulcer. | Associated injury. Steroid administration. Stress. CNS factors. | Monitor and record: Neurological status, vital signs. Signs and symptoms of gastric irritation – vomiting, pain anorexia, indigestion, haematemesis. Test nasogastric aspirate/emesis for presence of blood. Test stools for blood 3 x per week. Administer medications as ordered: Antacid. Administer milk as ordered. Decrease patient anxiety. Notify physician if any abnormality occurs. | Absence or early detection of gastro-intestinal bleeding. |
| **Communication** Impaired communication. | Inability of patient to communicate: Verbally: Aphasia. Dysarthria. Dysphasia. Intubated. Tracheostomy. Ventilation. Non-verbally. | TBI Speech deficit. | Avoid discussing diagnosis/prognosis over bedside. Assess and record level of consciousness. Develop effective nurse–patient relationship. Speak to patient. Explain procedures and treatment. Provide reassurance and support. Anticipate needs of patient. Establish and document means of communication: Provide: Call bell. Magic slate, pencil and paper if patient able to write. Communication board if patient is aphasic. Evaluate effectiveness of alternative means of communication. | Patient can communicate his/her needs to carers/family in manner appropriate to patient's level of consciousness and conceptual development. |

| Problem | Related factors | Nursing intervention | Goal |
|---|---|---|---|
| **Psychological/Cognitive** | | Obtain referral to SALT. | |
| Anxiety. | Patient/family anxiety. | Implement programme as indicated by SALT. | |
| Fear. | Actual injury. | Note and record patient's response and progress to therapy. | |
| Grieving. | Alteration in patient appearance. | Clinical nurse specialist/primary nurse to undertake patient/family counselling and support. | Reduction of anxiety with provision of sufficient information, explanation and encouragement. |
| | Behaviour problems. | Involve health team members. | Patient/family able to: |
| | Condition of patient. | Establish therapeutic relationship. | Discuss concerns |
| | Inability to communicate. | Establish rapport with patient and family. | Function appropriately. |
| | | Assess anxiety level of patient/family. | Support one another. |
| | | Encourage verbalisation of patient's/family's fears, anxieties, questions and reactions. | |
| Knowledge deficit. | Neurological deficit. | Provide realistic information. | Ability to establish realistic goals. |
| | Patient care required. | Answer questions realistically. | Sufficient information provided. |
| | Mechanical ventilation. | Explain at level of patient's/family's understanding. | Adequate ability to provide home health care or acceptance of discharge of patient to another institution. |
| | Progress. | Explain 'head injury' to patient/family: | |
| | Recovery. | Clinical appearance. | |
| | Sequalae of head injury. | Monitoring. | |
| | Patient's family may have insufficient information regarding patient's condition. | Investigations. | |
| | To provide home health care. | Pathology. | |
| | Regarding discharge planning, prognosis and recovery. | Recovery. | |
| | | Stages. | |
| | | Status. | |
| | | Treatment. | |
| | | Provide on-going explanation frequently and simply. | |
| | | Support family in dealing with the stages of head injury. | |
| | | Assist to accept the reality of the situation. | |
| | | Commence patient/family teaching as early as possible. | |
| | | Offer encouragement and support. | |
| | | Assess teaching/learning needs of patient and family. | |
| | | Assess family's/patient's readiness to learn. | |

*(Continued)*

**Table 23.1** (*Continued*)

| Nursing diagnosis | Potential problems | Possible cause/s | Planned intervention | Expected outcome (linked to timeframe) |
|---|---|---|---|---|
| | | | Begin teaching skills for home care slowly. | |
| | | | Motivate patient and family to learn. | |
| | | | Teach family about 'head injury' stages, after care/ prognosis. | |
| | | | Allow time to explain to patient's family. | |
| | | | Assess patient/family ability to carry out home health care. | |
| | | | Explain alternate forms of care for patient. | |
| | | | Make appropriate referrals. | |
| | | | Demonstrate use of aids/techniques. | |
| | | | Evaluate patient's ability to use aids/techniques. | |
| Behavioural disorders. | Aggression. Frustration. Manipulation. Non-compliance. | TBI | Early intervention of a neuropsychologist. | Normal acceptable behaviour patterns. |
| | | | Maintain an environment conducive to psycho-emotional wellbeing. | Resolution/modification of abnormal behaviour patterns. |
| | | | Early mobilisation. | |
| | | | Remain calm and tranquil. | |
| | | | Not to be offended by swearing/shouting. | |
| | | | Show patience/tolerance with patient. | |
| | | | Allow patient to verbalise feelings. | |
| | | | Assess functional level, cognitive ability/frustration/ aggression. | |
| | | | Seek cause of frustration/aggression. | |
| | | | Explain phase to patient/family. | |
| | | | Support patient/family through phase. | |
| | | | Counsel patient and family: Individual and group therapy. | |
| | | | Assist patient to adjust/accept limitations. | |
| | | | Apply appropriate discipline to patient. | |
| | | | Institute programme of behaviour modification. | |
| | | | Re-inforce good behaviour. | |
| | | | Stimulate positive outlook. | |
| | | | Encourage perseverance with tasks causing problems. | |
| | | | Administer medications as ordered. | |
| | | | Record and report alteration in behaviour patterns. | |

| Impaired thought processes. | Decreased intellectual ability. Lack of insight/reasoning. Poor assimilation of facts. | TBI | Maximise intellectual ability. | Early intervention of a neuropsychologist. Maintain an environment conducive to psycho emotional well-being. Assess and record patient's ability to comprehend. Talk to patient at his/her level. Assess patient's ability to understand injury. Institute educational programme gradually. Improve learning ability. Refer for individual/group therapy. |
|---|---|---|---|---|
| Cognitive alteration. | Altered: Attention. Memory. Mentation. Power of concentration. Reading and writing skills. | TBI. | Maximise cognitive functioning. | Provided intracranial pressure is within normal limits, active motivation and stimulation of the patient is imperative. Refer patient to neuropsychologist and other health services for evaluation of cognitive ability. Collaborate with health team and institute a programme of cognitive retraining as soon after the injury as possible. Re-orientate to time, place and person. Utilise techniques to improve memory, concentration, reading and writing ability. Employ individual and group therapy. Relieve anxiety and fear. Counselling. Cognitive remediation. Individual psychotherapy. Group psychotherapy. Behaviour modification. Cognitive behaviour therapy. Improve body image, self-concept, feeling of worth, self-confidence and self-esteem. SALT. Remedial reading, writing and arithmetic. Improve memory. Effective interpersonal relationships and communication. |

(Continued)

**Table 23.1** (*Continued*)

| Nursing diagnosis | Potential problems | Possible cause/s | Planned intervention | Expected outcome (linked to timeframe) |
|---|---|---|---|---|
| | | | Expect that the patient has learning potential. | |
| | | | Incorporate all five senses. | |
| | | | Make the information to be learned meaningful: | |
| | | | Show how teaching and learning relate to real-life situations. | |
| | | | Combine demonstration and explanation. | |
| | | | Allow time for a response. | |
| | | | Proceed from the simple to the complex. | |
| | | | Present information in small logical steps. | |
| | | | Introduce graded series of perceptual motor tasks. | |
| | | | Teach components separately rather than collectively. | |
| | | | Use over-learning in the past to benefit the patient's present situation. | |
| | | | Provide repetition and rehearsal. | |
| | | | Use cues and memory aids. | |
| | | | Provide positive feedback. | |
| | | | Reward positive behaviour. | |
| | | | Recognise achievement. | |
| Alteration in self- concept. | Altered self-image. Decreased self-esteem. Altered personality. | TBI | Assess patient's self-concept. | Maintain self-esteem. Belief in self-worth. |
| | | | Encourage verbalisation. | |
| | | | Encourage and reinforce self-care. | |
| | | | Accept patient. | |
| | | | Institute measures to encourage/maintain positive outlook. | |
| | | | Assist client to adapt self-image. | |
| | | | Behaviour modification. | |
| | | | Offer positive reinforcement. | |
| | | | Avoid negative criticism and judgement. | |
| | | | Encourage, support and counsel patient and family. | |
| | | | Obtain referral to social services and neuropsychological services. | |
| | | | Create job/educational opportunities. | |

| | | | |
|---|---|---|---|
| Alteration in parenting. Role alteration. | TBI. Cognitive deficits. | Assess and note family structure. Involve significant others in patient management and rehabilitation. Encourage verbalisation by patient/family/siblings. Allow patient to achieve maximal independence. Encourage patient and family to accept/adjust to new family patterning. Patient and family counselling. | Stable family environment. Stable support system. |
| Maladaptive coping pattern. | Cognitive/ psychological/ emotional deficits. Related to: Decreased intellect. Immaturity. Non-acceptance of injury. Personality/ behaviour pattern altered. | Assess intellectual level. Plan programme at patient's intellectual level. Support and counsel patient and family. Behaviour modification. Utilise system of token economy. | Adequate coping. |
| **Thermoregulation** Alteration in thermoregulation. | TBI. Alteration in metabolic functioning. Hyperthermia. Blood in CSF. Hypothalamic disturbance. Infection. | Monitor and record neurological status and vital signs including temperature hourly. Seek cause of hyperthermia. Prevent temperature elevation of 40°C. Attempt to reduce temperature: Tepid sponge. Wet sheet. Wet sheet and fan (do not direct fan at patient). Ice packs. Cold bath. Record methods used to control temperature. Administer medication as prescribed: Salicylic acid. NSAIDs Largactil. Ensure sufficient nutrition and adequate fluid intake. Measure and chart intake and output. Notify physician of elevation of temperature. Reassure and support patient and family. | Absence or resolution of temperature. Normothermia (37°C). Temperature reduction. Cease shivering. |

(*Continued*)

**Table 23.1** (*Continued*)

| Nursing diagnosis | Potential problems | Possible cause/s | Planned intervention | Expected outcome (linked to timeframe) |
|---|---|---|---|---|
| **Comfort** Alteration in comfort. | Decubitus ulcers. Depression. Discomfort. Extracranial injuries. Incontinence. Irritability. Pain. Poor body alignment. | GCS < 13/15 Cognitive deficit | Allow for sleep and rest. Monitor restlessness. Ensure head not twisted. Utilize bed accessories to maximise comfort. Keep patient clean and dry. Ensure bed is crease and crumb free. Turn and position patient 2–3 hourly. Position pillows correctly. Support limbs when positioning. Reassure and support patient. Record signs of discomfort. Administer analgesia if ordered. | Comfort of patient. Minimum discomfort of patient. |
| **Fluids** Inability to maintain body fluids | Fluid volume alteration | Dehydration. Diabetes insipidus. Electrolyte imbalance. Overhydration. Sodium and water retention from overproduction of aldosterone. Use of osmotic diuretic agents. | Humidify inspired oxygen. Prevent hyperthermia. Administer fluids according to physician's prescription. Calculate and replace fluid and electrolyte requirements daily according to the needs of the patient. Ensure patient receives prescribed fluid and electrolyte requirements. Monitor: Neurological status. Vital signs and CVP. Signs of dehydration/overhydration. Monitor and record all intake and output 1–6 hourly. Administer fluids via enteral or parenteral routes. Administer medications as ordered by physician: Mannitol. Furosemide. | Maintain body fluid homeostasis. Fluid intake ± 1500 mls/24 hours. Fluid output ± 1500 mls/24 hours. Maximum therapeutic effect. Maintain electrolyte balance. Potassium (3.5–5.0 mEq/L) Sodium (135–145 mEq/L) Calcium (3.5–5.0 mEq/L) |

| Nursing diagnosis | Related factors | Nursing interventions | Expected outcomes |
|---|---|---|---|
| | | Electrolytes. Monitor effects and side effects. Monitor serum electrolytes as needed 6 hourly/daily/weekly. Monitor haemoglobin and haematocrit. | Maintain normal haemoglobin and haematocrit. Normal Hgb: male 13–16 gm/100 ml female 12–14 gm/100 ml Haematocrit: male 42–50% female 40–58% |
| | | Monitor serum glucose level. | Normal serum glucose: 3.9 to 5.5 mmol/L |
| | | Monitor serum osmolality. Test all urine output (as ordered). Test urine specimens for Specific Gravity. Notify physician of any fluid or electrolyte imbalance. | Normal urine output: ±30 ml/hour SG 1010–1025. |
| Fluid volume deficit. | Inadequate fluid intake. Inadequate humidification of inspired air. Diabetes insipidus. | Assess level of patient's hydration. Assist with insertion of CVP. Calculate fluid requirement of patient. Humidify inspired air. Measure and chart all intake and output. | Adequate hydration. Easily suctioned secretions. Moist mucus membrane. Good skin turgor. |
| Diabetes insipidus. | TBI. | Measure and chart intake and output hourly. Test all urine specimens for Se (±1001). Monitor for signs and symptoms of dehydration. Maintain normal serum sodium. Notify physician. Administer PFDP or Pitressin as ordered. | Prevent/detect/treat as early as possible. SG 1010–1025. |

*(Continued)*

**Table 23.1** (*Continued*)

| Nursing diagnosis | Potential problems | Possible cause/s | Planned intervention | Expected outcome (linked to timeframe) |
|---|---|---|---|---|
| **Nutrition** | | | | |
| Nutritional alteration | Impairment of digestion. Poor nutritional state. Malnutrition. | Anorexia. Difficulty in swallowing: CNS cause. Tracheostomy tube. Presence of nasogastric tube. Extracranial injuries. Hypercatabolism. Hyperthermia. Inadequate caloric intake. Inability to digest food. Negative nitrogen balance. Nil per mouth. Paralytic ileus. Prolonged stay in hospital. Unconscious state. Vomiting. | Calculate and record patient's daily kilojoule requirements (2500–5000 cals/24 hours – acute phase). Counteract hypercatabolism and negative nitrogen balance. Establish means of feeding patient: Enteral feeding: oral or nasogastric tube. Parenteral hyperalimentation. Offer mouthwash and cloth prior to and after meals. Offer nourishment as ordered. Make food and meal times as appetising as possible. Encourage patient to take meals. Assist with feeding. Monitor serum glucose level. Monitor Hct and Hgb. Weigh patient daily (if possible) and notify physician if there is any significant weight loss (>1 kg/24 hrs in adults). Administer vitamins and electrolytes as ordered. Measure and chart patient intake. | Adequate nutritional status. Appropriate weight gain. Adequate subcutaneous fat. Adequate wound healing. Normal haemoglobin level. Appropriate BMI. |
| | Hyperglycaemia related to: Hyperalimentation. Shock. Glucose metabolism. | TBI. | Monitor and record kilojoule and fluid intake. Control hyperalimentation. Check serum glucose levels. Monitor urine output. Test urine specimens for glucose and ketones. Administer medication as ordered: Insulin. Prevent hyper/hypoglycaemia. Notify physician. | Blood glucose levels within normal limits (3.9 to 5.5 mmol/L) |

**Elimination**

| | | | | |
|---|---|---|---|---|
| Impairment of kidney function. | Decreased urine output. | Acute renal failure. CNS dysfunction. Dehydration. Hypertension. Renal calculi (prolonged bedrest). Trauma to bladder, kidney at time of injury. Unconscious state. Urinary tract infection. Use of medications. | Monitor and record vital signs. Monitor and record fluid intake and output 1–6 hourly. Prevent renal failure with early resuscitation and rehydration of trauma patient. Prevent dehydration from occurring by administering fluids as prescribed. Calculate requirements on daily basis. Monitor laboratory studies for indices of renal function. Ensure adequate means of urinary elimination. Test urine specimens. Perform Specific Gravity. Administer medications as prescribed. Avoid nephrotoxic drugs. Prepare patient and assist with diagnostic/operative procedures: Intravenous pyelogram. Suprapubic urostomy. | Normal urinary output. (>0.5 ml/kg/hr for adult). Absence of renal failure. Kidney function within normal limit. Values within normal limits. Uric acid. 1–6 mg/100 ml. Serum creatinine. 1–2 mg/100 ml. Urea. 10–20 mg/100 ml. |
| Impairment of urinary elimination. | Incontinence. Retention of urine: Unconscious state. Urinary obstruction. | GCS < 13/15. | Measure and chart urine output 1–6 hourly. Ensure patient is clean and dry at all times. Establish route for urinary elimination: Urinary catheter. Condom/sheath drainage. Perform catheter/condom care 1–6 hourly and when necessary. Maintain aseptic technique during urogenital care. Secure catheter: Inner thigh in female. Laterally to the thigh or to the abdomen in males. Explain means of urinary elimination to patient and family. Restrain patient if necessary. | Adequate urinary elimination. Absence of urinary incontinence. Absence of compression of peri-scrotal angle. Absence of injury to urethra by inadvertent removal of catheter. |

*(Continued)*

**Table 23.1** (*Continued*)

| Nursing diagnosis | Potential problems | Possible cause/s | Planned intervention | Expected outcome (linked to timeframe) |
|---|---|---|---|---|
| Alteration in bowel elimination. | Paralytic ileus. | Shock. | Assess and record patient's ability to digest. | Resolution of paralytic ileus. |
| | | | Monitor and record bowel sounds and passage of flatus. | |
| | | | Insert nasogastric tube. | |
| | | | Commence intravenous therapy. | |
| | | | Commence enteral feeding once bowel sounds have been noted, gastric balance (<150 mls) and graded fluids have been implemented. | |
| | | | Measure and chart intake and output 1–2 hourly. | |
| | Diarrhoea. | Bed rest. | Monitor bowel actions daily. | Adequate bowel action. |
| | Constipation. | Medication. | Commence bowel retraining programme as soon as possible. | Absence of diarrhoea. |
| | Impacted faeces. | Enteral feeds. | Encourage mobility as soon as possible. | Avoid constipation. |
| | | | Ensure balanced nutritional food, fluid and electrolyte intake. | Absence of anal/buttock excoriation. |
| | | | Avoid pure sugar feeds. | Resolution of diarrhoea. |
| | | | Avoid straining at stool. | |
| | | | Increase roughage intake. | |
| | | | Perform abdominal massage as means of bowel stimulation. | |
| | | | Avoid manual removal if possible. | |
| | | | Ensure patient clean, dry and comfortable at all times. | |
| | | | Apply barrier cream. | |
| | | | Test stools for occult blood. | |
| | | | Administer medications as ordered: Bulk binders, laxatives, aperients. Codeine Phosphate. | |
| | | | Send specimen for culture and sensitivity if infection suspected. | |
| | | | Notify physician of change in bowel habits. | |

**Hygiene**

| | | | | |
|---|---|---|---|---|
| Alteration in self-care activities. | Inability to maintain general body hygiene. Lack of cleanliness. Offensive body odour. | Head injury GCS < 13/15 Cognitive deficit. Physical deficit. | Comprehensive assessment of the patient by the multidisciplinary team. Set up prophylactic protocol to prevent contractures, malnutrition, skin breakdown, respiratory and urinary tract infections, deep vein thrombosis and sensory deprivation. Encourage independence in all aspects of self-care. Assist the patience to achieve maximum independence in activities of living. Physical conditioning to increase strength and range of motion. Training/instruction in self-care techniques. Use of assistive devices. Use of adaptive equipment. Assess and record the patient's ability to wash. Encourage, assist and teach patient to wash. Bath the patient in bed daily if unable to mobilise. Use mechanical lift to mobilise patient. Mobilise to bathroom if possible by ±10 days. Shave patient as required. Clean hair once per week. Clean nails when necessary. Refer patient to specialist services: Physiotherapist. Occupational therapist. Podiatrist. Hairdresser. | Independence/minimal dependence in self-care activities. Socially acceptable. Maintenance of own body hygiene. Improve patient appearance. |

(*Continued*)

**Table 23.1** (*Continued*)

| Nursing diagnosis | Potential problems | Possible cause/s | Planned intervention | Expected outcome (linked to timeframe) |
|---|---|---|---|---|
| | Inadequate eye hygiene:<br>Blindness.<br>Corneal ulceration.<br>Drying of cornea.<br>Infection.<br>Keratitis. | Head injury.<br>GCS < 13/15.<br>Cognitive deficit.<br>Decreased tear production.<br>Loss of blink reflex.<br>Ptosis of upper lid. | Assess and record patient's ability to produce tears/ clean/ close/open/ blink eyes.<br>Examine eyes at frequent intervals for early signs of irritation and inflammation.<br>Position patient's head correctly.<br>Protect eyes from injury and corneal irritation.<br>Explain eye cleaning procedure to patient.<br>Maintain aseptic technique.<br>Swab eyes with saline 2–4 hourly.<br>Administer medication as ordered.<br>Instil Chloramphenicol drops 4 times per day and at night.<br>Lubricate eyes 2–4 hourly using:<br>Methyl-cellulose, mineral oil or liquifilm tears.<br>Tape eyes if patient not blinking.<br>DO NOT PAD EYES.<br>Notify physician of any signs of infection, ulceration, swelling, oedema. | Patient accepts responsibility to perform own eye hygiene.<br>Maintains integrity of eyes.<br>Eyes free of complications. |
| | Inadequate oral hygiene:<br>Anorexia.<br>Dental care.<br>Dirty mouth.<br>Discomfort.<br>Gastritis.<br>Gingivitis.<br>Halitosis.<br>Stomatitis. | Confused state.<br>Endotracheal intubation.<br>Multiple trauma.<br>Nil per os.<br>Unconscious state.<br>Use of mechanical ventilation.<br>GCS < 13/15.<br>Cognitive deficit. | Assess state of patient's oropharynx.<br>Assess and record patient's ability to clean own mouth.<br>According to condition of mouth, use:<br>Dirty mouth:<br>Glycerine thymol solution.<br>Hydrogen peroxide 1:4.<br>Dry mouth:<br>Lemon juice.<br>Explain procedure to patient.<br>Try and obtain patient's co-operation.<br>Assist and encourage patient to clean own mouth.<br>Perform oropharyngeal care 2–4 hourly.<br>Maintain surgically clean technique.<br>A mouth gag or wooden peg may be required.<br>Do not injure patient. | Clean mouth.<br>Patient able to perform and accept responsibility for own oropharyngeal hygiene. |

| Problem | Cause | Nursing intervention | Expected outcome |
|---|---|---|---|
| | | Moisten lips. Brush teeth and rinse twice daily. Clean teeth. Clean dentures twice daily. Perform oropharyngeal suctioning utilising an oral airway. Protect mouth corners from injury. Report and record any mouth lesions. | |
| | Inadequate nasal care: Nasal infection. Nasal ulceration. GCS < 13/15. Cognitive deficit. | Observe nose for signs and symptoms of infection or ulceration. Perform nasal care 4 hourly. Maintain surgically clean technique. Secure nasogastric tube to forehead. Check position 4 hourly. Avoid traction on nares. Change nasogastric tube once per week. | Absence of injury to nose. |
| **Skin integrity** Impairment of skin integrity. | Abrasions, Lacerations. Wound. Actual injury. Surgical intervention. Therapeutic sites. GCS < 13/15. Cognitive deficit. | Assess patient for presence of bruises, haematomas, abrasions and lacerations. Monitor patient for signs and symptoms of wound infection or wound drainage. Debride and/or cleanse wounds using aseptic technique. Insert sutures if required. Re-apply dressing as ordered. Remove sutures as ordered: Scalp wound 3–5 days. Body wound 7–10 days. Administer medication as ordered – vitamins, antibiotics, drying agents. Notify physician of change in patient status. | Adequate healing of wounds. Abrasions free of infection. |

*(Continued)*

**Table 23.1** *(Continued)*

| Nursing diagnosis | Potential problems | Possible cause/s | Planned intervention | Expected outcome (linked to timeframe) |
|---|---|---|---|---|
| | Decubitus ulcers | GCS < 13/15. Cognitive deficit. Restlessness. Lack of movement. Abnormal movement. | Assess and record skin integrity, circulation and potential pressure sites 2 hourly. Mobilise patient as soon as possible. Employ at least 2 staff to turn/lift/position patient 2 hourly. Use: Bed accessories. Cradles. Mechanical lift to alter patient's position. Mechanically mobile bed. Correct mattress. Sheep skin. Ensure patient clean and dry and bed free of creases. Avoid friction. Protect the skin from moisture and injury: • Harden the skin by regular application of spirits. • Nurse's nails must be short. • Prompt cleaning of incontinent patient imperative. • Protect patient from self-injury on bedrails/bed end. • Ensure adequate hydration and nutrition of patient. If a decubitus ulcer is present: Keep dry. Monitor for signs of infection. Use aseptic technique to dress decubitus ulcer. Record and report presence of decubitus ulcer. | Integrity of skin maintained. Absence of decubitus ulcers. Resolution of decubitus ulcer. |
| | Tetanus. | Infected wound Lack of immunisation | Clean wound thoroughly. Check whether patient requires anti-tetanus prophylaxis. Record the administration of anti-tetanus prophylaxis. Discharge planning regarding subsequent regimen for tetanus prophylaxis. | Prevention of tetanus. |

| | | | | |
|---|---|---|---|---|
| **Dressing**<br>Altered ability to clothe himself/herself:<br>• Dressing.<br>• Putting on trousers.<br>• Doing up laces. | Inability to clothe himself/herself. | Head injury.<br>GCS<13/15.<br>Cognitive deficit. | 1 Assess and record patient's ability to clothe himself/herself.<br>2 Encourage, assist and teach patient to clothe himself/herself.<br>3 Show patience with patient.<br>4 Dress patient in own clothes. | Independence in dressing. |
| | Unable to reach area.<br>Unable to use arms/legs effectively.<br>Unable to select appropriate clothes for outside temperature. | TBI.<br>Hemiplegia.<br>Hemiparesis.<br>Poor posture.<br>Spasticity.<br>Decreased mobility. | Patient to be safe during dressing.<br>Colour co-ordinate clothes with labels.<br>Use clothes with Velcro fasteners/zips.<br>Allow patient to select clothes.<br>Facilitate patient to dress independently.<br>Teach appropriate dressing technique:<br>Start with affected limb/side first.<br>Encourage independence with dressing.<br>May need to sit when dressing.<br>Use aids for dressing.<br>Refer to OT, physiotherapist as required. | Patient able to dress independently. |
| **Mobility**<br>Impairment of mobility. | Contractures.<br>Foot drop.<br>Muscle wasting.<br>Renal calculi.<br>Spasticity. | CNS dysfunction.<br>Hemiplegia.<br>Decreased motivation.<br>Depression.<br>Increased muscle tone.<br>Poor positioning.<br>Unconscious state.<br>Cognitive deficit. | Assess and record patient's ability to mobilise.<br>Involve physiotherapist and occupational therapist as soon after admission as possible.<br>Active and passive exercises and breathing.<br>Mobilisation, development of seating, standing and balance.<br>Initiate a programme of graded exercise on admission.<br>Encourage mobilisation of patient as early as possible – up in bath and chair.<br>Use aids to mobility:<br>Walker.<br>Utilise bed accessories:<br>Bed cradle.<br>Foot board.<br>Monkey chain.<br>Correct Mattress.<br>Sheep skin.<br>Tilt table.<br>Use mechanically mobile bed and lift to alter position of patient. | Restore fitness, motivation and elevate mood.<br>Absence of complications of mobility.<br>Maximum mobilisation and independence.<br>Promote mobilisation and prevent contractures. |

*(Continued)*

**Table 23.1** (*Continued*)

| Nursing diagnosis | Potential problems | Possible cause/s | Planned intervention | Expected outcome (linked to timeframe) |
|---|---|---|---|---|
| | | | Teach patient/family about mobilisation and limb exercises. Perform passive range of motion exercises to arms and legs 2–4 hourly if patient at bed rest. Put all limbs through range of movements 2–4 times a day. Encourage active limb exercises as soon as possible. Position and turn patient 2 hourly. Place footboard at end of bed. Posture limbs in good alignment in optimal position of maximum function. Avoid pressure or trauma to calves. Maintain body alignment by use of pillows/splints. Apply splints correctly. Remove and re-apply 4 hourly, as instructed. Protect patient from superficial nerve injury. Apply ice packs to decrease muscle tone. Administer medication as ordered: Nitrazepam. Botox. Ensure adequate nutrition, fluid and electrolyte balance. Monitor and record: Intake and output. Signs and symptoms related to complication of immobility such as: Chest pain. Haemoptysis. Red skin. Shortened achilles tendon. Swollen calf. Re-assure and support patient. | Absence of deformity, contractures, footdrop. Absence of deep vein thrombosis. Decrease spasticity. |

| | | Show patience with patient. Sport and recreational activities. Remedial gymnastics. Notify physician staff of patient's status. | |
|---|---|---|---|
| Deep vein thrombosis. Pulmonary embolism. | Inadequate venous return. Incorrect positioning. Alteration in clotting factors. Bed rest. TBI. | Monitor and record: Vital signs. Manifestation of DVT and pulmonary embolism. Fluid and electrolyte balance. Perform range of motion exercises 2–4 hourly. Encourage mobility. Avoid trauma to calves. In susceptible patients use anti-embolic stockings. Perform chest physiotherapy and breathing exercises 2–4 hourly. Notify physician. Administer medication. | Prevention or early detection of deep veined thrombosis and pulmonary embolism. |
| Abrasions. Contractures. Ischaemia of limb. Nerve palsy. | Limitation of movement by restraints. | Check hospital policy regarding restraint. Decide on objective of restraint: Prevent patient from reaching nasogastric tube. Apply elbow splints. Apply body restrainer below level of chest and at the back, or use simple body jacket. Use padded leather wrist restrainer. NOTE: Bandaging: use reinforced padding and crepe bandage. If both bandages are secured to the same side of the bed, the patient will remain in the lateral position. To avoid permanent damage to limbs, exercise care in choice and application of restraints. Frequently re-evaluate need for restraint. Chart presence and type of restraint selected. Check 2–4 hourly for proper placement and effectiveness of restraint, skin integrity, circulation, discolouration and swelling. | Normal state of restrained limb. No injury from use of restrainer. Specific limitation of mobility. Prevent patient from jumping out of bed. Curb arm movements. Maximum immobility of part according to need. |

(*Continued*)

**Table 23.1** (*Continued*)

| Nursing diagnosis | Potential problems | Possible cause/s | Planned intervention | Expected outcome (linked to timeframe) |
|---|---|---|---|---|
| | | | Apply restraints to no more than three limbs at one time. | |
| | | | Restrain limb in position of maximum function. | |
| | | | Release, exercise extremity and re-apply 2–4 hourly. | |
| | | | Explain use of restraints to patient's family and friends. | |
| | | | Notify physician of occurrence of injury. | |
| | | | Injury/accident statement to be written, according to hospital policy. | |
| **Spiritual** Altered matters of spirituality. | Anger. Depression. Lack of interest. | TBI. | Recognise patient's religious beliefs. Call in services of religious minister, if requested by patient. | Maintenance of belief/faith. |
| **Social** Alteration in socialisation patterns. | Social isolation. | | Social rehabilitation of patient imperative. Assess social situation of patient. Assist patient to adjust to new lifestyle/altered living conditions/environment or family situation. Encourage active participation of friends and family in programme. Encourage and support patient through alteration in socialisation patterns. Encourage friends to visit patient. Positive re-inforcement. Behaviour modification. Individual/group therapy. Make referrals. Graded introduction to family, home and social environment Use of day programmes. Support group for patients and families. Encourage family to join social organisation: HEADWAY. Association for Disabled. | Social integration. Acceptable social behaviour. |

| Patient problem | Related to | Nursing action | Expected outcome |
|---|---|---|---|
| Impaired home management. | | Assess patient's ability to maintain home. Refer patient to social services, occupational therapist, building officer, neuropsychologist. | Adequate home management. |
| **Leisure/Recreation** Altered ability to undertake leisure and recreation. | Fatigue. Frustration. Boredom. | Assess patients ability to return to previous pursuits. Introduce recreational activities early in programme. Enable patient to join group for recreational activities whilst in unit. Facilitate patient to undertake therapeutic recreational activities. Maintain interest in leisure/recreation through magazines, books, TV. Arrange for patient to undertake activities. Teach patient new activities. Teach patient different ways of undertaking activities. Manage frustration/depression/anger in relation to activities undertaken. Refer to social worker, social clubs and voluntary organisations. | Return to previous leisure/recreation activities. Undertaking new leisure/recreation activities. Within 12 months post-head injury. |
| **Sexual** Sexual health needs. | TBI. Fatigue. Impotence. Vaginal dryness. Hypersexuality. | Encourage warm relationship with spouse/partner. Behaviour modification programme for overt sexual dysfunction. See Chapter 26. | 'Normal' sexual health needs and relationship with spouse/partner. |
| **Vocational/educational** Lack of vocational/educational advancement. | TBI. Physical deficits. Cognitive deficits. Intellectual deficits. Social behaviour. Incorrect placement. Loss of employment. Missed educational opportunities. Related to: Actual injury. Lack of motivation. | Vocational: Early contact and assessment of the patient is imperative. Early job assessment is essential. Early contact with the employer must be established. Correct placement of the patient, at the appropriate time in the rehabilitation programme, is essential. | Maximum independence in employment and education. |

*(Continued)*

**Table 23.1** (*Continued*)

| Nursing diagnosis | Potential problems | Possible cause/s | Planned intervention | Expected outcome (linked to timeframe) |
|---|---|---|---|---|
| | | | Assess functional level of patient and ability to return to employment/school. Encourage further learning. Adjust learning to level of patient. Improve cognitive skills. Esteem as well as independence must be increased. Provide adequate educational/vocational facilities. Provide further learning opportunities for patient. Utilise behaviour modification. Utilise hospital and community resources. Employ vocational rehabilitation officer and educational officer. Evaluate patient at regular intervals. Use a system of token rewards to stimulate production and promote appropriate behaviour. Evaluate progress at regular intervals. Education: Enable the clinical nurse specialist to teach, plan and evaluate patient education. Employ educational therapists. Use appropriate teaching strategies. Have educational facilities available. Memory and perception training are important aspects of education. Use teaching aids. Use blended learning. | |

**Rest/sleep**

| | | | |
|---|---|---|---|
| Altered rest and sleep. | Fatigue. Hyperactivity. Pain/discomfort. Depression. Recovery of function. Easily fatigued. | Encourage patient to use bedroom only for rest/sleep. Ensure environment is safe. Schedule activities to include rest and sleep. Pace patient activities. Allow sufficient time between activities. Encourage patient to be active during the day. Maintain restful environment. Ensure comfortable and supportive bed. Use relaxation techniques. Do not overstimulate before rest/sleep. Do not use medication to aid sleep unless other methods have failed. Avoid alcohol consumption. | |

**Other**

| | | | |
|---|---|---|---|
| Potential for infection. | Chest infection. Intracranial infection: Brain abscess. Encephalitis. Meningitis. Wound infection. Thrombophlebitis. Urinary tract infection. | Monitor and record neurological status and vital signs 1–2 hourly. Monitor and record: Wounds. IV sites. Signs and symptoms of infection/inflammation. Prevent precipitating factors: Pulmonary congestion/aspiration/urinary retention. Maintain aseptic technique for relevant procedures: Catheterisation. Tracheostomy care. Wound care. Monitor WBC levels. If infection present: Seek cause and site of infection. Institute measures to promote resolution of infection source. Obtain specimen for culture. Monitor wound culture results. Treat hyperthermia. Notify physician of any signs of infection. Administer medication/treatment as ordered. | Absence or resolution of infection. Normal value: WCC 3500 to 10500 cells/mcL (microlitre). |

# ACTIVITIES

## Activity 23.1

### Scenario

You are the Registered Nurse working in a unit. The patient, Mrs Jones, has had a closed head injury with a GCS 12/15. She is waking up slowly. Her husband informs you that he would like to make love to his wife. He asks if you could you please arrange for an intrauterine device to be inserted so that the next time he takes her home on weekend leave they can make love.

*How do you manage the situation?*

## Activity 23.2

### Scenario

You are the Registered Nurse working in a unit. The patient, Mrs Smith, 35 years old, has had a closed head injury with a GCS 12/15. She is due to go home on weekend leave. She has requested that she start the contraceptive pill in case 'something happens' and she does not want to fall pregnant.

*How do you manage the situation?*

## Activity 23.3

### Scenario

You are working as a Staff Nurse on the head injury unit. You have been asked to put up an intravenous line on a restless patient who has a head injury as his line has become dislodged. You know that you are not competent to insert an intravenous line.

*How do you manage the situation?*

## Activity 23.4

### Scenario

You are working on a busy head injury unit. You, and another staff nurse, have been allocated to care for six specific patients who are undergoing half hourly neuro-observations. The unit is very busy and you are behind with all the care that is required to be completed. You notice that the other Staff Nurse writes down the neurological observations without assessing the patient.

*How do you manage this situation?*

## Activity 23.5

### Scenario

You are looking after Mr Freesling, 32 years old. He has had a closed head injury and his current GCS is 12/15. Whilst you are working with him his wife arrives in the unit. She talks to him and asks him to sign some papers that she has brought with her. The papers relate to his finances and sale of a house.

*How do you manage the situation?*

## Activity 23.6

### Scenario

Mr Patel, 28 years old, has had a moderate head injury. He is very angry that 'we are keeping him in hospital' as he wants to go home. He says his wife can and will look after him. He will tell her what to do.

*How do you manage the situation?*

## Activity 23.7

### Scenario

Mr Naidoo, 30 years old, has had a severe head injury. He is improving slowly and his GCS is now 12/15. He has a gag, cough and swallow reflex and is on a nutritional regimen to introduce solid foods. You have been asked to observe him for any signs of aspiration.

*List these signs.*

## Activity 23.8

### Scenario

Mr Vosloo, 48 years old, has had a moderate head injury. The multidisciplinary team are planning for his discharge. He wants to be discharged to home but his wife is insistent that he must go to residential care as she will not be able to manage him at home. He still insists he wants to go home and is very angry with his wife as she 'does not want him'.

*How do you manage the situation?*

# Chapter 24
# Prognosis and Patient Outcome

*Zuhair Noori[1] and Nadine Abelson-Mitchell[2]*

[1]Croydon Healthcare Trust, London, UK
[2]School of Nursing and Midwifery, Faculty of Health, Education and Society, Plymouth University, Devon, UK

## INTRODUCTION

Along the patient's journey, it is essential to assess their progress. In order to ensure cost-effective and efficient evidence-based care, care needs to be outcome-based. Health professionals need to focus on the outcomes rather than on the process alone. Purchasers of healthcare and accrediting bodies now expect outcomes to be written in advance and the achieved outcomes compared to expected outcomes. Thereafter, if there are differences, these need to be justified (DH 2011c).

The long-term effects of traumatic brain injury can have serious detrimental effects on patients, families and society (Ackery *et al.* 2007; Langlois *et al.* 2006; McAllister *et al.* 2001; United States of America Department of Health and Human Services 1998). Of those with moderate head injuries, 63% remain disabled one year after the incident and 85% of those with severe head injuries. Of these, 79% suffer persistent headaches, 59% have memory problems and 34% of previously employed persons are still unemployed. Reports have indicated that '30% or more of patients, who are discharged from hospital in less than two days without apparent complications, have significant morbidity at three months' (BSRM 1998: p. 35–36). Gordon *et al.* (1995) show a significant correlation between age, type and severity of injury with good recovery rates in 55% of severely injured patients.

Mild injury can have long lasting sequelae such as cognitive deficits, deficits of memory, thought processing, concentration and judgement (Cassidy *et al.* 2004; Guerrero *et al.* 2000). Repeated head injury has a cumulative effect and leads to traumatic encephalopathy (Schulz *et al.* 2004).

People with moderate head injury often suffer residual physical, psychological, cognitive and behavioural symptoms.

Depending on the length of time in coma, patients with severe head injuries tend to have more serious physical deficits. The longer the coma and PTA, the poorer the outcome in terms of physical and social functioning (Annoni *et al.* 1992). Most patients with mild traumatic brain injury still harbour persistent troublesome symptoms one year thereafter. Those with minor injury (GCS 13–15) may have moderate to severe disability at 12 months (47%) with 33% never returning to work. For moderate injuries (GCS 9–12), 45% have moderate to severe disability. For severe injuries (GCS ≤8), 48% have moderate to severe disability and only 14% have a good outcome at 12 months (Thornhill *et al.* 2000).

## FACTORS PREDICTING PROGNOSIS AFTER HEAD INJURY

Many authors are in agreement regarding factors that may predict outcome after head injury.

These factors include:

- Pre-injury status is regarded as more important than injury severity (Novack *et al.* 2001).
- Pre-injury status, measures of working memory and cognitive flexibility in predicting functional independence (Hart *et al.* 2003).
- The timely and appropriate initial treatment of TBI.
- The severity of the brain injury as measured by the GCS (Lenartova *et al.* 2007).
- The GCS score is the best predictor for neuropsychological functioning (Lannoo *et al.* 2000).
- The duration of unconsciousness is as important as GCS.
- 'Time to command' is a more powerful predictor of outcome after severe brain injury than 'time to motor localization' (Whyte *et al.* 2001).
- Age: school age children and young adults (<45 years) achieve a better outcome than infants or older patients (>60 years) (Lenartova *et al.* 2007; Richmond *et al.* 2011). With regard to the GCS, age is the most important predictor (Lannoo *et al.* 2000).
- Lack of pupillary light reaction and dilatation reflect worse outcomes as these features are associated with brain swelling and herniation.
- Pupillary reactivity is the most important predictor for quality of life (Lannoo *et al.* 2000).
- Brain CT scan findings are a significant predictor of outcome in mild traumatic brain injury. Midline shift, mid-brain compression and vertical herniation of brain stem worsen the prognosis of severe TBI. The presence of either a midline shift greater than 5 mm or a subcortical contusion on acute CT scan is associated with a greater need for assistance with ambulation, ADLs and global supervision at rehabilitation from discharge. Patients with bilateral cortical contusions require more global supervision but no additional need for assistance with ambulation and ADLs (Englander *et al.* 2003).
- Intracranial bleeding, in particular epidural haematoma, subdural haematoma and subarachnoid bleeding worsen prognosis (Perel *et al.* 2009).
- Associated multiple trauma, musculo-skeletal or internal abdominal injury worsen outcome (Wenden *et al.* 1998).
- Hyperglycaemia post-TBI is related to poor outcomes and the use of mild hypothermia is related to better outcomes (Zhao *et al.* 2011: p. 311).
- Hypotension is related to poor outcomes (Lenartova *et al.* 2007).
- Worse prognosis for patients who have been assaulted (Wenden *et al.* 1998).

In general, poor prognostic factors include low GCS on admission, non-reactive pupil(s), older age, co-morbidity and CT scan findings, including midline shift (MRC CRASH trial collaborators 2008; Murray *et al.* 2007; Valadka *et al.* 2000). Factors such as ICP, blood glucose levels and CT scan findings, may assist in predicting mortality but not morbidity (Lannoo *et al.* 2000).

## OUTCOME MEASURES

The majority of outcome measures are professionally directed and there is no clear agreement as to how to measure outcome (BSRM 2008b; Rice-Oxley and Turner-Stokes 1999). As there are numerous types of measures to assess outcome, the BSRM have compiled a 'basket' of recommended measures (BSRM 2008b). Depending on the purpose of the assessment, it is important to select a valid and reliable measure that is able to detect changes in the patient's level of function. Whichever measure is selected, it is important to ensure that personnel are trained to use them correctly. The method of reporting, and analysis of the outcome measures, is also important.

Patient outcome may be measured with regard to the following:

- Functional outcome.
- Length of hospital stay (Cowen *et al.* 1995).
- Return to work.
- Quality of everyday life (Anderson and Burckhardt 1999).
- Programme delivery.

Examples of measures used within rehabilitation settings to measure outcome include:

- Glasgow Outcome Score (GOS) (Jennett and Bond 1975).
- Functional Independence Measure (FIM) (Granger *et al.* 1986).
- Functional Independence Measure + the Functional Assessment Measure (FIM + FAM) (Turner-Stokes *et al.* 1999b).
- Barthel ADL index (Mahoney and Barthel 1965; Wade and Collin 1988).
- Neurological Outcome Scale for Traumatic Brain Injury (NOS-TBI) (Wilde *et al.* 2010).

The FIM is the standard instrument utilised by the American rehabilitation industry and worldwide (Hoeman 2008). The FIM + FAM is commonly used in the UK to measure patient outcome (Barnes 1999; Turner-Stokes *et al.* 1999a; Turner-Stokes *et al.* 1999b). Turner-Stokes *et al.* (1999b) recommend that the FIM should be used as an interprofessional tool that includes at least three different disciplines.

## RETURN TO WORK

Return to work is used to determine outcome (Lippert-Grüner *et al.* 2002). Return to work and professional integration is determined by a number of factors including physical deficits, behaviour and speech deficits (Lippert-Grüner *et al.* 2002) as well as post-injury reading ability (Malec and Basford 1996).

After intensive rehabilitation the rate of return to work can vary from 60–80% (Malec and Basford 1996: p. 198). Return to work is possible if a patient-centred approach to assessment and placement, as well as specific strategies such as vocational guidance, counselling and on-the-job training, are used to enhance return to work (O'Brien 2007). Attending vocational rehabilitation is important as a predictor in determining vocational outcomes after neurotrauma (Johnstone *et al.* 2003). If a person is having difficulty obtaining gainful employment it may be beneficial for them to attend vocational rehabilitation services, where available, undertake voluntary work, take up alternative leisure activities or seek further education (Johnstone *et al.* 2003; McCabe *et al.* 2007). Lack of progress with return to work may lead to isolation and despair. Patients with a brain injury may be offered employment at a lower level, thus affecting their earning potential and job satisfaction.

There are numerous strategies that can be used to aid 'return to work' (see Chapter 23).

## QUALITY OF EVERYDAY LIFE

Instead of concentrating on recovery in terms of functional outcomes, outcomes that affect quality of everyday life should be considered (Johnston and Miklos 2002). Objective and subjective features enable the measurement to be more comprehensive and useful.

## CONCLUSION

In conclusion, maximising patient outcome is the goal of health management. The care received along the patient journey must enhance the final outcome. Delays in obtaining rehabilitative intervention affect final patient outcome (Andelic *et al.* 2012).

---

### Activity 24.1

**Scenario**

Kerry, a 20 year old student, has been in the unit for the last 2 months. She was admitted as a result of an unintentional drug overdose after going out clubbing. She is currently in a persistent vegetative state (GCS 3/15).

Her parents are convinced she is going to wake up shortly and are determined to take her home when she is ready to be discharged from hospital.

**Exercise**

1. Describe how you will manage this situation.

# Chapter 25
# Dying and Death

*Zuhair Noori[1] and Nadine Abelson-Mitchell[2]*

[1]Croydon Healthcare Trust, London, UK
[2]School of Nursing and Midwifery, Faculty of Health, Education and Society, Plymouth University, Devon, UK

## INTRODUCTION

TBI is a major cause of death in most developed nations and it continues to increase (Faul *et al.* 2010; Zink 2001). In mild TBI the fatality rate is 0.1% (Klauber *et al.* 1989), in severe TBI the fatality rate ranges from 30–50% (Greenwald *et al.* 2003) up to 90% (Peek-Asa *et al.* 2001). Patients who survive an accident present at major trauma centres, intubated and ventilated. Between the time of accident and arrival in the Emergency Department some develop brain failure due to progressive deterioration or inevitable complications, in spite of appropriate management (Moppet 2007).

An event that health professionals need to be able to discuss openly, when the need arises, is death. Experienced, trained staff, with clinical knowledge and ability, need to be able to discuss and communicate these issues clearly and empathetically (Spotlight 2010). Kubler-Ross's writings on death and bereavement will enable practitioners to understand the bereavement process in order to support families and carers at this time (Kubler-Ross and Kessler 2005).

There is much discussion regarding the withdrawal of treatment in patients with TBI in vegetative states (Grubb 1997; Pope John Paul II 2004). In cases of prolonged vegetative state of more than one year, and in the absence of an advanced directive, the issue of withdrawing the nutrition and hydration that is maintaining such life may be considered (Casarett *et al.* 2005). 'Many consider that indefinite survival in a vegetative state is of no benefit to the patient and that there is no moral or legal obligation to continue life-sustaining treatment, including artificial nutrition and hydration' (Jennett 2005: p. 537).

The implementation of standard palliative care policies and guidelines can prevent ethical conflicts and enhance the end-of-life care for patients with TBI in ICU (Royal College of Physicians, National Council for Palliative Care, British Society of Rehabilitation Medicine 2008). In these situations, recording the patient's management enhances clear communication and consistency in the care of patients whose management includes withdrawal of life support. Palliative care can be started straight away for patients in a permanent vegetative state. This care includes observation for signs of further recovery, the need for slow stream rehabilitation as well as musculoskeletal and cardio-respiratory passive fitness (Jennett 2002). There is a risk, albeit small, of applying criteria of a vegetative state to a patient and missing higher awareness states, such as minimal consciousness, which can result in regaining more awareness in the future (Andrews *et al.* 1996).

The above situation is in contrast to patients with intact cognitive cortical function who are confirmed to be conscious and alive, yet have no cortical physical function nor breathing. These patients are supported with artificial breathing for many years, for example as in locked-in-syndrome (Bauby 1997).

## THE FAMILY

Throughout the patient's end of life journey it is important to regularly inform the family about the situation, to involve them in decision-making and prepare them for the process of mourning, bereavement and counselling, if required. The decision protocols regarding the management of the patient, including the protocol for assessing brain death should be explained thoroughly. The family members require opportunities to question, consider, discuss and accept the injured person's predicament.

When brain death is suspected, it is necessary to share this with the family as soon as possible. Hope is important; false hope interferes with the mourning process and raises unrealistic expectations.

---

### Reflection

Whilst working in a neurosurgical head injury unit I was asked to see the mother of an 18 year old boy who had had a severe head injury. His GCS score was 3/15. He had been in the unit for two weeks and had not shown much improvement. At the interview, while discussing her son's progress, or lack thereof, the mother stated the following 'He would have been better off dead. Why don't you just leave him to die?' I was taken aback by her response and had to think quickly because this was the last thing that I was expecting. I asked her why she thought he would be better off dead. She stated 'this is not the son that I know. If I can't have him back like he was I'm not sure that I want him at all'. After a long discussion and in summary, my response was as follows: 'your son did not die in the accident. He is very much alive. At this stage, we cannot tell you what the outcome will be. All I know is that we will do all that is possible to ensure that he reaches his maximum potential, irrespective of what this level turns out to be.' It made me realise that early family counselling and communication is imperative, the little improvements that we notice need to be shared with the family. The family need to be involved from the outset in the patient's management. Every achievement needs to be praised in an attempt to maximise recovery and enable the family to come to terms with the situation.

---

## BRAIN DEATH

The team have to decide whether there is potential for recovery of brain function. If not, and brain death is confirmed using the appropriate protocol, the patient will be certified as being 'brain dead'. Certification of brain death may take place at the time of the accident, after admission to A&E, in an ICU situation or at a later stage. After a few days or weeks in ITU it may become clinically clear that there is evidence of brain death. When the clinical assessment indicates that brain death has occurred, a decision is taken to diagnose and confirm brain death. There is much debate regarding the definition and criteria for brain death (DuBois 2011; Miller and Truog 2009; Wijdicks *et al.* 2010).

Even in patients with brain death, certain functions such as hormonal control, temperature control, wound healing, the ability to fight infections and skin growth still continue (Halevy and Brody 1993; Miller and Truog 2009: p. 186). There is therefore argument over whether one can use the term 'whole brain failure' in these circumstances, and consideration that there is cessation of different brain functions at different times.

### Definition

Brain stem death is the 'irreversible loss of the capacity for consciousness, combined with irreversible loss of the capacity to breathe'. The irreversible cessation of brain stem function will produce this state and 'therefore brain stem death is equivalent to the death of the individual' (RCP 1995: pp. 381–382). When assessment of the brain stem reveals permanent loss of function interpreted as a loss of cortical function (cognitive function of awareness, communication, etc.) as well as autonomic vegetative function (breathing, awake–sleep cycles), a decision is taken to stop all artificial support of breathing and circulation. This state of loss of brain stem function is called 'brain stem death', which equates to traditional and legal death in spite of there being continuity of circulation (heart beating and blood pressure maintenance) and breathing through the agency of mechanical support only (Miller and Truog 2009; UKTransplant (No Date)). It is usually total brain failure (which includes the brain stem) that confirms brain death. Brain death is defined as '3 clinical findings necessary to confirm irreversible cessation of all functions of the entire brain including the brainstem: coma (with a known cause), absence of brainstem reflexes, and apnea' (Wijdicks *et al.* 2010: p. 1911). De Groot *et al.* (2010) stress the importance of not delaying the diagnosis of brain death.

## Background

Brain death raises legal, ethical and moral issues (Webb and Samuels 2011; Wijdicks *et al.* 2010). International guidelines have been developed (Miller and Truog 2009), aimed at protecting patients, enhancing public confidence and protecting healthcare professionals from misunderstanding and conflict of interest (Rodriguez-Arias *et al.* 2011). With regard to brain stem death there are variations in policies and procedures between different countries in Europe (Bell *et al.* 2004) and the USA (Jennett 2002; Miller and Truog 2009; Wijdicks *et al.* 2010).

## Assessment of brain death

The assessment includes brain stem death criteria, which in the UK are founded on clinical assessment rather than confirmatory investigation, of which the gold standard is cerebral angiography (Bell *et al.* 2004). The use of ancillary tests does not replace a good neurological examination and these tests are not really needed to confirm brain death unless there is some doubt (Wijdicks *et al.* 2010).

The brain stem death test guidelines have numerous components:

- Confirmation of the condition that has caused the brain stem death.
- Positive exclusion of confounding reversible factors.
- Identifying the professional who will undertake the test.
- Performing the test.
- Details of the test.
- Timing.

## Pre-requisites to confirming brain death

It is incumbent on the health professional team to ensure that the current state of the patient is due solely to the brain damage and not due to other correctable factors. The essence of brain stem death testing (BSDT) is to exclude other causes of unresponsiveness, such as reversible brain stem suspension of function, e.g. from extreme hypothermia, especially when the accident has occurred during winter and there is the possibility of periods of long exposure to cold, severe intoxication with alcohol, recreational or other drugs such as sedatives, depressants or muscle relaxants at any time in the management plan, as well as severe disturbance of electrolyte or blood glucose levels.

The variations in the process of performing the BSDT in different countries depends on professional judgement:

- How long to wait for the sedative effect to dissipate?
- How many times is the test to be repeated and by whom?
- What are the accepted values for electrolytes, blood glucose and temperature?

USA guidelines for testing for brain stem death entail exclusion of severe disturbances of electrolyte, acid-base or endocrine systems (Jennett 2002). The guideline does not specify the range of these disturbances, yet it demands that a temperature not lower than 32 °C is necessary to validate the BSDT result. In addition, it dictates a temperature of not more than 36.5 °C is necessary to validate the apnoea test component of the brain stem death criteria. The UK guidelines (Academy of Medical Royal Colleges 2008) do not refer to this minimum temperature for the reflex test nor do they mention 36.5 °C for the apnoea test. In cases of doubt, short-term correction of these parameters before the test should be undertaken. If there is still doubt, then as a confirmatory investigation, either cerebral angiography or cranial ultrasonography should be undertaken to confirm cessation of cerebral blood flow to the brain.

There are numerous protocols for determining brain death (Wijdicks *et al.* 2010: p. 1914–1916). The basics of the protocols are as follows:

Pre-requisites include:

- Establishing the cause of the irreversible coma.
- Maintaining a core temperature of >36 °C.
- Maintaining a normal systolic blood pressure ≥100 mm Hg.
- Undertaking a neurological examination. In some areas it is necessary for two practitioners to undertake separate examinations.

**Based on the above tests the clinical findings of brain death are:**

- GCS: 3/15.
- No independent breathing.
- No gag reflex.
- No eye movement after performing caloric tests.
- No purposeful or semi-purposeful movement.
- No corneal response.
- No papillary reaction.
- No occulo-cephalic reflex.
- No vestibular-cephalic reflex.
- There may be an iso-electric EEG.

## Brain stem death assessment

Brain stem death test components include the following that MUST be assessed:

- Level of consciousness.
- Ability of the patient to breathe independently.
- Gag and cough reflex by stimulation of the throat by either a tongue depressor or laryngoscope.
- Caloric test (infusion of ice water of 50 ml into each ear and note the response of the eye). The normal response should be nystagmus.
- Response of limbs to painful stimuli.
- Additional neurological examination, i.e. papillary reaction to light.
- Absence of limb movement to application of pain. (Spinal cord injury explanations for limb paralysis need to be excluded.)
- There is a special need to rule out locked-in-syndrome, with loss of most of the functions of the brain stem, yet maintenance of cortical function.

(Academy of Medical Royal Colleges 2008)

After confirming brain death it is important to consider whether the patient is suitable for organ donation. Timely discussion with the family and organ donation team about organ transplantation is essential. The family may decide to donate the patient's organs or there may be an advance directive, donor card or registration.

The family will be distressed, but may find solace in the idea that the organs can be used to save the life of others. Requesting permission for organ donations must be undertaken by suitably trained health professionals in a kind and considerate manner. There must be no coercion if the family refuse permission. Should permission for organ transplantation be granted, the vital functions will be maintained until the organs have been harvested. It is important for the family to understand that the patient has suffered irreversible brain death and that removal of the organs will not cause death (Miller and Truog 2009).

## CONCLUSION

Brain death occurs where there is irreversible loss of function of the cerebrum, cortex and brain stem, no recovery of cognitive function and no response to external stimuli, except for spinal reflexes (www.uktransplant.org.uk).

Dying and death are very personal experiences. Here is a poem that will help those considering difficult decisions to come to terms and face the situation.

'On Dying'
'I sit and wait with you
at the portals of eternity
and wonder at your quiet courage
and your strength.
No cry crosses your lips
except when blessed sleep has claimed you
for a short moment.
No complaint
no plea for mercy
no wondering as to why.
I'm humbled by your dignity
I'll try to live
as bravely as you die . . .'

Margaret A Campbell, R.N., Worcester, Mass
(Source unknown).

## ACTIVITIES

### Activity 25.1

#### Scenario

A 24 year old male patient has been admitted to the ICU with a GCS score of 3/15. You have been allocated as his key worker. CT scan shows severe cerebral oedema. He is ventilated, on intracranial pressure monitoring and is sedated. His wife asks if she can please see you as she wishes to discuss his condition.

#### Exercise

1. Discuss how you will prepare for this session.

## Activity 25.2

### Scenario

A 30 year old male patient has been admitted to the ICU with a GCS score of 3/15, is non-responsive and has fixed and dilated pupils. You have been allocated as his key worker. CT scan shows severe cerebral oedema and an intracranial haemorrhage. He is unable to maintain his ventilation and has been placed on a ventilator, as well as intracranial pressure monitoring. The doctor has informed the wife that the patient has the clinical manifestations of brain death. The doctor has scheduled a meeting with his wife and mother and, as key worker, you need to be present at the discussion.

### Exercise

1. Discuss how you will prepare for this session.

## Activity 25.3

### Scenario

A 22 year old male patient has been admitted to the ICU with a GCS score of 3/15. The doctor has confirmed that the patient has brain death and has approached the subject of organ donation. His mother asks if she can please see you as she wishes to discuss the situation.

### Exercise

1. Discuss how you will prepare for this session.

# Section 5
# NEUROREHABILITATION

## INTRODUCTION

This section is the ultimate stage of the patient's journey. It has been designed to empower health professionals in neurotrauma practice with knowledge applicable to neu-rorehabilitation, discharge planning, living in the community and legal matters. In the Appendices, a chapter with additional resources for professionals, patients, families and carers has been included.

---

### Key objectives

On completion of this section you should be able to achieved the following:

- Manage the sequelae of neurotrauma.
- Define neurorehabilitation.
- Debate concepts of rehabilitation.
- Discuss principles of rehabilitation.
- Identify neurorehabilitation techniques relevant to your practice.
- Utilise rehabilitation techniques to manage difficult behaviour.
- Debate the role of early stimulation programmes.
- Define discharge planning.
- Evaluate factors that enable effective discharge planning.
- Describe the role of family and carers in neurorehabilitation.
- Investigate community outreach resources.
- Identify local, national and international resources for community-based rehabilitation.
- Empower patients on their journey to wellness and health in the community.

---

### Ethical/legal considerations

Debate the ethical issues related to this section.

Consider and apply the legal and ethical issues high-lighted in these chapters to neurotrauma practice:

- Mental capacity.
- Consent.
- Vulnerable adults.
- Disability.
- Discrimination.
- Ethics of research.

# Chapter 26
# Sequelae of Neurotrauma

*Nadine Abelson-Mitchell*

School of Nursing and Midwifery, Faculty of Health, Education and Society, Plymouth University, Devon, UK

## INTRODUCTION

This so-called 'silent epidemic' is the main cause of morbidity, mortality and disability in the population below 40–45 years of age (Alexandrescu *et al.* 2009; Chua *et al.* 2007). It is also the leading cause of loss of years of productive life and is a social problem to which governments do not pay sufficient attention (Baldo *et al.* 2003; Basso *et al.* 2001; Bruns and Hauser 2003; Greenwald *et al.* 2003).

Post-head injury, the patient may suffer from various sequelae or consequences of the injury. It is necessary for health professionals caring for neurotrauma patients to be cognisant of the sequelae experienced by neurotrauma patients, their families, carers and the community in order to plan appropriate services for patients with neurotrauma (Roy *et al.* 2002). The sequelae may range from temporary and mild to permanent and severe sequelae. Management of the sequelae are described throughout the book, the sequelae themselves are summarised in this chapter.

The actual sequelae will:

1. Be particular to the individual patient
2. Be influenced by the patient's pre-existing health status and social practices
3. Depend on the nature, site and extent of the injury
4. Depend on the length of unconsciousness
5. Depend on the period of PTA
6. Depend on available resources
7. Be affected by the level of care received by the patient.

Families report that it is not the physical deficits but the neurobehavioural and cognitive deficits that are the most trying. Children who have suffered mild TBI may continue to suffer from neuropsychological sequelae in adulthood (Hessen *et al.* 2007).

> **Implications for practice**
>
> Astute observation will detect some of these sequelae early in the patient's journey. This will enable proactive programmes of management to be implemented to limit the extent and outcomes of the sequelae.

As there are so many sequelae of neurotrauma, these have been tabulated under the headings: physical, psychological, social, vocational and educational.

*Neurotrauma: Managing Patients with Head Injuries*, First Edition. Edited by Nadine Abelson-Mitchell.
© 2013 Blackwell Publishing Ltd. Published 2013 by Blackwell Publishing Ltd.

**Table 26.1** Sequelae of neurotrauma.

| Physical | Psychological | Cognitive | Social | Family | Economic/educational/vocational |
|---|---|---|---|---|---|
| Headache | Personality change | Post-traumatic amnesia (PTA) | Inappropriate behaviour in social situations | Change in role in family | Inability to return to work/education |
| Neurological deficit: Motor/Sensory | Lack of insight/reasoning | Poor memory | Isolation | Alteration in family relationships | ↓ family income |
| Seizure activity | Tiredness | Impaired concentration/attention | ↑ use of recreational drugs/alcohol | ↑ incidence of divorce or breakdown in relationships | Loss of work |
| Hemiplegia | Depression | Altered IQ | Impaired use of transportation | Need for carer | |
| Cranial nerve deficits e.g. anosmia; Changes in vision | Intellectual deficit | Changes in mood | | | |
| Post-traumatic hypopituitarism | Post-concussion syndrome | Labile emotions | | | |
| Vegetative state | Low self-esteem | Anxiety/irritability | | | |
| Locked-in syndrome | Lack of confidence | Aggression | | | |
| Pain | Sexual dysfunction | Disinhibition | | | |
| Cushing's ulcer | | Problems with language: Expressive dysphasia, Receptive dysphasia | | | |
| Malnutrition: Obesity, Underweight | | | | | |
| Inability to attend to self-care needs | | | | | |
| Complications of bed rest: Pressure sores, Deep vein thrombosis, Contractures | | | | | |
| Heterotopic ossification | | | | | |

(Das-Gupta and Turner-Stokes 2002; Deb and Burns 2007; Holsinger *et al.* 2002; Hudak *et al.* 2004; Langlois *et al.* 2006; Mitchell *et al.* 2010; Wilson 2008; Zampolini *et al.* 2012).

## ADDITIONAL INFORMATION ABOUT SOME SEQUELAE

### Cushing's ulcer

*Definition*

This is a type of stress ulcer that can occur in the oesophagus, lining of the stomach or duodenum (rare) in patients with a brain injury. The mortality rate from Cushing's ulcers is 50% (Alain and Wang 2008).

*Pathophysiology*

A Cushing's ulcer is an acute gastric ulcer that develops as a result of cerebral trauma or raised intracranial pressure. The exact pathophysiology of Cushing's ulcers is unclear.

The development of Cushing's ulcers may be related to:

- Hypersecretion of gastric acid.
- Delayed gastric emptying and gastric stasis.
- Possible ischaemia to the gastro-intestinal system (Daley *et al*. 2004; Skole *et al*. 2007).

*Signs and symptoms*

Signs and symptoms can vary from patient to patient:

- May be asymptomatic.
- Present with bleeding of the stomach or duodenum or an intermittent burning pain.
- Loss of appetite.
- Vomiting of blood.
- Blood in faeces.

### Risk factors for stress ulcers

In addition, patients with neurotrauma may have an increased risk of stress ulceration as they are subject to major physiological stress, caused by:

- Mechanical ventilation for >48 hours (Cook *et al*. 1994).
- Coagulopathy.
- Hypotension.
- Major surgery.
- Burns (Curling's ulcers).
- Renal or hepatic failure.
- Neurological risk factors include the extent of the injury, pre-existing disease, large haematomas, GCS<6/15 (Misra *et al*. 2003).

*Treatment*

Patients admitted directly to a neurosurgical ward may not receive gastric protection. This will depend on the patient's clinical presentation and cranial trauma. At risk patients in ICU will be treated with gastric protection of Ranitidine 50 mgs TDS intravenously. Prophylactic agents may include histamine receptor antagonists and proton pump inhibitors (Skole *et al*. 2007).

### Post-concussion syndrome (PCS)

Post-concussion syndrome usually occurs after mild head injury but can feature in moderate or severe head injury. The pathophysiological mechanism in moderate and severe head injury is unclear. PCS may be of short duration or could last for three to 12 months post-injury (Mittenberg and Strauman 2000; Satz *et al*. 1999). Many patients who experience PCS have normal MRI scans, CT scans and EEGs (Lewine *et al*. 1999).

Symptoms of PCS include headache, irritability, altered ability to concentrate and memory problems as well as fatigue, anxiety and depression (Perna and Geller 2000; Wade *et al*. 1998).

### Post-traumatic hypopituitarism

*Definition*

Pituitary homeostasis is necessary to maintain the patient's physical and psychological wellbeing and quality of life (Urban *et al*. 2005). Post-traumatic hypopituitarism relates to all hormones produced by the pituitary gland (see Chapter 12). It is suggested that growth hormone is most frequently affected (15%) (Klose *et al*. 2007a).

*Incidence*

Post-traumatic hypopituitarism occurs in 15% of patients who have suffered neurotrauma (Klose *et al*. 2007a).

*Risk factors include:*
- Severity of injury.
- ↑ Intracranial pressure.

*Symptoms*

These may occur soon after injury or sometime after the injury. Symptoms will relate to the particular hormone that is deficient such as:

- Growth hormone.
- ACTH.
- FSH/LH.
- ↑Cortisol.
- TSH.

The deficiency may be temporary or permanent (Klose *et al*. 2007b; Tanriverdi *et al*. 2006).

### Treatment

- Perform a neuro-endocrine evaluation.
- In the event of a permanent deficiency it may be necessary to replace and/or supplement the decreased hormones (Klose *et al.* 2007b; Urban *et al.* 2005).

## Heterotopic ossification (Das-Gupta and Turner-Stokes 2002)

### Definition

Heterotopic ossification occurs where there is an abnormal deposit of calcium in the soft tissues. This is of major importance in relation to joints, may result in lack of, or limited, movement and may be very debilitating.

### Incidence

Occurs in 10–20% of patients who have suffered neurotrauma.

### Symptoms

- Pain in area.
- Limited range of movement particularly hip, elbow and shoulder.

### Treatment

- Indomethacin for pain and inflammation.
- Physical therapy.
- Manipulation under anaesthetic.
- Surgical removal of affected area.

## Sexual health

Sexuality, which includes love and belonging, is an important consideration when looking at the holistic needs of patients.

It is important for suitably trained personnel to be able to discuss the sexual needs of the patient, spouse or partner. Patients and partners may be embarrassed to discuss sexuality therefore it is important that personnel are knowledgeable about sexuality and that educational material is freely available to patients, spouses or partners. Ensure the patient has a trusting relationship with the rehabilitation team to be able to discuss sexuality openly. The timing of the discussion regarding sexuality will be determined by the patient's attitude within the rehabilitation programme.

When taking a sexual history from the patient, spouses or partner, it is important to establish the pre-existing relationship, not only in terms of sex, but in terms of love, warmth and belonging. It is important to encourage the partner to demonstrate this love, warmth and belonging during the patient's recovery. Speaking to the patient, holding the patient's hands and maintaining a loving relationship is important in patient recovery.

### Anatomy and physiology

Sexuality involves the bilateral temporal lobes affecting the limbic system. Damage to the frontal, fronto-temporal, basal frontal lobes and medial septal lesions may result in changes in sexual function.

### Causes of sexual dysfunction

There are numerous causes of sexual dysfunction in a person who has had neurotrauma:

- Pre-injury sexuality.
- Actual physical damage to the brain.
- Endocrine problems associated with brain trauma.
- Any physical limitations or deficits.
- Cognitive deficits.
- Emotional disturbances.
- Interpersonal disturbances.
- Use of medication.

The psychological sequelae of head injury may have a large influence on the patient's sexuality. There may be a personality change or problems with attention, decreased speed of thought processing, learning and memory. There may also be a decreased ability to solve problems and a decreased reasoning ability. The patient may also experience fatigue and irritability, be confused and disorientated and there could also be mood lability, impulsiveness, disinhibition, depressive feelings or attention seeking behaviour, behavioural problems, emotional difficulties, interpersonal problems and aggression. All the fore-going will have a serious effect on any sexual relationship.

Altered sexuality may include difficulties within any stage of the sexual response cycle (desire, excitement, arousal, orgasm and resolution). The problem may relate to the frequency of sexual activity, hypersexuality, erectile dysfunction or inappropriate sexual behaviour. Inappropriate sexual behaviour may include activities such as inappropriate interpersonal contact, swearing and verbal harassment or public masturbation.

Inappropriate sexual behaviour is embarrassing for the patient, family, community and the personnel managing the patient. A programme to modify the patient's sexual behaviour should be developed with the patient and rehabilitation team.

## Aims of the programme

As sexuality does not only refer to the act of sex itself, it is important to consider all aspects related to sexual health.

Are there any triggers that spark the patient's sexual behaviour? These triggers could be as simple as seeing a girl in a bikini in a newspaper, or watching a video with hugging, kissing or sexual scenes. It could also be sparked by the spouse touching or not touching the patient. The triggers could relate to the company the patient is keeping, the environment in which the patient finds himself or an activity that the patient is undertaking.

## Management

It is important to ensure that patients, families, visitors and personnel are safe at all times. It may be necessary to arrange a period of observation in order to observe any triggers.

There are numerous techniques to stop unwanted behaviour. Ignoring the behaviour does not mean that the behaviour will stop. Introduce a programme of behaviour modification, which could include rewarding positive behaviour, promoting independence and teaching the patient more acceptable ways of behaving, including plans to avoid the negative manifestations of sexuality and the offering of various choices. Good behaviour will be rewarded and bad behaviour will have consequences that they need to accept – such as not being able to watch television or not being able to go out on pre-arranged activities. It may be possible to introduce a diversionary activity, exercises, sport, reading, going for a walk or introducing an activity that the patient enjoys. It may also be necessary to arrange counselling sessions and these can be arranged on an individual or a group basis, depending on the patient's needs.

If the patient is suffering from fatigue or a physical deficit it may be possible to teach them to select times for sexual activity when they are not tired, or are not in an inappropriate environment. In patients who are suffering from impotence or erectile dysfunction it is necessary to recommend that they try to decrease the number of times they try to initiate sex in favour of less frequent, but successful, sexual experiences. It may also be possible to

teach the patient different sexual techniques depending on their physical deficit.

Some of the medication that the patient receives may affect sexual function. It will be necessary to advise the patient that they should not stop taking medication without consulting a medical practitioner. If the team is aware of the problem, it may be possible to put the patient onto an alternative medication.

It is also important to protect the vulnerable person who has neurotrauma from sexual predation.

## CONCLUSION

On completion of the sexuality programme it is hoped that the patient will be safe, independent and can demonstrate appropriate social interaction and sexual behaviour.

---

### Activity 26.1

**Scenario**

Assess a patient who has been in the unit for the past two weeks for any potential short term or long term sequelae.

**Exercise**

1. Develop a plan of management to manage the sequelae.

---

### Activity 26.2

**Scenario**

A 28 year old male patient who is married with three children – aged 4 months, 2 years and 5 years – is to be discharged to home in the next two weeks.

**Exercise**

1. Assess the patient to determine any sequelae of the head injury.
2. Draw up, with him and his wife, a plan of management should these sequelae occur.

# Chapter 27
# Neurorehabilitation

*Zuhair Noori[1] and Nadine Abelson-Mitchell[2]*

[1]Croydon Healthcare Trust, London, UK
[2]School of Nursing and Midwifery, Faculty of Health, Education and Society, Plymouth University, Devon, UK

## INTRODUCTION

Rehabilitation is an area of health that is providing numerous opportunities and challenges for health professionals.

Renewed attention has been focused on the meaning and purpose of rehabilitation mainly due to patients demanding equitable and effective services from the time of the incident until final recovery (BSRM 2009; RCP 2010). There has been a paradigm shift in neurorehabilitation based on:

- An increased understanding of the re-organisation of the brain after injury.
- An appreciation of the chemical factors that promote learning and remodelling.
- Increased understanding of memory.
- The influence of evidence-based care on neurorehabilitation.
- The importance of reliable outcome measures for injury and treatment.

In terms of research, the BSRM (1998) and RCP (2010) recall a number of issues that identify rehabilitation as a unique discipline. Research into rehabilitation does not lend itself to randomised control trials and there are few longitudinal studies. The level of evidence is often based on 'best practice' by experts rather than higher levels of evidence. The research often involves a small number of patients, with diverse conditions and there is lack of agreement on rehabilitation techniques and outcome measures. The definition and interpretation of rehabilitation may also affect the research undertaken, and the level of rehabilitation provided to patients within a study may be determined by resources available rather than patient needs. Patients within rehabilitation often have complex disabilities and therefore may need to be treated as 'special cases'. The patient baseline may also change due, e.g. to spontaneous recovery, and therefore the results obtained cannot be authenticated as being due to the process implemented, because of the spontaneous recovery.

There is increasingly robust evidence for the effectiveness of rehabilitation in brain-injured populations (BSRM 1998; Chua *et al.* 2007; Rice-Oxley and Turner-Stokes 1999; Turner-Stokes *et al.* 2006; Turner-Stokes *et al.* 2008; Wilson 2008).

The number of people surviving neurotrauma and requiring rehabilitation is increasing as is the number of people with disability living in the community (BSRM 2008a; RCP 2010). Their diverse and complex rehabilitation needs require that professionals have specialist knowledge to meet their needs. Cost-effectiveness of multidisciplinary rehabilitation includes preventing costly complications, avoiding hospital re-admissions, reducing the length of stay of patients post-injury, reducing the cost of long-term care and enabling people with TBI to access work (BSRM 2008a; Turner-Stokes 2004, 2007; Turner-Stokes *et al.* 2006).

## DEFINITION OF REHABILITATION

Rehabilitation is defined by Waters and Luker (1996: p. 242) as:

'...the whole process of enabling and facilitating the restoration of a disabled person to regain optimal functioning (physically, socially, and psychologically) to the level that they are able or motivated to achieve.'

Using the outline of Donabedian (1996), rehabilitation is defined by Wade and De Jong (2000: p. 1386) as:

**'Structure**

A rehabilitation service comprises a multidisciplinary team of people who:

• Work together towards common goals for each patient.
• Involve and educate the patient and family.
• Have relevant knowledge and skills.
• Can resolve most of the common problems faced by the patients.

**Process**

Rehabilitation is an iterative, active, educational, problem solving process focused on a patient's behaviour (disability), with the following components:

• Assessment.
  The identification of the nature and extent of the patient's problems and the factors relevant to the resolution.
• Goal setting.
  Intervention, which may include either or both of (a) treatments, which affect the process of change; (b) support, which maintains the patient's quality of life and his or her safety.
• Evaluation – to check on effects of any intervention.

**Outcome**

The rehabilitation process aims to:

• Maximise the participation of the patient in his or her social setting.
• Minimise the pain and distress experienced by the patient.

• Minimise the distress of and stress on the patient's family and carers.'

From: Recent advances in rehabilitation, Wade, D.T. and De Jong, D.A. *British Medical Journal* 2000; 320 (7246). With permission from BMJ Publishing Group Ltd.

The World Health Organization (WHO) introduced its biopsychosocial approach to health when it published the International Classification of Function, Disability and Health (ICFDH), a positive approach to functional and structural impairment, activities and participation as well as impairment and activity limitation and participation restriction (WHO 2001). All of the ICFDH concepts are integral to the wellness model and Needs Approach Model described in this book. The ICFDH classification focuses on health and wellness rather than on disease as does the Needs Approach Model (Chapter 3). The term 'disability' includes dynamic interaction between the person, the environment, community and society. This classification describes core concepts of 'body function and structure', 'activity' and 'participation' that are important concepts in achieving human potential and independence through quality care and rehabilitation. Contextual factors, that may have an influence on body structure and functions, activity and participation, include 'environmental factors' that could be physical, social cultural or institutional as well as 'personal factors' such as gender, age, education and lifestyle (Rosenbaum and Stewart 2004; Wilson 2008). Participation includes psychosocial functioning, relationships with family and friends, work, leisure and community participation (Wilson 2008). The interaction of all concepts is described in the model, Figure 27.1 (WHO 2001).

## LEVELS OF REHABILITATION

The term 'rehabilitation without walls' aptly describes the need for rehabilitative intervention to take place as and when required (Barnes 1999a; RCP 2010). The Department of Health (RCP 2010: p. 8) and BSRM (2008a) suggest three levels of rehabilitation:

Level 1 **Tertiary specialist rehabilitation service**
  This service serves a population of 750 000 or more and deals with very complex needs.
Level 2 **District specialist rehabilitation service**
  This service serves a population of 250 000.
Level 3 **Local non-specialist rehabilitation teams**
  Services are provided within acute care settings, intermediate care or the community.

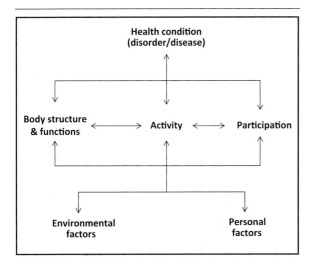

**Figure 27.1** The ICF Model. Copyright © 2001 International Classification of Functioning, Disability and Health. World Health Organization, Geneva. Reproduced with permission of the World Health Organization.

## SETTINGS FOR REHABILITATION

Rehabilitation should be included in all settings to meet the needs of the population, to reduce costs, maintain quality of care, realise patient outcomes and eliminate the need for re-admission (BSRM 2008a; RCP 2010).

In addition to the above levels as described by the Department of Health, with regard to public health, levels of rehabilitation are described in terms of primary, secondary and tertiary settings as:

- Primary rehabilitation includes health promotion and primary prevention of illness, including neurotrauma.
- Secondary rehabilitation takes place in acute hospitals and includes early stimulation programmes and preventive rehabilitation.
- Tertiary rehabilitation takes place in dedicated rehabilitation services, out-patient departments and community-based services including home-based programmes.

## REHABILITATION COSTS

Although it appears that the costs of rehabilitation are high the benefits to patients, families and society outweigh the costs (RCP 2010). A comparison of costs between countries cannot be undertaken as health services and resources differ. However:

- In the USA, Aronow (1987: p. 35) reports that it costs $1 000 000 to rehabilitate 60 patients.
- In the UK, Christensen *et al.* (2008) estimate that for a patient with blunt traumatic injuries the mean total hospital costs are £9 530 (median length of stay in critical care of four days, total hospital stay of nine days).
- According to RCP (2010: p. 41) for a patient with complex needs, following TBI, the costs of 6–18 months of rehabilitation is estimated at £300 000.
- Long-term care packages for patients with complex needs can cost ≥£1 500 per week (RCP 2010: p. 40).
- Each new patient will require £50 000–£150 000 per annum (RCP 2010: p. 40).

Resources for rehabilitation are limited. Decisions rely heavily on the process of diagnosis, interpretation of symptoms and who will benefit most from treatment. Decisions regarding access are also based on definitions of impairment and disablement. For the majority of people with traumatic brain injury early referral to rehabilitation results in a favourable outcome (RCP 2010). Yet, it is acknowledged that due to a limited number of services only a small proportion of people who could benefit from rehabilitation gain access to rehabilitation services (BSRM 2008a). Effective rehabilitation reduces patient dependency as well as the costs of continuing care (Turner-Stokes *et al.* 2006).

### Rehabilitation resources

Throughout the world, rehabilitation resources vary according to the requirements, infrastructure and finances of a particular country. According to the BSRM (BSRM 2009: p. 2) in the UK, the standard for rehabilitation is as follows:

- 6 rehabilitation medicine consultants per 1 000 000 population:
  - 3.6 for in-patient and out-patient services.
  - 2.4 for community services.
- 60 rehabilitation medicine beds per 1 000 000 population. The figure quoted by the Royal College of Physicians is 45–65/1 000 000 population (RCP 2010: p. 53). This equates to 15 beds per 250 000 population.
- The minimum size for an in-patient rehabilitation unit should be 20 beds.

## STAFFING FOR REHABILITATION

The British Society of Rehabilitation Medicine (BSRM 2009: p. 4–8) makes the following recommendations regarding staffing in rehabilitation (Tables 27.1 and 27.2):

**Table 27.1** Minimum staffing for district specialist in-patient rehabilitation service.

| Professional | For every 20 beds: | |
|---|---|---|
| **Medical staff** | 1.2 WTE consultant accredited in rehabilitation medicine | |
| | 2–3 WTE training grades (above FY) and/or 1.5 WTE trust grade doctors | |
| **Nurses** | 24–30 WTE | Plus |
| | (varies with dependency, but at least one third should have specific rehabilitation training) | Trained therapy assistants, technicians, engineers and other professions as appropriate to caseload |
| **Physiotherapists** | 4 WTE | |
| **Occupational therapists** | 4 WTE | |
| **Speech and language therapists** | 2–2.5 WTE | |
| | (depending on whether patients with tracheostomy are admitted) | |
| **Clinical psychologist/ counsellor** | 1.5–2 WTE | |
| | (depending on whether patients with severe behavioural problems are admitted) | |
| **Social workers/ discharge coordinator** | 1.5 WTE | |
| **Dietician** | 0.75–1.0 WTE (depending on proportion of patients on enteral feeding) | |
| **Clerical staff** | 3.0 WTE (dependent on caseload and throughput) | |

Note: These staffing levels support both the in-patient activity and associated outreach work including assessments, home visits, follow-up and case-conferences etc.

From British Society of Rehabilitation Medicine (2009). With kind permission from the British Society of Rehabilitation Medicine.

**Table 27.2** Minimum staffing provision for community specialist rehabilitation services.

| Professional | Number |
|---|---|
| Team leader/co-ordinator | 2 |
| Nurse specialists | 8 |
| Physiotherapists | 6 |
| Occupational therapists | 10 |
| Speech and language therapists | 4 |
| Clinical psychologists | 4 |
| Specialist social workers | 8 |
| Dietician | 2 |
| Technical instructors | 8 |
| Generic assistants | 8 |
| Consultants accredited in rehabilitation medicine | 2.4 |

From British Society of Rehabilitation Medicine (2009). With kind permission from the British Society of Rehabilitation Medicine.

**Nurse staffing**

According to the American Association of Rehabilitation Nurses (www.rehabnurse.org/advocacy/content/pcriteria.html) to achieve maximum benefit it is important to employ appropriately trained rehabilitation professionals. When determining nursing staff levels and skill mix the following factors need to be considered:

• Patient care needs and dependency.
• Number of nursing hours required per patient day.
• Discharges, admissions, transfers per day.
• Available technology.
• Unit structure (Association of Rehabilitation Nurses: www.rehabnurse.org).

The morale of the staff and job satisfaction are important in the recruitment and retention of personnel working within rehabilitation. Nurses working with brain injured patients have a higher level of psychological stress than those in general rehabilitation (Thorn 2000). It is therefore essential that management provide support to rehabilitation personnel by means of support groups, individual and group sessions and the introduction of fitness and wellness programmes.

Patient dependency ratings currently in use include the Northwick Park Dependency Score (Hatfield *et al.* 2003; Nyein *et al.* 1999; Turner-Stokes *et al.* 1998, 1999a; Williams *et al.* 2007) and the Barthel Index (al-Khawaja *et al.* 1997; Post *et al.* 2002; Turner-Stokes *et al.* 2010) amongst others.

## STANDARDS OF REHABILITATION PRACTICE

Standards for rehabilitation practice have been developed by the BSRM (2002). Standards for rehabilitation nursing practice have been established by the ARN (2008: p.19–33) to guide practice.

A summary of the ARN (2008 pp.19–33) Standards for Rehabilitation Nursing Practice is shown in Box 27.1.

## REHABILITATION CRITERIA

Many rehabilitation centres have set criteria for the admission of patients. These criteria vary from unit to unit and may include all or some of the following:

1. Medical condition and medical stability.
2. MRSA free status.
3. Patient's age <60 years old.
4. The extent of the injury.
5. The patient's level of consciousness.
6. Fitness to take part in programme.
7. The ability to manage physical needs such as incontinence.
8. Readiness for rehabilitation.
9. Availability of programmes.
10. Suitability of programmes.
11. Potential for recovery, especially where service providers are paid according to outcomes and results.
12. Potential to return to work.
13. Knowledge of possible discharge destinations to avoid bed blocking.
14. Finances.
15. Exclusion criteria may include aggression and non-compliance.

---

**Box 27.1** Standards of rehabilitation nursing practice

The rehabilitation registered nurse:
- Collects comprehensive data pertinent to the patient's health.
- Analyses assessment data when determining diagnoses or issues that affect the patient's health or success in the community.
- Identifies expected outcomes for a plan individualised to the patient.
- Develops a plan that prescribes strategies, alternatives and interventions to attain the expected outcomes.
- Implements the strategies and interventions identified in the plan.
- Co-ordinates care delivery.
- Employs strategies to promote health and a safe environment.
- Provides consultation to influence the identified plan, enhance the ability of others, and affects change.
- Uses prescriptive authority, procedures, referrals, treatment and therapies in accordance with state and federal laws and regulations.

- Evaluates the patient's progress toward attainment of outcomes.
- Systematically evaluates the quality and effectiveness of rehabilitation nursing practice.
- Evaluates their own nursing practice in relation to professional practice standards and relevant statutes and regulations.
- Interacts with and contributes to the professional development of peers, colleagues, and other healthcare providers.
- Ensures decisions and actions are determined in an ethical manner.
- Collaborates with the patient, family, and other healthcare providers in providing patient care.
- Uses research findings in practice.
- Considers factors related to safety, effectiveness, and cost in planning and delivering patient care.
- Provides leadership in the practice setting and the profession.
- Acquires and maintains current knowledge and competency in nursing practice.

From *Standards and Scope of Rehabilitation Nursing Practice*, pp. 19–33. American Association of Rehabilitation Nurses (ARN). Copyright © 2008 Association of Rehabilitation Nurses. Printed with permission.

## THE REHABILITATION PROCESS

The Needs Approach Model continues to be used within the rehabilitation setting and includes the same components as the rehabilitation process, namely:

1. **Assessment of the patient's needs**

   This involves history taking, physical examination, evaluating the results of investigations prior to establishing nursing diagnoses. In the rehabilitation setting the priority of needs will change (Abelson-Mitchell

and Watkins 2006). Additional elements of relevance in rehabilitation are reflected in Figure 27.2.

2. **Planning of care**

   The team, including the patient, family and the nurse, set goals and plan the patient's care. Planning care includes setting of specific immediate, intermediate and long-term goals as well as discharge planning. Planned care is developed within a framework of appropriate guidelines where these are available, for example Integrated Care Pathways (RCP 2010), National Service

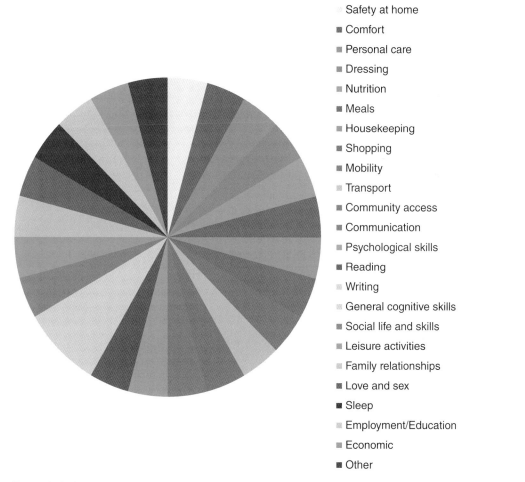

**Figure 27.2**   Extended Needs Approach Model. For a colour version of this figure, please refer to the plate section.

Frameworks (DH 2005a) and Skills for Health competencies (http://www.skillsforhealth.org.uk/). Setting realistic goals aids in the motivation of the patient (Wade 2005) and for patients and carers goal planning has psychological benefits.

3. The established plan is *implemented* in a specific timeframe.
4. The plan is *evaluated* in terms of the patient outcome and the plan itself.

## GOALS OF REHABILITATION

There are numerous goals of rehabilitation that can be summarised as follows:

- Facilitating, enabling and empowering patients to achieve and maximise their potential.
- Maximising self-determination, the restoration of function and optimising lifestyle choices.
- Ensuring adequate physical, behavioural, psychological and social functioning to enable the patient to return to the family, community, previous leisure activities and gainful employment, where possible.
- Enabling the patient to achieve his or her level of function by preventing complications, modifying the effects of disability and increasing independence.
- Helping people manage long-term health problems.

## CONCEPTS UNDERPINNING REHABILITATION

Certain concepts are basic to the rehabilitation effort:

1. Factors of relevance to patient rehabilitation include the gender of the patient, age, past experience, premorbid personality, psyche, anxiety level, the actual injury, the patient's socio-economic situation and environmental factors, as well as access to services.
2. It is necessary to believe in the value of human existence as well as the uniqueness and worth of people.
3. To be effective, rehabilitation must take place in a conducive environment.
4. The road to rehabilitation is not simple.
5. Rehabilitation is a dynamic, positive process (Barnes 1999a).
   Improvements, whether re-learning, compensation, adaptation or alteration in lifestyle, continue long after the formal rehabilitation process has been discontinued.
6. Rehabilitation is an opportunity for new initiatives, to be creative and to search for possibilities. Small changes and improvements in the patient are major events on the long road to recovery.

7. Correct timing for rehabilitation is imperative.
   Rehabilitation commences on the first day of the patients illness and should begin in parallel with, rather than in series with, medical care. Therapeutic treatment is most effective if it is initiated at the earliest opportunity during the first six months of convalescence.
8. Programming and scheduling are important considerations.
9. The client's attitude must be accepting of rehabilitation.
10. Honesty is imperative.
    Rehabilitation does not provide miraculous cures, but there are instances where patients with severe head injuries who, according to medical evidence should not have recovered, have made remarkable recoveries.
11. Hope is essential.
    False hope or setting unrealistic goals is unacceptable in rehabilitation practice. It is not always possible for the patient to return to their pristine state. What is effective for one person does not always work for another. In rehabilitation, there are no definitive answers, it is necessary to face harsh realities and sometimes rehabilitation efforts are not successful.
12. Accurate documentation, using standardised multidisciplinary records, is essential to record responses, progress of the patient, to allow for adjustment of the programme, for follow-up, programme evaluation and to ensure true collaboration (RCP 2010).

## PLANNING THE REHABILITATION PROGRAMME CONTENT

When planning rehabilitation programme content, it is important to consider the patient's needs. There is no agreement as to the rehabilitation interventions to be included in a rehabilitation programme (Wade 2005). Depending on the patients' needs, certain basic principles must be included in the programme (Abelson 1987; Audit Commission 2000):

- Maintenance of vital functions.
- Prevention of secondary disabilities.
- Improvement of physical fitness.
- Training in self-care activities.
- Training in activities of living.
- Ensuring effective stimulation and motivation for the patient to achieve maximum physical, psychosocial and emotional recovery.
- Ensuring maximum psychological functioning.
- Cognitive retraining.
- Maximising education and training.
- Maximising vocational training.
- Maximising social integration.

## SCHEDULING THE PROGRAMME

A daily schedule that can be adjusted weekly according to the patient's needs, detailing the amount of time spent in each department on each activity, must be discussed by the multidisciplinary team. The schedule of activities must combine basic maintenance and rehabilitation as well as exercise and training programmes. Time for rest, sleep and recreation must be included in the schedule (Audit Commission 2000). Short intensive periods of therapy have more effect than prolonged intermittent attendance (Abelson 1987).

## COMMUNITY-BASED REHABILITATION (CBR)

Along the journey, the patient may participate in community-based rehabilitation as part of the continuum of care for patients who have had neurotrauma (Abelson-Mitchell 2006; Das-Gupta and Turner-Stokes 2002; NICE 2007; RCP 2010).

### Developing a community-based rehabilitation programme

The development of community-based rehabilitation programmes within the current climate of user participation and patient choice, with an emphasis on community outreach, strengthens the need for effective, accessible and equitable community-based programmes (Audit Commission 2000; DH 2005a). Community-based rehabilitation programmes are used in any healthcare setting, such as a day centre or a residential facility, provided there is patient agreement, the rehabilitation techniques are appropriate to the setting and patient and appropriate resources are available. Such programmes may be funded by the NHS, private health insurance, employers, individual patients or a mix of these funding sources. In the UK, care in the community is an effective and efficient means of providing on-going rehabilitation (DH 2005a).

In the community, it is important to establish effective teams that include relevant personnel, the patient and family, to ensure that the right person is doing the right job at the right time. The personnel involved in the programmes will vary according to the needs of the patient. The team includes medical consultants, nurse consultants, Registered Nurses, staff nurses, neurologists, psychologists, social workers, allied health professionals and health care assistants. The scope of practice of the nurse enables the nurse to initiate, develop and prescribe community based rehabilitation programmes (American Association of Rehabilitation Nurses [ARN] and Rehabilitation Nursing Foundation [RNF] 2006; Association of Rehabilitation Nurses [ARN] 2008; Hoeman 2008; NMC 2008). A participative multidisciplinary approach is used to develop a community-based rehabilitation programme based on the Needs Approach Model. Nonprofessional personnel, family members and carers, play an important role in the community-based rehabilitation programme and are therefore provided with appropriate education and training to undertake a variety of activities, under the direct or indirect supervision of the rehabilitation team.

Preparing these programmes is challenging, requiring commitment to human potential, creativity, patience and determination on the part of the patient, family and multidisciplinary team.

### Purpose of CBR

- To value the patient as an individual who is an integral part of the system and participates in decision-making, when appropriate.
- To foster patient accountability and responsibility, where possible.
- To achieve maximum functional capacity and independence within a home environment or, if this is not possible, an alternative community setting.
- To provide opportunities to undertake multidisciplinary collaborative patient management in the community.
- To facilitate family and community re-integration and return to gainful employment, where possible, with minimal disruption.
- To consider outcomes affecting quality of everyday life.

The programme is based on the concepts of rehabilitation identified on p. 256 and uses an interprofessional problem-solving approach to assess, plan, implement and evaluate appropriate patient needs (DH 2005a; Semelyn *et al.* 1998).

### Assessment

Referral to the CBR service is from health professionals, social services or the patient's family. A nominated team member interviews the patient and family. The patient's readiness for rehabilitation, level of compliance and needs are assessed.

The patient must meet the criteria for CBR:

- Potential to benefit from the programme.
- Consent to participate in the programme.
- Appropriate family/carer support.

Specific rehabilitation needs are assessed using the Extended Needs Approach Model for CBR, designed for use with patients who have neurological disorders, at regular intervals throughout the programme (Abelson-Mitchell 1997; Abelson-Mitchell 2006).

The Extended Needs Approach model (Figure 27.2), based on the original Needs Approach Model, is divided into 24 activities of living relating to rehabilitation. These allow comprehensive assessment of a patient's level of functioning to enable appropriate planning and intervention within the home environment. Eight of these needs relate to physical wellbeing, two house management, two community access, nine psychosocial issues, two for finances and employment plus one other should other community-based needs be identified.

### Goals

The basis for individual goal setting is the generic community-based rehabilitation goals listed on p. 256 as well as those listed in Box 27.2.

Immediate, short- and long-term goals are determined. A chart is used to record overall daily, weekly and monthly goals that are reviewed, as necessary. When assessment and goal setting are complete, a detailed individualised programme is compiled and agreed by the patient and family. The programme is introduced to the patient and family and their written agreement, co-operation and commitment to participate are obtained (Abelson-Mitchell 2006).

### Planning

The programme is delivered in the patient's own environment over a period of one to twelve months, enabling rehabilitation to take place with as little disruption to home life as possible. When planning the programme, it is essential that a rigorous process is followed. The patient's individualised programme is developed on the basis of the determinants shown in Box 27.3.

Programme objectives are completed in relation to all identified needs (Box 27.4).

---

**Box 27.2  Goals of community-based rehabilitation**

Re-integration into family, community and society, return to work, leisure and social activities where possible.
Gaining independence in the home environment.
Building self-esteem and confidence.
Improving physical, psychological and social wellbeing in a familiar environment.
Continuing rehabilitation to achieve maximum potential.

---

**Box 27.3  Determinants of community-based rehabilitation**

Patient's physical wellbeing.
Patient's intellectual capacity.
Self-insight.
Level of motivation.
The sequelae of the injury.
Commitment of the family.
Level of training of carers.

From Abelson-Mitchell (2006). With kind permission from the British Journal of Neuroscience Nursing.

---

**Box 27.4  Programme content**

Maintenance of vital wellbeing.
Maximise independence.
Maximise wellness.
Effective motivation and stimulation in home environment.
Reality orientation.
Improvement of physical fitness.
Training in self-care activities and activities of living.
Maximum psychological functioning including self-esteem and self-belief.
Cognitive retraining.
Educational and vocational training.
Social integration.

From Abelson-Mitchell (2006). With kind permission from the British Journal of Neuroscience Nursing.

---

Objectives are specified to ensure that quality care, related to each need, is achieved. Once objectives have been set, the intervention for that need is determined and recorded. It is essential to ensure that the team, including the family and patient, are aware of the need to maintain safety at all times while carrying out the programme.

The multidisciplinary team adheres to the specific prescribed intervention. An example of safety needs, identified for a particular patient, are shown in Figure 27.3 and Figure 27.4.

A daily schedule is drawn up and adjusted as necessary. Figure 27.5 provides an example of a daily timetable for a patient who has been on the programme for four weeks.

During this daily programme, times for personal care, mobility and exercise, feeding and reality orientation, are included as well as time for rest, recreation and the family.

**Programme Objectives**

| Identified need: | Safety | Week 1 |
| --- | --- | --- |
| Patient: | Joanna | Date 28/02/2012 |
| Completed by: | NAM | Review date: Weekly |

| Date | Objectives | Time frame |
| --- | --- | --- |
| 28/2/2012 | To protect from physical/psychological harm | At all times |
| 28/2/2012 | Maintain safety | At all times |
| 28/2/2012 | Encourage independence within limitations | At all times |
| 28/2/2012 | Enable patient to feel safe within their home environment | At all times |
| 28/2/2012 | Perform risk assessment daily | At all times |

**Figure 27.3**  Extract of objectives related to the need: safety. From Abelson-Mitchell (2006). With kind permission from the British Journal of Neuroscience Nursing.

**Programme Intervention**

| Identified need: | Safety | Week 1 |
| --- | --- | --- |
| Client: | Joanna | Date 28/02/2012 |
| Completed by: | NAM | Review date: Weekly |

| Date | Intervention | Frequency |
| --- | --- | --- |
| 28/2/2012 | Maintain a safe environment | At all times |
| 28/2/2012 | Ensure bedrails in position, if necessary | When client at bed rest |
| 28/2/2012 | Remove lose carpets/rugs | At all times |
| 28/2/2012 | Ensure patient's shoes/slippers correctly fitted before mobilising | At all times |
| 28/2/2012 | When transferring use template | At all times |
| 28/2/2012 | Ensure sufficient personnel available for activities undertaken | At all times |
| 28/2/2012 | Do not injure when mobilising | At all times |
| 28/2/2012 | Reassure patient about progress regarding their safety | At all times |

**Figure 27.4**  Extract of prescribed intervention related to the need: safety. From Abelson-Mitchell (2006). With kind permission from the British Journal of Neuroscience Nursing.

The programme is implemented by the carer under the guidance of the rehabilitation specialist.

**Recording**

A multidisciplinary record is maintained to include the modalities of rehabilitation required by the patient including the goals, interventions, times and a section for progress notes (Figure 27.6). The record is completed daily by the team and is reviewed by the nurse consultant in consultation with other team members. Changes, trends or patterns are noted and relevant adjustments made to the programme in consultation with the patient, family and team.

**Evaluation**

The programme and patient need to be evaluated at regular intervals using multidisciplinary records. Initially this may be daily, weekly or monthly.

The effectiveness of the outcome, following community-based rehabilitation, is determined by characteristics such as the patient's profile, programme content and outcome measures (Evans and Brewis 2008). Research indicates that early discharge to home and community-based rehabilitation has improved patient outcome and satisfaction (Abelson-Mitchell 2006; Barnes and Radermacher 2003; McCabe *et al.* 2007).

**Proposed Timetable**

| Client: | Joanna | Date 28/02/2012 |
|---|---|---|
| Completed by: | NAM | Review date: Weekly |

| Time | Facilitate patient with activities: | Person |
|---|---|---|
| 07:00 | Bathing, skin care, dressing | Carer |
| | Standing exercise | |
| 08:00 | Sit in chair | Carer |
| 08:30 | Breakfast | Carer |
| 09:30 | Stimulation programme: | Carer |
| | Calendar, clock | |
| | Music 30 minutes | |
| 10:00 | Skin care | Carer |
| | Foot, toe, knee and wrist exercises | |
| | Breathing exercises | |
| 11:00 | Tea, toilet | Carer |
| 11:30–12:15 | Physiotherapy | Physiotherapist |
| 12:15–13:15 | Lunch | |
| 13:15–14:00 | Rest | Carer |
| 14:00–14:45 | Speech therapy | Speech therapist |
| 14:45–15:30 | Family time | |
| 15:45–16:30 | Occupational therapy | Occupational therapist |
| 16:30 | Family recreation | Family |
| | Dinner | Family |
| | Family time, stimulation programme | Family |
| 20:30–21:00 | To bed | Family |

**Figure 27.5** Extract of individualised timetable. From Abelson-Mitchell (2006). With kind permission from the British Journal of Neuroscience Nursing.

From a patient, professional and cost-effectiveness perspective, it is essential that local programme implementation is systematically evaluated and adapted, if necessary, to the local context. Nurse-led, community-based rehabilitation programmes, based on a needs approach, are an effective means of providing affordable, equitable, accessible rehabilitation to patients with neurotrauma.

The most effective rehabilitation occurs when there is a supportive family. It is important to ensure that patients are weaned from the programme appropriately and provided with a maintenance programme to ensure that abilities are retained and further developed (Abelson-Mitchell 2006).

**CONCLUSION**

Research into rehabilitation must be encouraged. Rehabilitation is hard work: it requires 100% commitment, focusing on the patient, the family and the community. The greatest reward is to see a patient who was unconscious and attending rehabilitation for weeks or months reintegrate into the family and community.

Reflection

'The ultimate test of the rehabilitation endeavour is the demonstrated ability of the individual to maintain what he has achieved and to use his potential capacities effectively for the duration of his life' (Anonymous).

Key points

- Ensure that appropriate resources are available.
- Rehabilitation is a component of integrated, holistic care.
- Rehabilitation involves a commitment to human potential.
- Rehabilitation has positive outcomes.
- Rehabilitation aims to maximise recovery.
- Family support is essential.

**Multidisciplinary Record**

| | | | |
|---|---|---|---|
| Client: | Joanna | **Date** | 28/02/2012 |
| Completed by; | NAM | **Review date:** | Weekly |

| Day/Time | Activity | Comments | Signature |
|---|---|---|---|
| 07:00 | Bathing/skin care<br>Dress for the day<br>Standing exercise | Keen to bathe herself today.<br>Well done. | HCA |
| 08:00 | Sit in chair | | Rehabilitation nurse consultant |
| 08:30 | Breakfast | Needed persuading to eat breakfast.<br>Ate with spoon. | HCA |
| 09:30 | Stimulation<br>programme<br>Calendar<br>Clock<br>Music 30 minutes | Orientated to time, place and person.<br>Able to tell time.<br>Recognise colours, pictures and names<br>of people from photos. | HCA |
| 10:00 | Skin care<br>Foot, toe, knee and<br>wrist exercises<br>Breathing exercises | No sign of redness or skin breakdown.<br>Completed series of foot and breathing<br>exercises with minimum prompting. | HCA |
| 11:00 | Tea, toilet | Able to manage cup independently.<br>Assistance required mobilising to toilet but<br>able to manage toileting independently. | HCA |
| 11:30-12:15 | Physiotherapy | Completed 8 minutes on exercise bicycle<br>without foot support. Leg muscle strength<br>improving. | Physiotherapist |
| 12:15-13:15 | Lunch | Ate well | HCA |
| 13:15-14:00 | Rest | Lying on bed reading magazine. | HCA |
| 14:00-14:45 | Speech therapy | Practised sounds and reading today. | Speech therapist |
| 14:45-15:30 | Family time | Played with children when they came<br>home from school. | Family member |
| 15:45-16:30 | Occupational<br>therapy | Quite animated today. Worked on cognitive<br>exercises. Please ensure left hand splinted<br>at night. | Occupational<br>therapist |
| 16:30 | Family recreation<br>Dinner<br>Family time<br>Stimulation<br>programme | Watched TV.<br><br>Sat in lounge with husband and mother.<br>Played 'scrabble'. | Family member<br>Family member |
| 20:30-21:00 | To bed | Quite tired after a full day. Good night. | Family member |

**Figure 27.6** An example of multidisciplinary record. Reproduced with permission of the British Journal of Neuroscience Nursing.

## Activity 27.1

### Scenario

A month ago Mr Jones, 21 years old, was in a motor vehicle accident. He suffered from polytrauma. His injuries included:

- Head injury with a GCS of 5/15.
- Fractured ribs 3, 4 and 5 on the right hand side for which he has been on a ventilator.
- Fractured pelvis.
- Fractured left femur which is pinned.
- His current functional ability is reported as:
  - Current GCS 9/15. Disorientated.
  - Left sided hemiparesis.
  - Difficulty with speech and eating.

### Exercises

1. Prepare a cognitive rehabilitation programme that can commence in the ward/unit as it will be some while before Mr Jones can be transferred to the Rehabilitation Unit.
2. In the accident Mr Jones' girlfriend, Samantha, was killed. Mr Jones keeps on asking you why Samantha has not been to see him. Describe how you will manage this situation.
3. Mr Jones family are most distressed at the lack of information that has been provided to them regarding head injuries. Describe how you will manage the situation and develop a resource for the family.

# Chapter 28
# Early Stimulation Programmes

*Nadine Abelson-Mitchell*

School of Nursing and Midwifery, Faculty of Health, Education and Society, Plymouth University, Devon, UK

## INTRODUCTION

Rehabilitation, using early stimulation programmes (ESPs), is an integral part of the patient's journey and needs to commence as soon after injury as is practicable (Andelic *et al.* 2012; Lippert-Grüner *et al.* 2002; Mitchell *et al.* 1990). Early stimulation programmes have been introduced into the management of head injured patients in an attempt to enable them to achieve maximum potential as well as maximum recovery in the shortest time period (Andelic *et al.* 2012; Bos 1997; Lippert-Grüner and Terhaag 2000).

There are a number of practitioners who acknowledge that there is no reliable evidence regarding the effectiveness of early stimulation programmes for head injured patients (Das-Gupta and Turner-Stokes 2002; Lombardi *et al.* 2002; Wood 1991). Das-Gupta and Turner-Stokes (2002: p. 655) and Wood (1991) suggest that ESP be introduced as it is 'therapeutic for the family'. Yet others believe that early stimulation is essential for head injured patients to maximise potential, especially in the light of new research related to neuroplasticity (Andelic *et al.* 2012; Bos 1997; Urbenjaphol *et al.* 2009). There is evidence that patients subjected to early intervention programmes have a far better discharge to home rate than those who did not (94 vs 57%) (Cope and Hall 1982).

## DEFINITION OF EARLY STIMULATION PROGRAMME

An individualised, comprehensive programme of stimulation, based on the patient's needs, that is introduced into the patient's programme whilst the patient is in a coma. Early stimulation programmes are formalised programmes that require patience and perseverance to ensure that the patient has the correct level of exposure to such a programme.

## BACKGROUND

The theoretical basis for introducing ESP is the belief that patients, whilst in a coma, suffer from sensory deprivation. It is this sensory deprivation that leads to a decrease in the mechanisms of information processing (Mitchell *et al.* 1990). Thus, the use of an enriched environment will aid physiological development and prevent deterioration of brain structures (Mitchell *et al.* 1990).

## OBJECTIVES OF INTRODUCING AN EARLY STIMULATION PROGRAMME (ESP)

1. To achieve the broader objectives of comprehensive rehabilitation by implementing the programme as soon as possible.

*Neurotrauma: Managing Patients with Head Injuries*, First Edition. Edited by Nadine Abelson-Mitchell.
© 2013 Blackwell Publishing Ltd. Published 2013 by Blackwell Publishing Ltd.

2. To provide the patient with every opportunity to achieve maximum potential and independence.
3. To promote neuroplasticity, by utilising areas of the brain that are damaged.
4. To establish additional/alternative networks through stimulation.
5. To improve awareness and alertness.
6. To improve blood flow to various areas of the brain.
7. To reduce the length of coma (Mitchell *et al.* 1990).

## SETTING UP THE ESP

The implementation of the early stimulation programme must be defined within the management plan, after discussion with, and agreement of, the multidisciplinary team and the family (Andelic *et al.* 2012; Lippert-Grüner and Terhaag 2000). Early stimulation programmes are labour-intensive and often require 1:1 stimulation. Families, friends and others, such as voluntary workers who have been trained, can participate in such stimulation programmes.

## CONTENT OF THE ESP

There is no agreed content of the stimulation programme and therefore this may vary within settings (Andelic *et al.* 2012; Lombardi *et al.* 2002; Vanier *et al.* 2002). For patients in a coma, all extraneous noises and all activities undertaken with the patient are regarded as stimulation. It is essential to consider the role of arousal, awareness, vigilance and habituation in the programme (Wood 1991). The most important aspect of the stimulation programme is to do no harm and cause no stress to the patient.

Use the Needs Approach Model (Chapter 3/Chapter 27) to determine the interests of the patient, any likes or dislikes that could be used within the stimulation programme. For example, the patient may have favourite smells, music, photos, sounds or books and all of these can be included in the stimulation programme. If the family is aware that the patient does not like a particular sensation, e.g. touching or rubbing his/her arms, this must be specifically excluded from the stimulation programme (Lippert-Grüner and Terhaag 2000).

Initially the ESP may be introduced for a few seconds or a few minutes in every hour or every two hours. Slowly the length of time spent on the ESP should be increased to about 15 minutes every hour. This may not always be possible due to the other needs of the patient. Observe and record the patient's responses to the various aspects of the stimulation programme. The patient may respond by moving a part of the body, by eye movements or by

### Top tips for early stimulation programmes

- Perform initial assessment of patient.
- Review programme daily/weekly.
- Ensure patient medically stable before implementing programme.
- Decrease noxious/environmental noise.
- Allow patient sufficient rest and sleep.
- Schedule stimulation programme for eventual maximum of 5–15 minutes per hour.
- Depending on the level of consciousness and needs of the patient the programme may include:
  - Reality orientation:
    - Use of calendar and clock.
    - Speaking to the patient about familiar aspects of daily life.
  - Sensory stimulation:
    - Use of familiar music at intervals throughout the day.
    - Use of colour charts or objects.
    - Use of photos.
    - Use of touch.
- Do not overstimulate.
- Note and document patient's response.
- Use music intermittently as part of stimulation programme:
  - Do not play music incessantly.
  - Definitely switch off music/radio at night.
  - When using music or a tape recorder the sound should be directed within the room.
  - Monitor the volume control.
  - If the patient is not in a private room use headsets that fit over the patient ears. Do not use headsets that fit directly into the patient's external auditory meatus.
  - Consider other patients in unit.
- Each patient to have their own Early Stimulation Programme with appropriate equipment. This equipment may be brought in from the family home. Please note any insurance issues.
- Touching/stroking the patients face is to be avoided because of the risk of introducing infection.

### Warning

In the presence of raised intracranial pressure, do not introduce any stimulation that will raise pressure, for example, music and loud noises. Limit the programme to speaking to the patient and gentle touch (not to the face).

producing tears or there may not be an obvious response. Lippert-Grüner *et al.* (2002) and Lippert-Grüner and Terhaag (2000) suggest the use of physiological monitoring to assess response to stimulation. Note the effect of the programme on intracranial pressure. If the patient is attached to a heart monitor or blood pressure monitor, note the patient's heart rate increase or decrease depending on the stimulation. It is important to note whether the patient is becoming distressed by the stimulation.

## SPECIFIC TECHNIQUES

There are specific techniques used for ESPs, including unimodal (one at a time) or multimodal (a number of different senses at the same time) stimulation of all senses, that vary depending on the needs of the patient (Bos 1997). Lippert-Grüner and Terhaag (2000) report the effectiveness of acoustic and tactile stimulation.

There are five senses that are included in the ESP:

- Hearing.
- Touch.
- Vision.
- Taste.
- Smell.

Examples of interventions that may be included:

Smell:
- Pleasant smells.
- Strong smells such as curry, cinnamon.
  NB: Check cough, gag, swallow reflex.
Taste:
- Favourite food, such as chocolate.
- Familiar food.
- Smell of food.
- Perfumes/aftershave.
Vision:
- Colours.
- Posters.
- Photos:
  - Family.
  - Friends.
  - Pets.
- Magazines.

Touch:
- Human touch.
- Stroke patients arm.
- Favourite objects.
- Feeling different textures.

Some centres have dedicated sensory stimulation units.

## HOW TO ENCOURAGE THE INVOLVEMENT OF FAMILY OR FRIENDS

Family and friends who visit the head injured person often do not know what to say or how to interact with the patient. By teaching them how to undertake various aspects of the programme, they are able to become directly involved by doing something constructive for the patient. After their visit they need to record their comments in the visitors' stimulation book.

Patient progress must be recorded in a care plan. The unit may also use visual progress charts and a family member, or the patient, may decide to keep a diary. Reviewing the diary with the patient at a later stage is a positive, albeit sometimes disturbing, experience.

---

### Activity 28.1

#### Scenario

Mrs Joanna Jones, 22 years old, has been admitted to the unit following a severe head injury.

Her injuries included:

- Head injury with a GCS of 5/15.
- Stable medical condition.

#### Exercises

1. Prepare an early stimulation programme for Joanna.
2. List the factors you will take into account when preparing the ESP.
3. Describe how you will assess Joanna's response to the programme.

# Chapter 29
# Discharge Planning

*Nadine Abelson-Mitchell*

School of Nursing and Midwifery, Faculty of Health, Education and Society, Plymouth University, Devon, UK

## INTRODUCTION

Discharge planning in neurotrauma is a multi-sectoral, multi-agency, complex process involving the patient, family, multidisciplinary team, as well as social and financial services. Effective discharge planning involves good communication, co-ordination of team effort, consideration of the needs of the patient and family, collaboration with individuals, agencies and organisations, being creative to find and utilise resources and finally maintaining integrity by doing the right thing for the individual and ensuring that the best possible outcomes will be achieved (Hunt and Levine 2006, National Leadership and Innovation Agency for Healthcare 2008, RCN 2004).

## WHAT IS DISCHARGE PLANNING?

Discharge planning commences on the day of admission and is continuous until discharge of the patient to the appropriate location. Discharge planning is about person-centred care that requires changing the patient's level of care from one of dependence to greater independence, where possible. Discharge planning involves getting the patient out of hospital to another location and may include plans for the patient's immediate, short-term and long-term future.

Active participation and ownership of the plan is essential to achieve positive outcomes. The family/carers will

need to be assertive, and be able to listen and accept compromise if necessary. Always consider what is best for the patient and aspire to achieve what is in the patient's best interest to achieve maximum potential.

## BENEFITS OF DISCHARGE PLANNING

There are a number of benefits of effective discharge planning (Shepperd *et al.* 2010) as it:

- Enables the patient to return to as normal a life as possible, as soon as possible.
- Encourages independence rather than dependence.
- Decreases the length of stay of the patient in hospital/rehabilitation centre.
- Relieves pressure on hospital beds (Bradley *et al.* 2006).
- Prevents/Decreases readmission to hospital.
- Decreases hospital costs.
- Aids in patient satisfaction (Shepperd *et al.* 2010).

## DISCHARGE PLANNING PROCESS

Discharge planning is defined as 'a process not an isolated event' (DH 2003: p. 2). Discharge planning is a process that involves a multidisciplinary approach, focusing on the patient and family. Discharge planning is part of the patient's journey and is determined using a holistic

*Neurotrauma: Managing Patients with Head Injuries*, First Edition. Edited by Nadine Abelson-Mitchell.
© 2013 Blackwell Publishing Ltd. Published 2013 by Blackwell Publishing Ltd.

approach. Once again, the Needs Approach Model can be used to determine discharge planning needs and outcomes (see Chapter 3/Chapter 27).

There are a number of phases included in discharge planning:

- Assessment of the patient's needs (see Appendix 2 for discharge planning assessment).
- Planning for the discharge.
- Implementing the plan.
- Review of outcomes.
- Discharging the patient.
- Follow-up after discharge.

## CRITERIA FOR DISCHARGE PLANNING

Criteria that may be considered when planning for discharge include:

Physical criteria:
- Level of consciousness (GCS).
- Stable vital signs.
- Incontinence.
- Physical care needs, e.g. wounds, means of feeding.
- Mobility.
- Level of independence.

Psychological criteria:
- Level of motivation.
- Mood.
- Aggression.

## SELECTING THE DISCHARGE DESTINATION

The discharge destination is determined mainly by the patient's needs. This could be home, another hospital, regional centre, rehabilitation centre or residential facility depending on the patient's needs, family circumstances and availability of appropriate resources. It may be necessary for members of the multidisciplinary team, the patient and family to make a home visit to assess resource requirements. The patient and family may also wish to visit any recommended facilities to enable them to make an informed choice regarding the patient's destination.

The patient and family need to be aware of the planned discharge date towards which the team are working as delays in discharge may have detrimental effects on the patient (Bryan 2010). To build confidence it may be possible to introduce days or weekends at home into the rehabilitation programme as part of the planning for discharge.

A pre-requisite for discharge planning is preparing the patient and family. The patient and family need to know how to implement all aspects of the discharge plan. Training is an important part of discharge planning. It is essential to assess the level of knowledge and competence of the carers. Carers may need to undertake specific tasks and may need to learn how to do the required tasks. To ensure a smooth transition to home, teaching and learning need to continue until the carers feel confident and competent to undertake the tasks. Teaching strategies that may be employed include demonstrations, use of equipment, books, pamphlets, web-based learning and experiential learning regarding various aspects of care that may be required.

## THE DAY OF DISCHARGE

The family may find the patient's discharge an emotional and stressful experience; therefore provide support to the family at discharge as they may be concerned about taking the patient home. Taking the patient home should be a joyful process rather than being seen as a burden to the family. Arrange the actual time and date of discharge with precision and provide a written plan and reassure the patient and carers that their needs have been considered.

Prior to discharge contact the patient's GP practice to notify them of the patient's impending discharge. On discharge, provide the patient with a letter for the GP.

## CONCLUSION

The discharge process needs to be fully planned. To ensure a seamless transition from hospital to home, effective discharge planning is essential.

## Top tips for discharge planning

- Commence as soon as possible after admission.
- Communication is key.
- Keep a notebook to record meetings, appointments, questions, phone numbers, etc.
- Identify multidisciplinary discharge team.
- Team to take ownership of process.
- Consider needs of patient on discharge.
- Be realistic, persistent and prepared.
- Do not be pressurised into actions.
- Make informed decisions and choices.
- Set realistic goals and outcomes.
- Specify a timeframe.
- Work within timeframe.
- Identify resources required, including community resources.
- Ensure all resources in place to enable effective discharge planning.
- Financial implications of discharge plan.
- Are carers required?
  - Consider needs of carers.
  - Consider health of carers.
- Consider carer capability.
- Number of hours of care required.
- Activities carer has agreed to undertake.
- Current employment pattern of carers.
- Financial implications for carers.
- What resources are available to support carers?
- Consider training needs of carers.
- Ensure people needed for care post-discharge are in place.
- How will patient reach discharge destination?
- Ensure written discharge plan.
- Provide date for follow-up.
- Provide emergency contact numbers.
- Document discharge plan.
- Provide means of documentation for patient or family to use at home to enable effective feedback on follow-up.
- Notify discharge destination of impending transfer.
- It is preferable not to discharge patients to their new placement on Fridays as resources are usually limited on weekends.

## Activity 29.1

### Scenario

Mr Brown, 31 years old, was involved in a road traffic accident. He has been in the ward for the past 6 weeks. He is about to be discharged to home. He presents with the following:

- GCS score 14/15.
- At times he is agitated. Right-sided weakness and short-term memory loss.
- He is on Paracetamol for pain.

### Exercises

1. Using a needs approach assess Mr Brown's needs.
2. Prepare a care plan for Mr Brown for discharge to home.
3. Consider any aspects that are of significance to patient rehabilitation and recovery in the home environment.

| Nursing diagnosis | Potential problems | Possible causes | Intervention | Outcome/Evaluation |
|---|---|---|---|---|
| | | | | |
| | | | | |

## Activity 29.2

### Scenario

Mr O'Connell, 51 years old, has been in the ward for the past 6 weeks. He is about to be discharged to home. Mr O'Connell has had a craniotomy for removal of a subdural haematoma after falling in the street.

He presents with the following:

- GCS score 14/15.
- At times he is agitated and aggressive.
- He is not always steady on his feet.

### Exercises

1. Using a needs approach assess Mr O'Connell's needs.
2. Prepare a care plan for Mr O'Connell's discharge to home.
3. Consider any aspects that are of significance to patient rehabilitation and recovery.

Utilise the following format:

| Nursing diagnosis | Potential problems | Possible causes | Intervention | Outcome/Evaluation |
|---|---|---|---|---|
| | | | | |
| | | | | |

## Activity 29.3

### Scenario

Charles, 18 years old, Steven, 19 years old, and Chris, 17 years old, were tombstoning (jumping off a height of 15 metres into the sea). They thought the water was deep enough.

Charles dived into the water and suffered an extradural bleed over the left parietal region as well as a fractured base of the skull with blood leaking out of his left ear.

He was in hospital for 6 weeks. He then attended a rehabilitation centre for 4 months. He is now going back home to live with his parents.

### Exercises

1. Using a needs approach assess his needs.
2. Prepare a care plan to discharge Charles to home.
3. Consider any aspects that are of significance to patient rehabilitation and recovery.

| Nursing diagnosis | Potential problems | Possible causes | Intervention | Outcome/Evaluation |
|---|---|---|---|---|
| | | | | |
| | | | | |

# Chapter 30
# Living in the Community

*Nadine Abelson-Mitchell*

School of Nursing and Midwifery, Faculty of Health, Education and Society, Plymouth University, Devon, UK

## INTRODUCTION

The goals of rehabilitation include the promotion of independence, social integration and return to work. Therefore, a person living in the community with a long-term condition, with residual cognitive and psychological difficulties, needs to be managed as effectively possible (Turner-Stokes *et al.* 2008). Social integration includes aspects such as satisfaction with quality of life, productivity and return to driving (McCabe *et al.* 2007). With a focus on living in the community, it is important to assess the patient within their own environment, work, home, education and leisure, as patients with neurotrauma are encouraged to return to their previous roles, relationships, lives, work and leisure activities, where possible.

## INTEGRATING INTO THE COMMUNITY

In recent years, legislation, such as the Human Rights Act 1998, Department of Health policies and the Equality Act 2010, have influenced society. Legislation has been introduced regarding access to buildings for people with disabilities and long-term conditions. An integral aspect of community management is the education of patients, families and the society to enhance tolerance and understanding of the abilities, capabilities and limitations of people after brain injury. The patient who has returned to the community may be perceived as being 'different' or 'not the same person'. It is important to empower the patient to inform the people in his environment of his ability to interact with them. It is important for patients, families and communities to facilitate and share available space and resources for mutual benefit and to improve the quality of life for all people. Patients and families need to seek out these resources and must be encouraged to participate and be actively involved in the community (Johnstone *et al.* 2003).

Many head-injured people lead unsatisfactory social lives. This can be because of their behaviour, attitudes and approach. Often they lose their friends and find it difficult to make new friends, resulting in social isolation and lack of self-esteem (McCabe *et al.* 2007). The introduction of a 'supportive relationship', a friend or buddy for the head-injured person, may help to resolve this situation (Johnson and Davis 1998).

Mobility and transport, post-injury, need to be considered. Driving post-head injury is an important aspect of social competence and independence. Many head-injured people wish to carry on driving post-injury (Leon-Carrion *et al.* 2005): 50% of people with a severe TBI and 75% of people with a moderate TBI return to driving (Perino and Rago [cited in McCabe *et al.* (2007)]). According to McCabe *et al.* (2007) there is a higher incident of collisions in drivers who have suffered a previous head injury. The key to driving post-head injury is whether the head-injured person is safe to drive and competent at driving. If people with head injuries wish to drive they need to be responsible drivers, have insight into their condition and limitations, undertake further examinations to assess driver competence and drive within the limits and requirements of the law (McCabe *et al.* 2007).

# Chapter 31
# Legal Matters

*Andrew Warlow[1] and Simon Parford[2]*

[1]Head and Spinal Injuries Unit, Wolferstans, Plymouth, UK
[2]Clinical Negligence, Wolferstans, Plymouth, UK

## INTRODUCTION

Throughout the patient journey it is vitally important to avoid the occurrence of real or potential medico-legal issues. A basic knowledge of legal matters will assist the professional to avoid some medico-legal pitfalls. Legal concepts of relevance to neurotrauma have been provided by experts in the field.

## COMPENSATION CLAIMS ARISING OUT OF HEAD INJURIES

Not all acquired brain injuries result in compensation claims. Far from it. Some, of course, are naturally occurring. Others arise out of pure accident where no-one is to blame for what happened except perhaps the injured person. It is only where the injury was directly caused by the negligence or breach of statutory duty imposed on a third party that there may be a claim for compensation. It is because of this that one of the first things a lawyer will consider when presented with a potential new client who has suffered head injury, is whether the accident which gave rise to the head injury was the direct result of the failure of a third party to exercise due care or to comply with a duty of care imposed by statute. A lawyer will therefore wish to establish the position in this connection as a matter of urgency. This is because the lawyer will

know that to establish liability it will be necessary to be able to produce evidence, whether in the form of statements, documents (such as records as to correct procedures to be followed), photographs or expert reports. In the case of witness statements particularly, it is important to establish the evidence as soon as possible after an accident because peoples' recollections fade fairly quickly and the sooner a witness gives written evidence the more reliable that evidence is likely to be considered.

Often, assistance can be obtained in establishing liability through the obtaining of an admission of liability from insurers or other legal representatives acting on behalf of the person at fault. Indeed, a lawyer will wish to make contact with such a representative as soon as possible, not only to seek an admission of liability but, in the case of insurers, to involve them in setting up rehabilitation for the client at the earliest possible opportunity. It appears to be generally accepted that the earlier rehabilitation can be put into place, the better the final outcome. This will usually be provided under what is known as the Rehabilitation Code of Best Practice, originally set up in 1999 but subsequently revised in August 2007. The object of this Code is to consider, so far as practical, whether early intervention, rehabilitation or medical treatment would improve the present or long-term situation, and then to

*Neurotrauma: Managing Patients with Head Injuries*, First Edition. Edited by Nadine Abelson-Mitchell.
© 2013 Blackwell Publishing Ltd. Published 2013 by Blackwell Publishing Ltd.

obtain an early independent needs assessment, which should be followed by appropriate treatment. This is considered to be one of the most important aspects of lawyer's work, because whilst compensation is very important, it pales against the benefit of good health. Indeed, it would be highly unlikely that one would encounter a client who has suffered serious head injury who would not much rather have had their pre-accident health and wellbeing than the compensation they subsequently received.

Of course, there are cases where the person at fault may not be insured. Whilst this is unlikely to be a problem in road traffic accident cases where there is provision for compulsory insurance and the Motor Insurers Bureau, a body set up by insurers, deals with claims against uninsured drivers (subject to exceptions), this is not so in other cases. One cannot get blood out of a stone and if a party at fault does not have insurance or other funds to meet a compensation claim then there is not going to be any point in bringing such a claim.

In the case of a head injury arising out of a criminal assault, compensation may be claimed under the Criminal Injuries Compensation Scheme, even if the person who committed the assault has no money. The present scheme provides for a tariff-based system of compensation for those who meet the appropriate criteria.

Enquiries into the circumstances giving rise to an accident, with a view to establishing liability, may take some time. They may involve the obtaining of records from the police or other agency, detailed inspection of where the accident happened or equipment involved, and expert reports. Therefore things don't always proceed as quickly as one would hope. In any event, it is at the forefront of the minds of all lawyers dealing with personal injury claims that proceedings must be commenced within three years of the date of the accident, failing which they will be statute barred. As is often the case, there can be exceptions to this. Also, the Court has a discretion to disapply this time limit. Further, the three years only starts from the date of the accident or from when the injured person first had the necessary knowledge of the injury or the negligence which caused it. Indeed, if the accident immediately caused the client to have, in the words of the relevant statute, 'unsound mind' the time period will not start to run whilst he or she is of unsound mind.

In this connection it may be relevant that the person who has suffered a head injury may, because of his or her injuries, lack the legal capacity necessary to manage their own affairs and/or bring a compensation claim. In that event, a Litigation Friend will need to be appointed to represent the head-injured person. This person must be somebody who

has no conflicting interest with the person they represent. In cases where liability is agreed and significant compensation is expected, it is advisable for the Litigation Friend to apply to the Court of Protection for the injured person to be made a Protected Party and for the Litigation Friend to be appointed to deal with the administration of the injured person's finances and conduct of their claim. Upon such appointment the Litigation Friend is known as a Deputy. The lawyer will take instructions from such person. There are, of course, costs involved in this and they will form part of the compensation claim.

Of course, the work of a lawyer in compensation claims must be paid for. Generally speaking (and as ever there are exceptions to this), the successful party in a claim for compensation is entitled to the payment of the majority of their legal costs and expenses from the unsuccessful party. This is all well and good if you are successful as a Claimant, but what if you are not? In that event, there will be a liability on the part of the injured person and/or their Litigation Friend/Deputy to pay not only their own lawyer's fees and expenses but also those of the other side. This would present, in many cases, an insurmountable hurdle to pursuing a claim for compensation. However, because of the introduction a few years ago of what are known as Conditional Fee Agreements, sometimes rather imprecisely referred to as 'No Win, No Fee Agreements', this problem can be overcome so far as the lawyer's own costs are concerned, because under such agreements, if the case fails, then the lawyer will not recover his or her fees. What then about the expenses incurred during the course of a claim and the other side's costs, both of which can be substantial? It is here that what is known as 'After The Event Legal Expenses Insurance' comes in. This strange creature is a form of insurance by which an insurer will cover these liabilities of the Claimant if the case fails. However, as with insurances generally there is a premium to be paid, but what makes this particular type of insurance unusual, is that often the premium can be paid at the end of the case. If the case is successful then the other side will be required to pay the premium, providing it is reasonable. If the case is not successful then the premium will be paid by the insurers themselves. This is all subject to the terms of the particular insurance provided.

Perhaps you will gain the impression from the last two paragraphs that the issue of costs in compensation claims is complicated. So it is. Further, the system is anticipated to change under legislation being taken through Parliament at the present time. At the moment it appears that these changes will take place sometime in April 2013. Unfortunately, at the present time, we don't know quite what the changes will be and these two paragraphs dealing with costs will, by then, be out-of-date.

Indeed, the law when it comes to compensation claims is a constantly-changing thing. It is important therefore that the lawyer handling the claim should be up-to-date with all the latest developments. It is also a substantial help if the lawyer is familiar with the impact of head injuries on victims of accidents and has a good understanding of head injury. This is because he or she will then have a much better appreciation of what the injured person and those close to him are going through and will therefore be able to provide more effective support. Not only will he have a greater awareness of the resources available to provide such support for as long as the head injury is likely to impact on the victim, which can often be for the rest of that person's life, but also he will have a greater knowledge of the best experts available to assess the nature and extent of the injuries suffered. In this way the victim's claim will be put forward to the best advantage with a view to maximising the compensation claimed and the help received en route. Helpful information about specialist personal injury lawyers can be found from the website of the Association of Personal Injury Lawyers (www.apil.org.uk). Also, Headway, The Brain Injury Association have a Directory of Head Injury Solicitors: information can be accessed from their website (www.headway.org.uk).

Finally, the legal process might sound as if it is a long-winded one. In fact, there is more and more emphasis on the importance of progressing claims as quickly as possible. Indeed, once Court proceedings have been commenced the management of cases is in the hands of the Court. They, in turn, are required to give effect to what is known as 'Overriding Objective' which, amongst other things, requires the Court to ensure that cases are dealt with expeditiously and fairly.

## BRAIN INJURY AND MEDICAL NEGLIGENCE

Brain injury can sometimes arise as a result of an error on the part of a member of the medical profession to provide appropriate care. Medical professionals owe what is known as a 'duty of care' to all patients and, if they fall below an acceptable standard of care (as measured by the legal tests established in *Bolam v Friern Hospital Management Committee* ([1957] 1 WLR 582) and *Bolitho v City* and *Hackney Health Authority* ([1998] AC 232), generally known as the 'Bolam Test', an injury may result.

Brain injury may result from inappropriate or negligent surgery or in connection with the provision of other treatment, but occurs far more commonly from delays in definitive diagnosis and errors occurring during post-operative management.

Whereas an individual who suffers a brain injury as a result of a road traffic accident, accident at work, a fall or an assault is likely to have been perfectly healthy prior to the event, in every case where medical negligence occurs the patient will already be under investigation or treatment for an underlying illness. Brain injuries may result from any number of injuries or medical conditions. In some cases, even with appropriate treatment, the patient will still have some residual degree of disability but in others, if a timely diagnosis is made and appropriate treatment provided, the patient may make a full recovery.

A number of the common areas of medical negligence where brain injury occurs or is exacerbated are dealt with below.

## HEAD INJURIES

The Royal College of Surgeons in England published a report in 1999 dealing with their concerns that some patients with head injuries die unnecessarily and other patients suffer long-term sequelae due to inappropriate management. The report highlighted inadequacies in the provision of head injury services for these patients, many of whom are initially, and sometimes exclusively, seen by relatively junior doctors. The National Institute for Health and Clinical Excellence (NICE) subsequently published guidelines for the triage, assessment, investigation and early management of head injury in infants, children and adults, in 2003, which were updated in 2007.

Head injuries occur in all age groups, with a peak incidence in males between the ages of 16 and 25 years and a second peak in the elderly, who have a high incidence of chronic subdural haematomas. The majority of head injuries in the UK are caused by road traffic accidents, falls and assaults (Jennett 1996).

Medical litigation usually arises from errors in the management of head injury patients occurring in accident and emergency departments and observation wards. In accident and emergency departments patients can be inappropriately reassured and discharged without the appropriate investigations or observations being undertaken, only to return within 24 or 48 hours in a moribund condition.

In other cases, where the patient is believed to have used, or admits to having used, recreational drugs (such as alcohol, hallucinogens and cannabis), it may be difficult to obtain a history and the patient's behaviour, and that of his companions, may be aggressive and disruptive.

However, before a patient's condition is attributed wholly to the effects of alcohol, a blood level should be taken and, if appropriate, the patient should be admitted for observation.

In the conscious head injured patient, a decision must be taken about whether or not a skull x-ray or CT scan should be undertaken immediately or whether the patient should be admitted for observation.

For patients admitted for head injury observation, the minimum acceptable documented neurological observations are:

- GCS (Glasgow Coma Scale).
- Pupil size and reactivity.
- Limb movements.
- Respiratory rate.
- Heart rate.
- Blood pressure.
- Temperature.
- Blood oxygen saturation.

Medical, nursing and other staff caring for patients with head injury admitted for observation should all be capable of performing these observations. Observations should be performed and recorded on a half hourly basis until a GCS equal to 15 has been achieved. The minimum frequency of observations for patients with GCS equal to 15 should be as follows, starting after the initial assessment in the Emergency Department: half hourly for two hours; then one hourly for four hours; then two hourly thereafter. If the patient with GCS equal to 15 deteriorates at any time after the initial two hour period, observation should revert to half hourly and follow the original frequency of observation.

If a patient is discharged following a head injury it is obligatory that they are in the care of a responsible adult and that head injury advice is given. This should not only be verbal advice, there should be a written head injury advice card. The details of the card should be discussed with the patient and their carer/s.

Unfortunately, there are occasions when the observations are not conducted or recorded appropriately by the nursing staff so that it is not possible to determine whether further investigations, specifically a CT scan, need to be performed and/or to ensure that it is performed at the appropriate time.

In addition there are occasions when a patient is discharged without there being a responsible adult to accompany them and/or without their having been provided with appropriate head injury advice.

## Case study

A young man, aged 23, went out for the night with his friends. He was drinking alcohol and during the latter part of the evening he fell down three stairs and struck his head on the floor.

An ambulance was called and he was taken to the Accident and Emergency Department of his local hospital, arriving at 22.30 hours. He had a scalp laceration and it was intended to undertake a skull x-ray but this proved to be impossible as the patient was unco-operative.

He was admitted to the Accident and Emergency observation ward for neurological observations, where he remained overnight. The nurses carried out their observations appropriately and recorded their findings. However they failed to notify the medical staff during the night that the patient had a fluctuating GCS, dropping to 9 at one point.

The next day, after spending the morning sleeping, the patient was seen by a consultant in the Accident and Emergency Department. The patient appeared co-operative and communicative and the Consultant, who had not seen all his notes, advised that he should be discharged home that afternoon – which is what occurred. No responsible adult was contacted to collect the patient from hospital but he was given a head injury advice sheet.

The following morning, the patient was found by his father lying face down on his bedroom floor. An ambulance was called and on arrival at the accident and emergency department at 08.00 hours, it was noted that the patient's GCS was 3, he was cyanosed and tachycardic. He was intubated and an urgent CT head scan was undertaken which demonstrated a left acute subdural haematoma. He was taken to theatre for evacuation of the haematoma.

It was alleged on the patient's behalf that there had been a failure to act upon the observations recorded during his first admission. The fluctuating GCS which dropped to 9 at one stage during the night should have resulted in the nursing staff alerting the medical staff immediately which would have resulted in the performance of an early CT head scan. This would have diagnosed the subdural haematoma and he would have been taken to theatre for evacuation of the haematoma before the catastrophic brain injury occurred.

The hospital admitted liability and the claim was settled.

## Subarachnoid haemorrhage (SAH)

The effects of delayed diagnosis of an aneurysmal SAH have been well documented. The consequence of such a delay is usually that the patient suffers a rebleed with increased morbidity and mortality. It has been shown that as a direct result of delay significantly more patients died or were severely disabled than those whose haemorrhage was diagnosed without delay (Neil-Dwyer and Lang 1997).

The majority of patients who suffer an SAH complain of a sudden headache which is quite unlike any headache they have previously experienced. While 2% of patients deny a headache having suffered an SAH and 40% of patients may have no confirmatory sign such as neck stiffness, the majority will give a history clearly indicative of a sudden intracranial event. It is the history of headache with its mode of onset, severity and persistence which is the single and most certain way of making a diagnosis of subarachnoid haemorrhage.

Medical litigation is usually pursued against the patient's General Practitioner for failure to consider a possible diagnosis of SAH and to immediately refer the patient to an A&E, or against NHS Trusts for the failure of the staff in the Accident and Emergency Department to correctly identify the possibility that the patient may have suffered a subarachnoid haemorrhage, discharging the patient without having arranged for appropriate investigations to be undertaken, specifically a CT scan and a lumbar puncture.

## Hydrocephalus

Hydrocephalus, both congenital and resulting from haemorrhage, is effectively treated by the insertion of a valved shunt system. This bypasses the blockage to the flow of cerebrospinal fluid and usually a ventriculoperitoneal shunt is used. However, endoscopic techniques for carrying out the ventriculostomy are increasingly preferred in appropriate cases.

Medical litigation usually revolves around delays in the original diagnosis of raised intracranial pressure and in recognising complications arising from the shunt insertion or the ventriculoscopic surgery.

Claims are usually pursued against the patient's General Practitioner for a failure to consider the possibility of raised intracranial pressure and immediately referring the patient to an A&E, or against the NHS Trusts for the failure of the staff in the A&E to correctly identify the possibility that the patient is suffering from raised intracranial pressure, discharging the patient without having arranged an appropriate investigation to be undertaken, specifically a CT scan.

Claims are also pursued against NHS Trusts for failures by nursing staff to properly observe and record their observations during the post-operative period with the result that an increase in raised intracranial pressure is not detected until it is too late, with catastrophic consequences.

### Case study

A young woman aged 25 had developed non-communicating hydrocephalus at the age of 16 after a TBI, and a VP shunt had been inserted. Everything was fine for approximately 10 years until her shunt became blocked.

The young woman developed signs of raised intracranial pressure. She attended the Accident and Emergency Department of her local hospital who initially reassured her and discharged her. However, after she returned 24 hours later, a CT scan was undertaken and she was immediately referred to the local neurosurgical centre where surgery was performed to replace the blocked shunt.

Post-operatively the nursing staff initially performed neurological observations and recorded their findings regularly. However, during the course of the night the nursing staff failed to undertake several neurological observations and/or to record their findings and they also failed to appreciate the significance of a lack of drainage of CSF, increasing blood pressure and increasing respiratory rate. As a result, medical staff were not called to review the patient until after the patient had suffered a sustained period of severe raised intracranial pressure which resulted in a catastrophic brain injury.

The hospital admitted liability and the claim was settled.

## Infection

Medical litigation arises from a delayed diagnosis and, less frequently, from the delay in commencing appropriate treatment after a diagnosis has been made.

The most frequent cause of litigation is the failure to diagnose meningitis with its sequelae. However, there are other circumstances where infection may result in brain injury if there is a delay in diagnosis or treatment, the most frequent of which are cerebral abscess and subdural empyema.

Claims relating to a failure or delay in the diagnosis of meningitis are usually against the patient's General Practitioner on the basis that there was a failure to consider the correct diagnosis and to make a timely or urgent referral to hospital.

Claims relating to a failure to diagnose and treat a cerebral abscess or a subdural empyema are usually against the patient's General Practitioner for failing to appreciate the need for further investigation of the patient's presenting symptoms and failing to refer the patient to hospital.

Claims against NHS Trusts are either for failures on the part of the staff in the A&E to appreciate the potential severity of the patient's condition and to arrange for appropriate investigations to be undertaken before discharge or, occasionally, for failing to prescribe appropriate antibiotics or to prescribe and/or administer appropriate antibiotics sufficiently promptly.

Whilst there are a number of well-known cardinal signs to assist in the diagnosis of meningitis, one of the difficulties in diagnosing a cerebral abscess is that the presenting symptoms tend to be non-specific. It tends to occur more commonly in males, with general symptoms of raised intracranial pressure in which the commonest features are headache, vomiting and nausea. Subdural empyema is less common than cerebral abscess. It affects males more than females and a common age at presentation is between 10–20 years old. The common presenting features are sinusitis, pyrexia, headache, neurological deficit, seizures, neck stiffness and less commonly swelling over the forehead and vomiting.

The main investigation for both cerebral abscess and subdural empyema is a CT scan, although in subdural empyema this may fail to demonstrate the pathology, particularly if contrast is not given and the scan quality is poor.

The most significant factors determining a good outcome in the treatment of both cerebral abscess and subdural empyema are early diagnosis and the clinical state of the patient at the time of surgery.

A delay in diagnosis and the commencement of appropriate treatment can result in a catastrophic brain injury which would otherwise have been avoided completely or the severity of which would have been reduced.

### Vegetative state and minimally conscious state

Patients who have suffered catastrophic brain injuries may be diagnosed as being in a vegetative state; such patients may live for many years, if provided with appropriate nursing care. However, there is a widespread consensus in many countries that survival for many years in a vegetative state is of no benefit to the patient and it is, therefore, appropriate to withdraw life-sustaining treatment once permanence is declared.

The decision to withdraw life-sustaining treatment can be a highly emotive one, with which the patient's family cannot agree, either with the medical professionals or amongst themselves.

In the UK the case of Bland (*Airedale National Health Service Trust v Bland* [1993] AC 789; [1993] 1 All ER 821) established that withdrawal of tube feeding from a permanently vegetative patient is lawful and this was confirmed in the unanimous decision in the House of Lords.

It is, therefore, of considerable concern that there are alarmingly high rates of misdiagnosis (40–43%) where patients in a minimally conscious state are wrongly diagnosed as being in a vegetative state (Gill-Thwaites 2006). It is essential that appropriate assessments are undertaken to determine the correct level of consciousness in such patients before decisions are made about their future treatment.

### THE COST OF BRAIN INJURY

The cost of brain injury resulting from medical negligence is huge both in human and financial terms. A productive member of society, in full-time employment, playing a full role in their family and community, may suddenly become entirely dependent upon others for the remainder of their life. Alternatively a child, who is still dependent, even from the time of their birth, may suffer a brain injury which significantly reduces or completely removes any quality of life for the whole of their life, however long that may be.

In human terms, it is a catastrophe not only for the person who has suffered the injury but also for their family and friends and others who may be dependent upon them in some way.

Nowadays, with advances in medical science and improvements in the quality of care provided, a person with a brain injury may have a very long, often near normal, life expectancy.

In financial terms, a person who has suffered a brain injury, particularly where a severe disability results, requires very substantial resources to be made available to support them and provide for their needs. These may include the provision of care and domestic assistance, medical treatment and therapies, suitable alternative accommodation, as well as adapted transport, aids and appliances and other items. Whether these resources are provided by the NHS and/or social services or an award of damages is made, the cost is likely to run into millions of pounds. It is not uncommon for awards of damages for a severely brain injured claimant to have a value of £5 million, or even £10 million or more.

# Chapter 32
# Meeting Tomorrow's Challenges

*Nadine Abelson-Mitchell*

School of Nursing and Midwifery, Faculty of Health, Education and Society, Plymouth University, Devon, UK

## CONCLUSION

Neurotrauma remains a major public health issue. Neurotrauma management continues to strive for the patient's maximum potential and independence as well as integration into the family and community with a contribution to the common good. The incidence of head injury is increasing as is the prevalence of neurotrauma in the community. Mortality has decreased but morbidity and sequelae of neurotrauma remain evident and require preventive management to ensure the patient is able to return to their family and community.

The acquisition of knowledge enables an understanding of the neurosciences, patient behaviour and community integration as well as the ability to develop as a confident and competent practitioner who has accepted the challenge of neurotrauma excellence. Nurses, who have acquired in-depth knowledge, will be able to assist the patient, family, carers and community along the patient journey in a positive manner and support the patient in his return to the family and community. Contained within this book are the elements necessary to enable those who have suffered a traumatic brain injury to regain their dignity and attain their maximum psychological and physical potential, through competent, comprehensive multidisciplinary management, including nursing.

The patients who have lost so much and whose greatest desire is be 'as they were' before the incident are the central focus of the multidisciplinary team, determine the continuing care needs and the contribution of team members to their on-going care in the community. The patient, family and carers need to be supported throughout the journey to ensure a seamless transition from injury to final placement. Families need to seek additional resources in order to cope with the newly created situation in which they find themselves.

The multidisciplinary team is made up of doctors, nurses, ambulance personnel, therapists, carers and family whose knowledge, expertise, experience and abilities are continually working towards improving the quality of care and the patient experience for people with TBI. Support via the multidisciplinary team and legal issues are described to enable professionals, patients and families to gain insight into the ethical and medico-legal issues facing patients with neurotrauma. This provides an opportunity to consider values and ethical issues appropriate to neurotrauma.

The management of the patient in primary, secondary and tertiary settings will affect outcome and the manner in which the patient settles within the environment. With all the discussion, research and concerns, little progress has been made towards the need to increase facilities for rehabilitation after the initial acute medical care has been concluded, as reflected in the carers' stories. There have been numerous government and private initiatives, including the drive for community-based rehabilitation services, but the outcome is that with a steadily expanding population and an increasing number of traumatic brain injured people, there remains a lack of facilities.

The challenge for the future is to continue with the development of the skills necessary to offer traumatic brain-injured persons their best chance of attaining maximum potential. Then, to actively seek ways and means of reducing the incidence of TBI.

The patient's journey continues until ultimate recovery has been achieved. This may continue for many years after the initial injury, provided appropriate management and resources are in place.

It is essential to encourage professionals and patients to meet the challenges of tomorrow.

# Section 6
# APPENDICES

# Appendix 1
# Pre-Admission Assessment

## INSTRUCTIONS

This form is to be completed by the Registered Nurse undertaking the pre-admission assessment in conjunction with the client, carer, family and referring unit.

The pre-admission assessment will be undertaken:

1. By the pre-admission co-ordinator (Registered Nurse).
2. Within 7 days of referral to the rehabilitation service.
3. A date and time for the assessment will be arranged with the referring unit.
4. Where applicable, the referring unit will arrange for the carer, family member and/or significant other to be present.

5. The referring unit will be notified of the decision to admit within 7 days of completion of the assessment.
6. Although a decision may be made to admit a client, the date of admission will depend on bed availability in the various units.

> **NOTE:**
>
> **At all times the Unit maintains a non-alcohol policy within the service.**

*Neurotrauma: Managing Patients with Head Injuries*, First Edition. Edited by Nadine Abelson-Mitchell.
© 2013 Blackwell Publishing Ltd. Published 2013 by Blackwell Publishing Ltd.

**PRE-ADMISSION ASSESSMENT**
**DEMOGRAPHIC DATA:**

| 1. | Name of client: | |
|---|---|---|
| 2. | Date of birth: | |

| 3. | Sex: | Male | Female |
|---|---|---|---|

| 4. | Client's home address:<br><br>Contact number: | |
|---|---|---|
| 5. | Medical diagnosis: | |

**REFERRAL AGENT:**

| 6. | Client's current placement:<br><br>Contact number: | |
|---|---|---|
| 7. | Person referring client:<br><br>Contact number: | |
| 8. | Length of stay in current placement: | |

| 9. | Reason for referral: | Assessment | |
|---|---|---|---|
| | | Intermediate | |
| | | Continuing | |
| | | Respite | |
| | | Other | |

10. Interdisciplinary team involvement

| Professional | Name | Contact no.: | Date of last review |
|---|---|---|---|
| Medical consultant | | | |
| General practitioner | | | |
| Nurse consultant | | | |
| Primary nurse | | | |
| District Nurse | | | |
| Health visitor | | | |
| Physiotherapist | | | |
| Occupational therapist | | | |
| Speech and Language Therapist | | | |

| Professional | Name | Contact no.: | Date of last review |
|---|---|---|---|
| Psychology | | | |
| Neuropsychology | | | |
| Dietician | | | |
| Social worker: | | | |

| 11. | Name of client's GP:<br><br>Address:<br><br>Contact number: | |
|---|---|---|

**FAMILY INFORMATION**

| 12. | Marital status: | |
|---|---|---|
| | Married | |
| | Living with partner | |
| | Separated | |
| | Divorced | |
| | Widowed | |
| | Other | |

13. No. and ages of children:

| | Number | Age | Sex |
|---|---|---|---|
| Nil | | | |
| 1 | | | |
| 2 | | | |
| 3 | | | |
| 4 | | | |
| 5 | | | |

14. Current employment:

15. Local contact details for next of kin

| Name: |
|---|
| Address:<br><br>Contact number: |

16. Short stay contact details for next of kin

| |
|---|
| Name: |
| Address: |
| |
| |
| Contact number: |

17. Date of initial contact:
18. Details of proposed respite:
18.1 Preferred date of admission.
18.2 Preferred length of stay.
18.3 Preferred date of discharge.

19. | Date of assessment: | |
    |---|---|

20. | Name/s of assessor/s: | |
    |---|---|

21. | Planned date of review: | |
    |---|---|

22. | Signature of assessor/s | |
    |---|---|

## PREVIOUS HEALTH HISTORY

23. | Date of injury/illness: | | | | | | | | |
    |---|---|---|---|---|---|---|---|---|

24. | Previous health history: |
    |---|
    | |
    | |
    | |
    | |
    | |
    | |
    | Mental health history: |
    | |
    | |

25. | Nature of current illness/injury: |
    |---|
    | |
    | |

**26.  SOCIAL PRACTICES:**

26.1
| Smoking | YES | | NO | |
|---|---|---|---|---|
| Quantity: | | | | |

| Client able to smoke: | |
|---|---|
| Without assistance | |
| Requires assistance | |

26.2
| Alcohol consumption | YES | | NO | |
|---|---|---|---|---|

| Substance | Frequency | Quantity |
|---|---|---|
| | | |
| | | |

26.3
| Non prescription drugs | YES | | NO | |
|---|---|---|---|---|

| Substance | Frequency | Quantity |
|---|---|---|
| Cannabis | | |
| Heroin | | |
| Ecstasy | | |
| Other | | |
| | | |
| | | |
| | | |

26.4
| Is client receiving treatment? | YES | | NO | |
|---|---|---|---|---|

| Treatment | Source | Frequency |
|---|---|---|
| Drug programme | | |
| General Practitioner | | |
| Counsellor | | |
| Other | | |
| | | |
| | | |
| | | |
| | | |

## CURRENT HEALTH STATUS

27. **LEVEL OF CONSCIOUSNESS**

| Glasgow Coma Scale Score | | |
|---|---|---|
| Eye opening | | 4 |
| Verbal Response | | 5 |
| Motor Response | | 6 |
| **Total** | | 15 |

| Comment (Explain alteration in findings): |
|---|

**28. COGNITIVE FUNCTION**

28.1
| Requires assistance with cognitive functioning | YES | | NO | |
|---|---|---|---|---|

28.2
| Cognitive deficits identified: | |
|---|---|
| Memory | |
| Concentration | |
| Attention span | |
| Reading | |
| Other (Specify): | |

**29. BEHAVIOUR**

29.1
| Requires assistance with behaviour | YES | | NO | |
|---|---|---|---|---|

29.2 Behaviour identified:
| | Information provided by: |
|---|---|
| Aggression | |
| Depression | |
| Mood swings | |
| Emotional lability | |
| Perseveration | |
| Wandering | |
| Other: | |

**30. Communication**

30.1
| Experiences problems with speech | YES | | NO | |
|---|---|---|---|---|

30.2
| Registered deaf | YES | | NO | |
|---|---|---|---|---|
| Registered blind | YES | | NO | |

30.3
| Able to communicate by means of: | |
|---|---|
| Oral speech | |
| Sign language | |
| Gestures | |
| Electronic device | |
| Other: | |

**31. SEIZURE ACTIVITY**

31.1
| Seizures present: | YES | | NO | |
|---|---|---|---|---|

31.2
| Type | Frequency | Treatment |
|---|---|---|
| | | |
| | | |
| | | |
| | | |
| | | |
| | | |
| | | |
| | | |
| | | |

**32. PRESENCE OF REFLEXES**

| Cough | |
|---|---|
| Swallow | |
| Gag | |
| Risk of aspiration | |

**33. Motor function**

| Location | Left | Right |
|---|---|---|
| **Upper limb:** | | |
| Paresis | | |
| Paralysis | | |
| Hemiplegia | | |
| Wasting | | |
| **Lower limb:** | | |
| Paresis | | |
| Paralysis | | |
| Hemiplegia | | |
| Wasting | | |

**34. MOBILITY**

34.1
| Requires assistance with mobility | YES | | NO | |
|---|---|---|---|---|

34.2
| Level of assistance required: | |
|---|---|
| Independent | |
| Independent with aids | |
| Independent with structure | |
| Requires assistance of 1 helper | |
| Requires assistance of 2 helpers | |
| Other: | |

35.

| **CSF LEAK:** | YES | | NO | |
|---|---|---|---|---|
| Location: | | | | |

36. **SENSORY FUNCTION**

36.1

| **Sensory deficits**: | YES | | NO | |
|---|---|---|---|---|

| **Location** | **Frequency** | **Treatment** |
|---|---|---|
| | | |
| | | |

37. **Summary of daily activity**

| TIME | ACTIVITY | PERSON RESPONSIBLE | COMMENT |
|---|---|---|---|
| 07:00–08:00 | | | |
| 08:00–09:00 | | | |
| 09:00–10:00 | | | |
| 10:00–11:00 | | | |
| 11:00–12:00 | | | |
| 12:00–13:00 | | | |
| 13:00–14:00 | | | |
| 14:00–15:00 | | | |
| 15:00–16:00 | | | |
| 16:00–17:00 | | | |
| 17:00–18:00 | | | |
| 18:00–19:00 | | | |
| 19:00–20:00 | | | |
| 20:00–21:00 | | | |
| 21:00–22:00 | | | |
| 22:00–23:00 | | | |
| 23:00–24:00 | | | |
| 24:00–01:00 | | | |
| 01:00–02:00 | | | |
| 02:00–03:00 | | | |
| 03:00–04:00 | | | |
| 04:00–05:00 | | | |
| 06:00–07:00 | | | |

**38.**    **List of common problems experienced by client**

| PROBLEM | FREQUENCY | LAST EXPERIENCED | MANAGEMENT |
|---|---|---|---|
|  |  |  |  |
|  |  |  |  |
|  |  |  |  |
|  |  |  |  |
|  |  |  |  |
|  |  |  |  |
|  |  |  |  |
|  |  |  |  |
|  |  |  |  |
|  |  |  |  |
|  |  |  |  |
|  |  |  |  |
|  |  |  |  |
|  |  |  |  |
|  |  |  |  |
|  |  |  |  |
|  |  |  |  |
|  |  |  |  |
|  |  |  |  |
|  |  |  |  |
|  |  |  |  |
|  |  |  |  |
|  |  |  |  |
|  |  |  |  |

**HEALTH NEEDS**

**39**    **Level of independence**

| | |
|---|---|
| Severe disability | |
| Moderate disability | |
| Mild disability | |
| Independent | |

**40.**    **NUTRITION:**

| | | |
|---|---|---|
| 40.1 | Height | |
| 40.2 | Body mass | |
| 40.3 | Daily Kilojoule intake | |

**40.4**    **Method of feeding:**

| Route | Type of Feed | Frequency |
|---|---|---|
| Oral | | |
| PEG | | |
| Other (Specify): | | |
|  |  |  |
|  |  |  |
|  |  |  |

40.5 **PROBLEMS EXPERIENCED WITH FEEDING IN THE LAST 4 WEEKS:**

| Type | Frequency | Treatment |
|---|---|---|
|  |  |  |
|  |  |  |
|  |  |  |
|  |  |  |
|  |  |  |
|  |  |  |
|  |  |  |
|  |  |  |
|  |  |  |

41. **SKIN INTEGRITY:**

41.1
| Presence of decubitus ulcers: | YES |  | NO |  |
|---|---|---|---|---|

41.2
| Site | Size (photograph) | Treatment |
|---|---|---|
|  |  |  |
|  |  |  |
|  |  |  |
|  |  |  |
|  |  |  |
|  |  |  |
|  |  |  |
|  |  |  |

41.3
| Presence of wounds | YES |  | NO |  |
|---|---|---|---|---|

| Site | Size (photograph) | Treatment |
|---|---|---|
|  |  |  |
|  |  |  |
|  |  |  |
|  |  |  |
|  |  |  |
|  |  |  |
|  |  |  |
|  |  |  |

41.4
| Presence of dribbling | YES |  | NO |  |
|---|---|---|---|---|

| Site | Management |
|---|---|
|  |  |
|  |  |

41.5
| Presence of skin sensitivity | YES |  | NO |  |
|---|---|---|---|---|

| Site | Management |
|---|---|
|  |  |
|  |  |

41.6
| Allergy to Elastoplast/ other plaster | YES |  | NO |  |
|---|---|---|---|---|

42. **Elimination**

42.1 **PRESENCE OF:**

| BLADDER INCONTINENCE | YES |  | NO |  |
|---|---|---|---|---|
| BOWEL INCONTINENCE | YES |  | NO |  |

42.2
| Management | Date of last tube change |
|---|---|
|  |  |

## 43.  Medication

43.1  **Ability to self medicate:**  YES ☐  NO ☐

43.2

| Name of drug | Dose | Route | Frequency | Date of last review |
|---|---|---|---|---|
|  |  |  |  |  |
|  |  |  |  |  |
|  |  |  |  |  |
|  |  |  |  |  |
|  |  |  |  |  |
|  |  |  |  |  |
|  |  |  |  |  |
|  |  |  |  |  |
|  |  |  |  |  |
|  |  |  |  |  |
|  |  |  |  |  |
|  |  |  |  |  |
|  |  |  |  |  |
|  |  |  |  |  |
|  |  |  |  |  |
|  |  |  |  |  |
|  |  |  |  |  |
|  |  |  |  |  |
|  |  |  |  |  |
|  |  |  |  |  |
|  |  |  |  |  |
|  |  |  |  |  |
|  |  |  |  |  |
|  |  |  |  |  |
|  |  |  |  |  |
|  |  |  |  |  |
|  |  |  |  |  |

44. **Current Health Intervention**

Tick (✓) activity required

| | Activity | Frequency | Resources | Specialised equipment | Site/Date of last tube change | Comment |
|---|---|---|---|---|---|---|
| | Orientation programme | | | | | |
| | Rehabilitation programme | | | | | |
| | | | | | | |
| | Neurological monitoring | | | | | |
| | | | | | | |
| | Fluids | | | | | |
| | | | | | | |
| | Nutrition | | | | | |
| | | | | | | |
| | Hygiene: | | | | | |
| |   Eye care | | | | | |
| |   Oropharyngeal care | | | | | |
| |   General hygiene | | | | | |
| |   Care of catheters/tubes | | | | | |
| |   Perineal care | | | | | |
| | | | | | | |
| | Skin integrity: | | | | | |
| |   Wound care | | | | | |
| |   Turning | | | | | |
| |   Prevention regime | | | | | |
| |   Decubitus ulcers | | | | | |
| | Elimination: | | | | | |
| |   Bowel care | | | | | |
| |   Bladder care | | | | | |
| | | | | | | |
| | Mobility: | | | | | |
| | | | | | | |
| | | | | | | |
| | | | | | | |
| | | | | | | |
| | | | | | | |
| | | | | | | |
| | | | | | | |
| | | | | | | |
| | | | | | | |
| | | | | | | |

## 45.    RISK FACTORS

The following environmental risk assessment must be completed:

All items in document in CAPITAL LETTERS (FONT 12) relate to risk.

Identify additional items according to client situation and findings.

Tick (✓) appropriate box. Add relevant information.

| KEY: | |
|---|---|
| 5 | High risk |
| 4 | Above average risk |
| 3 | Medium risk |
| 2 | Rising risk |
| 1 | Low risk |
| 0 | No risk |

| Risk | YES | | | | | NO | Additional requirements to be in place | | Details | |
|---|---|---|---|---|---|---|---|---|---|---|
| | 5 | 4 | 3 | 2 | 1 | 0 | YES | NO | Type | Available |
| **Safety:** | | | | | | | | | | |
| | | | | | | | | | | |
| | | | | | | | | | | |
| | | | | | | | | | | |
| **Environment:** | | | | | | | | | | |
| Room | | | | | | | | | | |
| Bed height | | | | | | | | | | |
| Lighting | | | | | | | | | | |
| Light switches | | | | | | | | | | |
| Heating | | | | | | | | | | |
| Windows: | | | | | | | | | | |
| Locks | | | | | | | | | | |
| Bedrails | | | | | | | | | | |
| Electric plugs | | | | | | | | | | |
| Flooring | | | | | | | | | | |
| Furniture | | | | | | | | | | |
| | | | | | | | | | | |
| **Infection control:** | | | | | | | | | | |
| MRSA | | | | | | | | | | |
| Hepatitis C | | | | | | | | | | |
| HIV/Aids | | | | | | | | | | |
| | | | | | | | | | | |
| **Level of consciousness:** | | | | | | | | | | |
| GCS 13–15 | | | | | | | | | | |
| GCS 9–12 | | | | | | | | | | |
| GCS <8 | | | | | | | | | | |
| | | | | | | | | | | |
| **Seizures** | | | | | | | | | | |
| Type | | | | | | | | | | |
| | | | | | | | | | | |

| Risk | YES | | | | | NO | Additional requirements to be in place | | Details | |
|---|---|---|---|---|---|---|---|---|---|---|
| | 5 | 4 | 3 | 2 | 1 | 0 | YES | NO | Type | Available |
| **Absence of reflexes:** | | | | | | | | | | |
| Cough | | | | | | | | | | |
| Swallow | | | | | | | | | | |
| Gag | | | | | | | | | | |
| | | | | | | | | | | |
| **Risk of aspiration** | | | | | | | | | | |
| | | | | | | | | | | |
| **Known allergies** | | | | | | | | | | |
| **To:** | | | | | | | | | | |
| | | | | | | | | | | |
| **Nutrition/Elimination:** | | | | | | | | | | |
| Diarrhoea/Constipation | | | | | | | | | | |
| Dehydration | | | | | | | | | | |
| **Behaviour:** | | | | | | | | | | |
| Issue | | | | | | | | | | |
| Self-harm | | | | | | | | | | |
| Abscond | | | | | | | | | | |
| Inappropriate | | | | | | | | | | |
| Violence | | | | | | | | | | |
| | | | | | | | | | | |
| **Mobility:** | | | | | | | | | | |
| Use of stairs | | | | | | | | | | |
| **Falls** | | | | | | | | | | |
| | | | | | | | | | | |
| **Equipment:** | | | | | | | | | | |
| | | | | | | | | | | |
| **Medication:** | | | | | | | | | | |
| | | | | | | | | | | |
| **Other (Specify):** | | | | | | | | | | |
| | | | | | | | | | | |
| Skin integrity | | | | | | | | | | |
| Skin sensitivity | | | | | | | | | | |
| Sensitivity to elastoplast | | | | | | | | | | |
| Dribbling | | | | | | | | | | |
| | | | | | | | | | | |
| | | | | | | | | | | |
| | | | | | | | | | | |
| | | | | | | | | | | |
| | | | | | | | | | | |

**46.  SUMMARY OF FINDINGS**
**Diagnosis**
**GCS**
**Family**
**Placement**
Risk

| Client problem | Potential outcome |
|---|---|
|  |  |
|  |  |
|  |  |
|  |  |
|  |  |
|  |  |
|  |  |
|  |  |
|  |  |
|  |  |
|  |  |
|  |  |

**Signature:**

**Glasgow Coma Scale**

| Category | Score | Symbol if unable to test |
|---|---|---|
| **EYE OPENING** |  | e |
| Spontaneous | 4 |  |
| To command | 3 |  |
| To pain | 2 |  |
| Nil | 1 |  |
| **VERBAL RESPONSE** |  | t |
| Orientated | 6 |  |
| Confused | 5 |  |
| To pain | 4 |  |
| Inappropriate | 3 |  |
| Incomprehensible | 2 |  |
| Nil | 1 |  |
| **MOTOR RESPONSE** |  |  |
| Obeys command | 5 |  |
| To pain | 4 |  |
| Localises | 3 |  |
| Withdraws | 2 |  |
| Nil | 1 |  |
| **TOTAL** | /15 |  |

# Appendix 2
# Discharge Report

**INSTRUCTIONS**

This form is to be completed by the client's Key Worker/ Home Manager/Registered Nurse in conjunction with the client, carer and family, where appropriate.

The discharge report will be prepared:

1. By the client's Key Worker/Home Manager/Registered Nurse.
2. Within 7 days of discharge from the rehabilitation service.
3. A date and time for discharge will be arranged with the transferring unit/family.
4. Where applicable, the key worker will arrange for the carer/family member/significant other to be present.

**SECTION A**
**DEMOGRAPHIC DATA:**

| | | | | | |
|---|---|---|---|---|---|
| 1. | Name of client: | | | | |
| 2. | Date of birth: | | | | |
| 3. | Sex: | | Male | | Female | |

4. Client's home address:

Contact number:

5. Medical diagnosis:

6. Date of injury/illness:

**DISCHARGE AGENT:**

7. Person responsible for client's discharge:

Contact number:

8. Length of stay:

*Neurotrauma: Managing Patients with Head Injuries*, First Edition. Edited by Nadine Abelson-Mitchell.
© 2013 Blackwell Publishing Ltd. Published 2013 by Blackwell Publishing Ltd.

9. 
| Name of client's GP: |  |
| Address: |  |
| Contact number: |  |

10. 
| Date of discharge: |  |

11. 
| Planned date of follow-up: |  |

12. 
| Name/s of person/s preparing discharge report: |  |

13. 
| Signature of person/s preparing discharge report: |  |

## SECTION B
## FAMILY INFORMATION

14. Marital status:

| Married |  |
| --- | --- |
| Living with partner |  |
| Separated |  |
| Divorced |  |
| Widowed |  |
| Other |  |

15. Local contact details for next of kin

| Name: |
| --- |
| Address: |
| Contact number: |

## SECTION C
## PREVIOUS HEALTH HISTORY

16. 
| Previous health history: |
| --- |
| Mental health history: |

## SECTION D
## CURRENT HEALTH STATUS

17. **Level of consciousness**

| **Glasgow Coma Scale Score** | | |
| --- | --- | --- |
| Eye opening |  | 4 |
| Verbal Response |  | 5 |
| Motor Response |  | 6 |
| **Total** | | 15 |

| Comment (explain alteration in findings): |
| --- |

18 **Overall level of independence**

| Severe disability |  |
| --- | --- |
| Moderate disability |  |
| Mild disability |  |
| Independent |  |

19.  **List of common problems currently experienced by client**

| PROBLEM | FREQUENCY | LAST EXPERIENCED | MANAGEMENT |
|---------|-----------|------------------|------------|
|         |           |                  |            |
|         |           |                  |            |
|         |           |                  |            |
|         |           |                  |            |
|         |           |                  |            |
|         |           |                  |            |
|         |           |                  |            |
|         |           |                  |            |
|         |           |                  |            |
|         |           |                  |            |
|         |           |                  |            |
|         |           |                  |            |
|         |           |                  |            |

20.  **Summary of daily activity**

| TIME | ACTIVITY | PERSON RESPONSIBLE | COMMENT |
|------|----------|--------------------|---------|
| 07:00–08:00 |  |  |  |
| 08:00–09:00 |  |  |  |
| 09:00–10:00 |  |  |  |
| 10:00–11:00 |  |  |  |
| 11:00–12:00 |  |  |  |
| 12:00–13:00 |  |  |  |
| 13:00–14:00 |  |  |  |
| 14:00–15:00 |  |  |  |
| 15:00–16:00 |  |  |  |
| 16:00–17:00 |  |  |  |
| 17:00–18:00 |  |  |  |
| 18:00–19:00 |  |  |  |
| 19:00–20:00 |  |  |  |
| 20:00–21:00 |  |  |  |
| 21:00–22:00 |  |  |  |
| 22:00–23:00 |  |  |  |
| 23:00–24:00 |  |  |  |
| 24:00–01:00 |  |  |  |
| 01:00–02:00 |  |  |  |
| 02:00–03:00 |  |  |  |
| 03:00–04:00 |  |  |  |
| 04:00–05:00 |  |  |  |
| 05:00–06:00 |  |  |  |
| 06:00–07:00 |  |  |  |

## 21.   DISCHARGE REPORT BASED ON NEEDS APPROACH

**Client need**

Include:

1. Level of independence for each activity of living
2. Risk factors
3. Interdisciplinary team involvement
4. Relate to specific intervention for client need

|   | **Specific intervention** | **Client need** |
|---|---|---|
| 1. | Level of independence | **Maintaining a safe environment** |
| 2. | LOC<br>Orientation programme<br>Cognitive rehabilitation programme<br>Behaviour<br>Seizure activity<br>CSF leaks<br>Sensory deficits<br>Reflexes | **Mentation** |
| 3. | Vital signs | **Haemodynamic** |
| 4. | Speech deficits<br>Means of communication | **Communication** |
| 5. | Respiratory support | **Breathing** |
| 6. | Body mass<br>Method of feeding<br>Eating programme<br>Eating habits | **Eating and Drinking** |
| 7. | Presence of incontinence:<br>Bowel<br>Bladder<br>Use of protective appliances<br>Diarrhoea<br>Constipation | **Elimination/Continence/Bowel habits** |
| 8. | General hygiene<br>Eye care<br>Oral hygiene<br>Perineal hygiene<br>Care of catheters/tubes | **Personal Hygiene and Dressing** |
| 9. | Clothing<br>Environmental temperature<br>Patient's temperature | **Controlling Body Temperature** |

| 10. | Motor function<br>Turning<br>Transferring<br>Use of assistive devices | **Mobilising** |
| 11. | Presence of wounds<br>Decubitus ulcers<br>Dribbling<br>Allergy<br>Skin sensitivity | **Skin integrity** |
| 12. | | **Comfort** |
| 13. | | **Expressing Sexuality** |
| 14. | | **Sleeping** |
| 15. | | |
| 16. | Behaviour<br>Mood<br>Depression<br>Aggression | **Mental Health Requirements** |
| 17. | | **Sexuality** |
| 18. | Spiritual beliefs<br>Cultural aspects | **Spiritual** |
| 19. | Attendance at workshop | **Vocational** |
| 20. | | **Education** |
| 21. | Social practices:<br>Smoking<br>Alcohol consumption<br>Use of recreational drugs<br>Activities programme<br>Socialisation programme | **Social** |

**22.  Medication**

22.1

| Ability to self medicate: | YES | | NO | |
|---|---|---|---|---|

22.2

| Name of drug | Dose | Route | Frequency | Date of last review |
|---|---|---|---|---|
| | | | | |
| | | | | |
| | | | | |
| | | | | |
| | | | | |
| | | | | |
| | | | | |
| | | | | |
| | | | | |
| | | | | |

**23.  Signature/s:**

**Patient:**

**Carer:**

**Family:**

**Named key worker:**

**Date of report:**

# Activity Answers

Dear Reader,

I hope you have enjoyed undertaking the activities in this book.

I have included the answers to the activities in this section:

1. Answers to the anatomy and physiology quiz including references to page numbers in the text.
2. For answers to assessments, please refer to Chapter 18.
3. For solutions to activities in Chapters 4 and 24, please refer to Table 23.1.

4. For answers to care scenarios, please refer to Table 23.1.
5. Other answers are included in this section.

I have deliberately not included all answers to some of the activities as these need consideration and debate and there may be numerous possible answers.

I did not want to make it too easy. If you would like specific answers, please contact me via email on namconsultants@aol.com.

Best of luck with the activities.

Nadine Abelson-Mitchell

**CHAPTER 12 ANSWERS**

**Anatomy and physiology quiz**
You will need to find the answers to the quiz on the following pages:

| Section | Questions | Page numbers |
|---|---|---|
| THE SCALP | a. What are the names of the five layers of the scalp? | 74 |
| | b. What are the purposes of each layer? | 74/75 |
| | c. Why is a scalp laceration likely to bleed profusely? | 75 |
| | d. Why is a patient who has a scalp laceration that becomes infected likely to develop a brain abscess thereafter? | 75 |
| THE SKULL | a. How would you describe the superior aspect of the skull? | 75 |
| | b. How would you describe the lateral aspect of the skull? | 76 |
| | c. How would you describe the posterior aspect of the skull? | 76 |
| | d. How would you describe the inferior aspect of the skull? | 82 |
| | e. How would you describe the sutures of the skull? | 76 |
| | f. What are the purposes of the sutures? | 76 |
| | g. If the sutures do not develop normally, what condition may arise? | Craniosynostosis |
| | h. Examine the base of the skull and state the path for the following: | |
| |    i.  spinal cord | 78 Fig. 12.3 |
| |    ii.  internal carotid artery | 94 |
| |    iii. meningeal artery | 80 |
| |    iv. vagus nerve. | 93 |
| THE MENINGES | a. The meninges consist of 3 layers. | |
| | b. How would you describe each layer of the meninges? | 82–84 |
| | c. How would you describe the falx cerebri and the falx cerebelli? | 83 |
| THE VENOUS DRAINAGE OF THE BRAIN | a. Describe the venous drainage of the brain using the following table: NAME    LOCATION    FUNCTION | 90 |
| | b. How would you differentiate between the two groups of sinuses? | 91 |
| | c. Draw a schematic representation of the venous drainage of the brain. | 97 |
| THE NEURONE | a. What is the definition of the term 'neurone'? | 84 |
| | b. How would you describe the basic structure of each part of a neurone? | Tortora & Derrickson 2011 p. 450–454 |
| | c. What are the functions of each part of a neurone? | Tortora & Derrickson 2011 p. 450–454 |
| | d. List four types of neurones that are to be found in the CNS? | Tortora & Derrickson 2011 p. 450–454 |

*(Continued)*

| Section | Questions | Page numbers |
|---|---|---|
| THE AUTONOMIC NERVOUS SYSTEM | a. What two systems make up the autonomic nervous system? | 100/101 |
| | b. How would you describe the sympathetic nervous system in terms of its structure, function, and location? | 101 |
| | c. How would you describe the parasympathetic nervous system in terms of its structure, function and location? | 100/101 |
| | d. What are the outflows of the: | |
| |    i.  sympathetic nervous system? | 101 |
| |    ii.  parasympathetic nervous system? | 101 |
| THE PITUITARY GLAND | a. How would you describe the location of the pituitary gland? | 90 |
| | b. List the hormones found in the following pituitary glands: | 91 Table 12.2 |
| |    i.  posterior pituitary gland | |
| |    ii.  anterior pituitary gland. | |
| | c. What are the functions of each hormone listed? | 91 Table 12.2 |
| ACID-BASE BALANCE | a. State the normal arterial blood gas values. | 124 |
| | b. How does the body maintain homeostasis? | 103–106 |
| | c. Describe respiratory acidosis. | 106 and 125 |
| | d. Describe metabolic acidosis. | 106 and 125 |

## CHAPTER 18 ANSWERS

### Activity 18.4

*Scenario*

The direct and consensual light reflex.

*Procedure*

Using a penlight torch shine the light into the patients left eye.

*Questions*

1. **What do you expect to happen?**
   - The normal response is that the pupil on the left eye reacts by contracting in size to the bright light source.
   - Now look at the right eye, the normal response is that the pupil on the right eye reacts by contracting in size to the bright light source in the left eye. This is the consensual light reflex.
2. **Why does this occur?**
   See Chapter 18 Assessment p. 149.
3. **What happens if the patient is blind?**
   If the patient is blind, i.e. damage to CN II there will be no response as the optic nerve cannot pick up the stimulus to send back to the Occulomotor nerve. See diagram on p. 303 item marked 1 for site of lesion.
4. **What is hemianopia and physiologically why does it occur?**

Hemianopia (hemianopsia) is a visual field defect in which there is loss of vision in either the right or left on both sides of the eye.

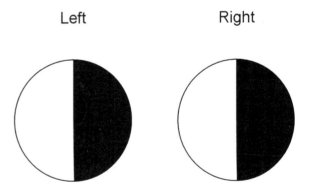

Left                              Right

5. **What is homonymous hemianopia and why does it occur?**
   Homonymous hemianopia e.g. Right-sided homonymous hemianopia

   A lesion in the left involving both fibres in the left optic tract results in loss of vision to the right in the nasal and temporal visual fields, therefore loss of vision on the right side of the visual fields. This will result in the person seeing half an image in both eyes. See diagram on p. 303 marked 2 for site of lesion.

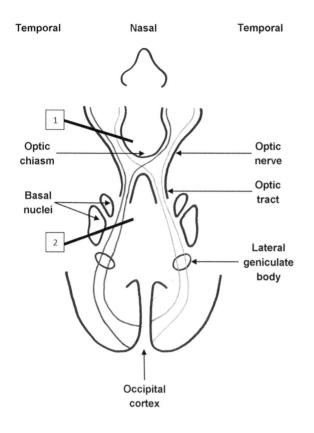

Temporal      Nasal      Temporal

1

Optic chiasm

Optic nerve

Optic tract

Basal nuclei

2

Lateral geniculate body

Occipital cortex

## CHAPTER 20 ANSWERS

### Scenario 1 – John Smith

John Smith is a 19 year old, previously fit, man who was accidentally hit on the head with a golf club. There was no loss of consciousness and he walked into the ED. On examination his GCS was 15 and he had no neurological deficit. He did, however have a stellate laceration of his forehead. A CT showed a depressed fracture underlying this laceration but no other intracranial injury. He needs to be transferred to the neurosurgical unit 30 miles away for this to be debrided and for the fracture to be elevated.

1. *How will you organise this?*
   This needs to be done in conjunction with a senior doctor in the ED and the neurosurgeons. You need to know:
   • Where is he going? Which ward? What is the name of the doctor accepting the patient?
   • What is the degree of urgency? *You are told: as soon as reasonably possible but it does not require a blue light ambulance* (emergency).

• What potential complications may occur over the next 90 minutes (the time you estimate that it will take to get him to the neurosurgical unit)? *You are told that as there is no brain injury on the CT, complications are unlikely but that a compound depressed fracture is a known risk factor for a grand mal seizure.* The basic principle for any transfer is to anticipate all possible problems and act to prevent them, if possible, and to ensure that you have the personnel and equipment to deal with them if they occur. Thus you need to ask whether he should have prophylactic anticonvulsants (e.g. Phenytoin) before transfer. He should have an IV cannula sited and whoever accompanies the patient should take an anticonvulsant with them (e.g. Lorazepam, Diazepam).

2. *Who should accompany the patient?*
   This is likely to be an uncomplicated transfer but the person accompanying the patient should be capable of dealing with a grand mal convulsion and giving an anticonvulsant. He can probably be accompanied by a paramedic.

   A paramedic ambulance has been booked and will arrive in 10 minutes: *what else do you need to consider?*
   • Has his next of kin been informed? He can do that himself, if necessary.
   • All his notes, observation sheets and pathology results will need to go with him. Check that the neurosurgical unit can access the scans and x-rays via an electronic link. If not, he will need to take these with him (either electronic copies on a disk, or hard copies).
   • There may be a transfer document to be filled in.
   • The ambulance crew will need to be briefed about where to go, the risk of fitting etc.

### Scenario 2 – Judith Brown

Judith Brown is a 54 year old woman who has been involved in a road traffic crash. Her main injury is a head injury. On arrival she had a GCS of 12 (E3, M5, V4) with no localising signs. A CT has shown multiple contusions. When she returned from CT, her GCS had fallen to 10 (E2, M5, V3). She still has no localising signs. The CT of her neck, chest, abdomen and pelvis showed no injuries. She does, however, have an obvious open fracture of her left tibia and a swollen right foot but neither of these has been x-rayed yet. Her cardiovascular system is stable.

It has been decided that she needs to be transferred to the neurosurgical unit 60 miles away and she has been accepted by the neurosurgeons there who have asked that she be transferred as soon as possible.

1. *What needs to be done before she is transferred?*
   - A GCS of 8 or below is usually considered an indication for intubation and ventilation. Her GCS of 10 would not normally be an indication (in itself) for intubation but her GCS is falling and might reduce further over the next two hours which you think is a realistic time before she gets to the neurosurgical unit. There is almost certainly an indication for her to be intubated and ventilated before transfer to avoid a difficult intubation in the back of an ambulance or helicopter. If this is done, the neurosurgeons need to be told.
   - In view of the deteriorating level of consciousness, advice should be sought as to whether she should be given anything (e.g. Mannitol) to reduce her intracranial pressure.
   - A urinary catheter will need inserting at some time, especially if it is decided to use Mannitol which is an osmotic diuretic.
   - A normal CT of the cervical spine does not completely exclude a neck injury and so a decision needs to be made as to whether to continue with cervical spine immobilisation.
   - The compound fracture of the tibia needs to be cleaned, dressed and put into plaster to stabilise it and prophylactic antibiotics should be given. The right foot should be splinted in plaster. If there is time, these can be x-rayed before transfer but as x-rays will not alter the immediate management in this hospital, this is not essential. If they are not x-rayed, this fact should be passed on to the receiving hospital.
   - Next of kin should be informed.
   - There may be a transfer document to be filled in.
   The patient is intubated and stabilised on a ventilator and an arterial line is inserted. The patient remains cardiovascularly stable and blood gases are satisfactory. It is decided that neck immobilisation will be continued until the patient is assessed by a neurosurgeon. The fractures are immobilised in plaster, a urinary catheter and gastric tube have been inserted.

2. *Should this patient be transferred by ambulance or helicopter?*
   There is no right answer as this will depend on:
   - Availability of a helicopter.
   - The location of a landing site at your hospital and the receiving hospital.
   - Urgency of the case.
   - Estimated travel times.
   - Time of the day.

3. *It is decided to transfer the patient by ambulance. Who should accompany the patient?*
   As the patient is intubated and ventilated, the patient should be accompanied by someone who can manage this, usually an anaesthetist. They will need support from a nurse who is competent to manage the various pieces of medical equipment that will go with the patient.

4. *What equipment will be needed?*
   There will usually be a bag containing all the equipment for a transfer and the ambulance will be able to provide equipment as well, but you will need:
   - Full airway equipment including equipment for intubation should the endotracheal tube displace.
   - Ventilator with bag-valve-mask as a back up.
   - Monitoring including heart rate, blood pressure, pulse oximetry, capnography.
   - IV fluids.
   - Syringe driver(s).
   - Spare batteries.
   - Drugs.
   - Simple dressing material.
   - All notes, observation sheets, pathology results, x-rays and scans (if not available to the receiving hospital electronically).

5. *The nurse accompanying the anaesthetist has never done a hospital transfer before and asks what else they should take.*
   Explain that hopefully the ambulance will be able to bring you back. However it may be re-tasked to an emergency and may not be able to do so, so be prepared to return under your own steam and take:
   - Warm clothes.
   - Mobile phone.
   - Money and/or credit card for food, drink and fares.
   - Any medication that you are on, that may need to be taken within the next six hours.

## CHAPTER 21 ANSWERS

### Activity 21.1

You are working in an emergency department when, with no prior warning, an ambulance arrives with a young man who has been involved in a motorcycle crash. His name is unknown. You receive the following ATMIST handover:

**A**ge: unknown but looks in his late teens.
**T**ime of accident: about 40 minutes ago.

**M**echanism: the patient was riding his motor cycle very fast when a car pulled out of a side road. The motorcycle hit the car and the rider was thrown over the car, landing in the road at least 10 metres away. He then slid along the road. His helmet was cracked.

**In**juries: he has clearly had a head injury and also appears to have a fractured right femur.

**V**ital **S**igns: at scene his GCS was 7 (E2, V2, M3), pulse 80, BP 120 systolic.

**T**reatment: his neck has been immobilised on a spinal board with a cervical collar and head blocks. He is tolerating an oropharyngeal airway and has been given oxygen.

1. *What are you going to do?*
   - This patient is seriously injured and you need help. Urgently call for medical and nursing help and ask someone to bleep the trauma team urgently.
   - Move the patient to the resuscitation room.
   - Make a mental note to ask the ambulance crew why no advanced warning was given and to stress the importance of such a warning. However, now is not the time to do this.

2. *Three ED doctors and three ED nurses respond immediately to your call for help. How will they be used?*
   - All should put on personal protective equipment and lead aprons.
   - The most senior ED doctor will take charge and will lead the primary survey.
   - Another ED doctor, assisted by a nurse, will take charge of the airway and ventilation.
   - The third doctor will gain IV access and take bloods.
   - One nurse should remove all the clothing with scissors.
   - The third nurse can set up monitoring and can start to prepare the drugs and fluids that will be required.

   As soon as possible, the patient should be removed from the spinal board either by log-rolling or by the use of a scoop stretcher.

   *Further information*:

   The primary survey reveals:

   **A**irway: the patient is tolerating an oropharyngeal airway. With this in place, the airway is patent.

   **B**reathing: RR 12, there is bruising over the left lower chest but there is good air entry on both sides of the chest. Oxygen saturation 97% on oxygen at 15 litres per minute via a mask with a reservoir bag.

   **C**irculation: heart rate 70 beats per minute, BP 160/80. There is no evidence of external blood loss.

**D**isability:
   - Conscious level. Eyes: no response to painful stimulus (PS). Verbal: no sound to PS. Motor: left side has abnormal flexion to PS and right side extends to PS.
   - Pupils equal and react to light.
   - Blood sugar 7 mmol/L.

**E**xposure: the patient has been fully stripped. The only obvious injury is a deformity of the right thigh suggestive of a fractured femur. Pulses in the right foot are present.

3. *What is the GCS?*

   The GCS is 5. (E 1, V 1, M 3) – the left side is M 3, the right side is M 2 but for calculating the GCS, one takes the better of the two sides.

4. *What do these observations tell you?*

   He has clearly got a severe head injury. The GCS was 7 and is now 5 so his condition has deteriorated. There is a difference between the two sides indicating a localised brain injury. His blood pressure has gone up and his heart rate has gone down since he was first seen. This may indicate rising intracranial pressure.

5. *For things to run smoothly, it is necessary to plan ahead: what will need to be done over the next 15 minutes (or shorter time if possible)?*
   - The patient will need intubation. This will require:
     - Intubating equipment (laryngoscope, endotracheal tube, bougie, tie, etc.) to be at hand.
     - Anaesthetic drugs to be made ready.
     - The collar will need to be removed prior to intubation and replaced with somebody doing manual in-line immobilisation.
     - Another person will need to apply cricoid pressure.
     - Once intubated, the patient will need capnography and will be connected to a ventilator. The collar will need to be reapplied.
   - An arterial blood gas sample will be taken to assess ventilation and acid-base balance.
   - If not already done, two IV cannulae will be inserted and bloods taken for full blood count, urea and electrolytes, clotting, bedside blood sugar and group and save. (If the patient was female, a pregnancy test would be taken.)Bottles will need to be labelled and sent to the laboratory. (The hospital should have a policy for the safe management of unknown patients.) An IV infusion of warmed crystalloid will be started.
   - At this stage, the best care of the brain is close attention to the airway, breathing and circulation but in

view of the deteriorating level of consciousness, the trauma team leader may request Mannitol to be given. Also

- Chest and pelvic x-rays will need to be taken in the resuscitation room. This should be done simultaneously with the rest of the resuscitation. The radiographer may need to be assertive to get the x-rays done.
- If any injuries are identified on the chest and pelvic x-rays, these may need treatment.
- The team leader may wish to do a FAST scan to exclude intra-abdominal bleeding.
- A traction splint should be applied to the right leg.
- He will probably also have an arterial cannula inserted and will, at some stage, require a urinary catheter and a gastric tube.
- The patient needs an urgent CT of the head and cervical spine. Because the mechanism has a potential for causing other serious injuries and his decreased level of consciousness means that these cannot be excluded clinically, he will also have a CT of the chest, abdomen and pelvis with reformats of the scans to provide images of the whole spine (a pan-CT). This will need organising.
- Safe transfer to CT will need to be organised.

6. *The patient is now in CT with a team of ED and ITU doctors and nurses. You are still in the ED. What else is likely to be needed when he returns from CT?*
   - He is still unknown and it is important to try to identify him. Get someone to search his belongings for any form of identification. Failing that, the police should be able to help (but don't forget that the motorcycle he was riding may not belong to him).
   - When he has been identified, relatives will need to be informed (probably via the police) and will come to the department and someone will need to talk to them to obtain details of his medical history, medications etc. and also to talk to them about the prognosis.
   - The police will arrive and will want information. In particular, they will be interested in a prognosis as if he dies (which is a definite possibility), this will change the way they investigate the crash.
   - He will need a secondary survey including a log roll (if this was not done when he came off the spinal board).
   - If a catheter and gastric tube were not passed earlier, this will need doing now.
   - A further arterial blood gas will be required.
   - He will need x-rays of his femur (and any other areas where injuries are identified during the secondary survey).

- He will almost certainly need to be transferred to a neurosurgical intensive care unit and this will need organising.

## Activity 21.2

It is 10am and you are working in an emergency department when you get a phone call from an ambulance crew to warn you that they are bringing you a 72 year old woman who has fallen down stairs and who has a severe head injury. They will be with you in 10 minutes.

1. *What further information do you need?*
   The following ATMIST mnemonic indicates what you already know and what you still need to know

| | |
|---|---|
| **A**ge | 72 |
| **T**ime of injury | ? |
| Time of arrival | 10 minutes |
| **M**echanism | Fall down stairs |
| **I**njuries | Head injury (but are there any other injuries?) |
| Vital **S**igns | ? |
| **T**reatment | ? |

*Further information from the ambulance crew:*
The time of the injury is unknown, she has no other obvious injuries, her vital signs are pulse 60, BP 160/100, RR 16, GCS 14. They have dressed a scalp laceration and have immobilised her on a spinal board with a cervical collar and head blocks.
*Comment:*
They said she had a severe head injury because she had a nasty scalp laceration but the GCS of 14 is not indicative of a severe head injury.
*Further history:*
When the ambulance crew arrives they give some further history. Her name is Mrs. Mary Jones and she was found at the bottom of the stairs by a carer. She was in her night clothes and it is uncertain how long she has been there but she could have been there all night.
*Initial assessment* reveals:
**A**irway: patent and breathing normally.
**B**reathing: RR 16, good air entry on both sides of the chest and no evidence of chest injury. Oxygen saturation 96% on air.
**C**irculation: she has clearly lost some blood from her scalp laceration but it is no longer bleeding. Her heart rate is still 60 beats per minute and her BP is still 160/100.

Disability: her GCS is E4, M6, V4. She is confused and does not know where she is or what day it is. She is unable to give a history. Her pupils are equal and react to light and she will move all four limbs to command.

There is no other obvious injury. She is log-rolled off the spinal board onto the ED trolley while maintaining in-line manual immobilisation of her cervical spine and the cervical collar and head blocks are replaced.

2. *What thoughts are going through your mind about this patient's injury?*

She has clearly had a head injury as she has a scalp laceration.

She has carers coming to her house. Why? What other medical problems does she have? What medication is she on?

Did she have a mechanical fall or, in view of her age and presumed other medical problems, did she 'collapse' as a result of a medical problem?

She has a GCS of 14: is this as a result of her head injury or (because of other presumed medical problems) is this normal for her? Until we get more information, we must assume that this is the result of the head injury.

She may have sustained other injuries in the fall.

If she has been on the floor all night, she may be hypothermic.

3. *How could you get further information?*

There are a variety of ways to obtain further information. The ambulance crew may have further information and should have brought in any medication. Hopefully they will have contact details of the carer who should have more information including contact details for the patient's family. Old hospital notes of records of previous ED visits may be helpful as will a telephone call to the patient's GP.

4. *What investigations will be needed?*

The following investigations will be needed:

- Blood sugar to exclude hypoglycaemia.
- 12 lead ECG may give clues to any medical cause for a collapse.

- Chest x-ray to exclude a chest injury occurring in the fall and to detect any associated medical problems.
- Pelvic x-ray. Although there is no clinical evidence of a pelvic or hip injury, fractures of the neck of the femur are common in the elderly and are easily missed. A pelvic x-ray should be done based on the mechanism of injury.
- CT scan of the head.
- Imaging of the cervical spine – either cervical spine x-rays or a CT.
- X-rays of the thoracic and lumbar spine should be considered in a patient who has fallen down stairs.
- Other investigations depending on her associated medical problems.

All investigations are normal and it turns out that Mrs Jones has dementia. When the collar is removed, she has painless neck movements. A full secondary survey reveals no other injury. The carer comes in and says that she is almost her normal self except that she is more subdued than normal. Her scalp wound is glued and it is recommended that she is admitted for head injury observations for 24 hours before being referred to the health care of the elderly team to investigate the cause of the fall and for an assessment as to whether she is safe to return home.

5. *When doing head injury observations, what signs would indicate that she was developing an intracranial haematoma?*

The first sign of raised intracranial pressure would be a decreasing level of consciousness. Other signs might include:

- Rising blood pressure and a falling heart rate.
- Dilatation of first one, then both, pupils.

# Additional Resources

While preparing this book, the editor has come across many excellent resources that she would like to share with you. These will provide additional information.

## BOOKS

BMJ Group and the Royal Pharmaceutical Society of Great Britain (2011) *British National Formulary*. BMJ Group/Pharmaceutical Press, London.

Branch, R. and Willson, R. (2010) *Cognitive Behavioural Therapy for Dummies*. 2nd edn. John Wiley and Sons Inc., Chichester.

Cifu, D.X. and Caruso, D. (2010) *Traumatic Brain Injury*. Demos Medical Publishing, New York.

Edlow, J.A. and Selim, M.H. (2011) *Neurology Emergencies*. Oxford University Press, Oxford.

Greaves, I., Porter, K.M. and Ryan, J.M. (2009) *Trauma Care Manual*. 2nd edn. Hodder Arnold, New York.

Hickey, J.V. (2008) *The Clinical Practice of Neurological and Neurosurgical Nursing*. 6th edn. Lippincott Williams and Wilkins, Philadelphia.

Jallo, J. and Loftus, C.M. (2009) *Neurotrauma and Critical Care of the Brain*. Thieme Medical Publishers, New York.

Nair, M. and Peate, I. (Eds) (2009) *Fundamentals of Applied Pathophysiology: An Essential Guide for Nursing Students*. Wiley-Blackwell. John Wiley & Sons, Chichester.

Payne, M. (2000) *Teamwork in Multiprofessional Care*. Palgrave, Basigstoke.

Pollard, K.C., Thomas, J. and Miers, M. (2010) *Understanding Interprofessional Working in Health and Social Care*. Palgrave Macmillan, Basingstoke.

Powell, T. (2004) *Head Injury: A Practical Guide*. Revised edn. Speechmark Editions, London.

Selladurai, B. and Reilly, P. (2007) *Initial Management of Head Injury: A Comprehensive Guide*. McGraw Hill Medical, Australia.

Whitfield, P., Thomas, E.O., Summers, F., Whyte, M. and Hutchinson, P.J. (2009) *Head Injury: A Multidisciplinary Approach*. Cambridge University Press, Cambridge.

Wilson, B.A., Gracey, F., Evans, J.J. and Bateman, A. (2009) *Neuropsychological Rehabilitation: Theory, Models, Therapy and Outcome*. Cambridge University Press, Cambridge.

Woodrow, P. (2012) *Intensive Care Nursing*. 3rd edn. Routledge, Oxford.

# HELPFUL WEBSITES

## Further information for health professionals and the public
*General information (all websites correct and operational as of August 2012)*

| Website | Organisation | Information |
|---|---|---|
| www.dh.gov.uk | Department of Health | Provides material which is primarily for use by health and social care professionals, academics and other interested parties. |
| www.drugs.com | Drugs.com | Information regarding pharmaceutical agents. |
| www.rxlist.com | Rxlist.com | Information regarding pharmaceutical agents (USA). |
| http://www.npc.co.uk/ | National Prescribing Centre | Information regarding pharmaceutical agents. |
| www.nhs.uk/medicine-guides | NHS | Information regarding pharmaceutical agents (UK). |
| www.nhsdirect.nhs.uk | NHS Direct | Provides reliable information on conditions, treatments and local services. |
| www.divine.vic.gov.au | DiVine | An on-line community. It is for and by people with a disability. The website is published by the Victorian Government, Australia. |
| www.who.int | World Health Organization (WHO) International | Responsible for providing leadership on global health matters, shaping the health research agenda, setting norms and standards. |
| www.healthfinder.gov | Healthfinder.gov (US Department of Health and Human Services) | Find information and tools to help you and those you care about stay healthy. |
| www.bnf.org | British National Formulary (BNF) | Provides UK healthcare professionals with authoritative and practical information on the selection and clinical use of medicines in a clear, concise and accessible manner. |
| www.nice.org.uk | National Institute for Health and Clinical Excellence (NICE) | Provides independent, authoritative and evidence-based guidance on the most effective ways to prevent, diagnose and treat disease and ill health, reducing inequalities and variation. |
| www.cochrane.org | The Cochrane Collaboration | An international network that works together to help healthcare providers, policy-makers, patients, their advocates and carers, make well-informed decisions about healthcare, based on the best available research evidence, by preparing, updating and promoting the accessibility of Cochrane Reviews. |
| www.npsa.nhs.uk | National Patient Safety Agency (NPSA) | Leads and contributes to improved, safe patient care by informing, supporting and influencing the health sector. |
| www.mind.org.uk | MIND | The leading mental health charity for England and Wales. |

| Website | Organisation | Information |
| --- | --- | --- |
| www.crusebereavementcare.org.uk | CRUSE | Promotes the well-being of bereaved people and enables anyone bereaved by death to understand their grief and cope with their loss. |
| www.ltcas.org.uk | LTCAS (Long-term conditions alliance Scotland) | Aims to provide a voice for the people who live with long-term conditions in Scotland. |
| www.anatomyatlases.org | Anatomy Atlases | A digital library of anatomy information, including diagrams and pictures. |
| www.patients-association.com | The Patients Association | Better access to accurate and independent information for patients and the public. |
| www.pals.nhs.uk | Patient Advice and Liaison Services | Ensures that the NHS listens to patients, their relatives, carers and friends, answers their questions and resolves their concerns as quickly as possible. |
| www.dh.gov.uk/health/category/policy-areas/social-care/ | UK Social Services | Works to define policy and guidance for delivering a social care system that provides care equally for all, while enabling people to retain their independence, control and dignity. |

### *Specific neuro websites*

| Website | Organisation | Information |
| --- | --- | --- |
| www.biausa.org | Brain injury in the United States (BIAA) | Nationwide brain injury advocacy organisation. |
| www.birt.co.uk | Brain Injury Rehabilitation Trust (BIRT) | Helps people regain the skills lost as a result of brain injury. |
| www.headinjury.com | Brain Injury Resource Center | Services and resources reflect the best practices in the field of traumatic brain injury. |
| www.brainhelp.co.uk | BrainHelp | Addresses the challenges as a result of brain haemorrhage or brain injury for patients, families and carers. |
| www.brake.org.uk | Brake | Aims to reduce road accidents, provide road safety advice, and supports victims injured on the road. |
| www.differentstrokes.co.uk | Different Strokes, UK | Provides a free service to younger stroke survivors throughout the United Kingdom. |
| www.headway.org.uk | HEADWAY – The Brain Injury Association | The charity that works to improve life after brain injury. |
| www.headwaydorset.org.uk | HEADWAY Dorset | Promotes a wider understanding of brain injury and provides information, advice and support to people with brain injuries, their families and carers. |

*(Continued)*

| Website | Organisation | Information |
|---------|--------------|-------------|
| www.ncepod.org.uk | National Confidential Enquiry into Patient Outcome and Death (NCEPOD) | To assist in maintaining and improving standards of medical and surgical care for the benefit of the public by reviewing the management of patients. |
| http://www.ninds.nih.gov/disorders/tbi/tbi.htm | National Institute of Neurological Disorders and Stroke, US (NINDS). | Conducts and supports research on brain and nervous system disorders. |
| www.neuropat.dote.hu | Neuroanatomy and neuropathology on the Internet | A searchable directory compiled for health professionals. |
| www.neuroguide.com | Neuroguide.com | Website which lists the best neuroscience resources on the Web. |
| www.neuroland.com | Neuroland | Website containing neuroscience resources and links to useful neuroscience websites. |
| www.neural.org | Neurological Alliance | Policy in neurological rehabilitation, links to multiple government and charity organisations. |
| www.spinal.co.uk | Spinal Injuries Association | Spinal injuries, services and support, community chat zone, news and research, links to other research sites, experience of SCI. |
| www.alz.org | The Alzheimer's Association | Global voluntary health organisation in Alzheimer's care and support. |
| www.braintrauma.org | The Brain Trauma Foundation (BTF) | Dedicated to improving the outcome of TBI patients worldwide by developing best practices guidelines, conducting clinical research, and educating medical professionals and consumers. |
| www.encephalitis.info | The Encephalitis Society, UK | Set up by people affected by encephalitis. |
| www.mayoclinic.com | The Mayo Clinic | A nonprofit worldwide leader in medical care, research and education for people from all walks of life. |
| www.stroke.org.uk | The Stroke Association, UK | Solely concerned with combating stroke in people of all ages. |
| www.med.harvard.edu/aanlib | The Whole Brain Atlas | Website that contains illustrations of the normal brain and many neurological conditions by means of neuro-imaging techniques. |

## Nursing

| Website | Organisation | Information |
|---------|--------------|-------------|
| www.rehabnurse.org | Association of Rehabilitation Nurses (ARN) | ARN's mission is to promote and advance professional rehabilitation nursing practice through education, advocacy, collaboration and research to enhance the quality of life for those affected by disability and chronic illness. |
| http://www.nanda.org/ | NANDA International | Using nursing diagnoses provides a framework for evidence-based clinical decision making. |
| www.sexualhealth.com | SexualHealth.com | Offers expert information on matters related to sexual health. |

*Wellness*

| Website | Organisation | Information |
|---|---|---|
| www.uncg.edu/ced/jemyers/ wellness/docs | Myers JE and Sweeney TJ Wellness | The Wheel of Wellness. |
| http://www.nationalwellness.org/ index.php?id_tier=2&id_c=25 | The National Wellness Institute | A non-profit organisation promoting wellness globally. |
| http://www.thewellspring.com/ | The Wellspring | Comprehensive collection of wellness writings and resources, presented by John W. Travis. |
| www.wellnesscontinuum.com | Travis and Ryan | The Wellness Continuum. |

*Discharge planning*

| Website | Organisation | Information |
|---|---|---|
| www.caregiving.org | The National Alliance for Caregiving | A non-profit coalition of national organisations focusing on issues of family caregiving. |
| www.nfcacares.org | The National Family Caregivers Association (NFCA) | Educates, supports, empowers and speaks up for the more than 65 million Americans who care for loved ones with a chronic illness or disability or the frailties of old age. |
| www.uhfnyc.org | The United Hospital Fund New York (US) | A non-profit health services research and philanthropic organisation whose primary mission is to shape positive change in healthcare for the people of New York. |

# Glossary

**Advanced directive**: A legal document wherein a person states their decisions regarding end-of-life care. Can also include living wills and power of attorney.

**Carer**: Named person responsible for care of patient.

**Epidemiology**: 'the study of the distribution and the determinants of disease and problems of health, disease or injuries in human populations' (Barker 1982: p. 1).

**Family**: Family members, partners and significant others.

**Head injury**: 'definite history of a blow to the head, a laceration to the scalp or head, or altered consciousness no matter how brief' (Jennett and Teasdale 1977, cited in Palmer 1998: p. 31).

**Mild brain injury**: GCS ≥13–15.

**Moderate brain injury**: GCS ≥9–12/15.

**Nurse**: In the text when referred to in the female gender, this represents all genders.

**Patient**: A person who has sustained a head injury. In the text when referred to in the male gender, this represents all genders.

**PTA**: Duration of memory loss until return of the clear and normal memory.

**Severe brain injury**: GCS ≤3–8/15.

*Neurotrauma: Managing Patients with Head Injuries*, First Edition. Edited by Nadine Abelson-Mitchell.

# References

Abelson, N. (1982) Observation of the neurosurgical patient. *Curationis*, 5 (3), 32–37.

Abelson, N. (1987) *The comprehensive care of the moderate and severely head injured patient. Volume I.* A thesis submitted to the Faculty of Medicine, University of the Witwatersrand, Johannesburg, in fulfilment of the requirements for the degree of Doctor of Philosophy. Unpublished PhD thesis. University of Witwatersrand.

Abelson-Mitchell, N. (1997) A strategy for rehabilitation – a nursing perspective. *Professional Nursing Today*, 1 (3), 26–29.

Abelson-Mitchell, N. (2006) A model for rehabilitation in the community: A client–needs approach. *British Journal of Neuroscience Nursing*, 2 (3), 116–123.

Abelson-Mitchell, N. (2008) Epidemiology and prevention of head injuries: Literature review. *Journal of Clinical Nursing*, 17 (1), 46–57.

Abelson-Mitchell, N. and Watkins, M.J. (2006) Rehabilitation after traumatic brain injury: A survey of clients' needs and service provision in one English region. *British Journal of Neuroscience Nursing*, 2 (6), 295–304.

Academy of Medical Royal Colleges (2008) *A code of practice for the diagnosis and confirmation of death.* Academy of Medical Royal Colleges, London.

Ackery, A., Hagel, B.E., Provvidenza, C. and Tator, C.H. (2007) An international review of head and spinal cord injuries in alpine skiing and snowboarding. *Injury Prevention*, 13 (6), 368–375.

Agency for Healthcare Research and Quality (2004) *Rehabilitation for traumatic brain injury* [Online]. Available at: http://archive.ahrq.gov/clinic/epcsums/tbisumm.htm#Contents (accessed 24 September 2012).

*Airedale National Health Service Trust v. Bland [1993] AC 789; 1 All ER 821.*

Alain, B.B. and Wang, Y.J. (2008) Cushing's ulcers in traumatic brain injury. *Chinese Journal of Traumatology*, 11 (2), 114–119.

Alexandrescu, R., O'Brien, S. and Lecky, F.E. (2009) A review of injury epidemiology in the UK and Europe: some methodological considerations in constructing rates. *BMC Public Health*, 9 (1), 1–22.

Allum, J.H.J., Bloem, B.R., Carpenter, M.G., Hulliger, M. and Hadders-Algra, M. (1998) Proprioceptive control of posture: A review of new concepts. *Gait and Posture*, 8 (3), 214–242.

Al-Khawaja, I., Wade, D.T. and Turner, F. (1997) The Barthel Index and its relationship to nursing dependency in rehabilitation. *Clinical Rehabilitation*, 11 (4), 335–337.

American Association of Rehabilitation Nurses (ARN) (2003) *Health Policy and Advocacy. Position Statement. Ethical issues* [Online]. Available at: www.rehabnurse.org/advocacy/content/pethical.html (accessed 24 September 2012).

American Association of Rehabilitation Nurses (ARN) (2008) *Standards and scope of rehabilitation nursing practice.* Association of Rehabilitation Nurses, USA.

*Neurotrauma: Managing Patients with Head Injuries*, First Edition. Edited by Nadine Abelson-Mitchell.
© 2013 Blackwell Publishing Ltd. Published 2013 by Blackwell Publishing Ltd.

American Association of Rehabilitation Nurses (ARN) and RNF (Rehabilitation Nursing Foundation) (2006) *Evidence–based rehabilitation nursing: Common challenges and interventions*. Association of Rehabilitation Nurses and Rehabilitation Nursing Foundation, USA.

American College of Surgeons Trauma Committee (2008) *Advanced trauma life support for doctors*, 8th edn. American College of Surgeons, Chicago, Il.

Andelic, N., Bautz-Holter, E., Ronning, P., et al. (2012) Does an early onset and continuous chain of rehabilitation improve the long–term functional outcome of patients with severe traumatic brain injury? *Journal of Neurotrauma*, 29 (1), 66–74.

Andersen, T.E., Árnason, Á., Engebretsen, L. and Bahr, R. (2004) Mechanism of head injuries in elite football. *British Journal of Sports Medicine*, 38 (6), 690–696.

Anderson, K.L. and Burckhardt, C.S. (1999) Conceptualization and measurement of quality of life as an outcome variable for health care intervention and research. *Journal of Advanced Nursing*, 29 (2), 298–306.

Andersson, B.J., Ortengren, R., Nachemson, A. and Elfstrom, G. (1974) Lumbar disc pressure and myoelectric back muscle activity during sitting. *Scandinavian Journal of Rehabilitation Medicine*, 6 (3), 104–114.

Andersson, E.H., Björklund, R., Emanuelson, I. and Stålhammar, D. (2003) Epidemiology of traumatic brain injury: A population-based study in western Sweden. *Acta Neurologica Scandinavica*, 107 (4), 256–259.

Andrews, K., Murphy, L., Munday, R. and Littlewood, C. (1996) Misdiagnosis of the vegetative state: Retrospective study in a rehabilitation unit. *British Medical Journal*, 313 (7048), 13–16.

Annoni, J.M., Beer, S. and Kesselring, J. (1992) Severe traumatic brain injury – epidemiology and outcome after 3 years. *Disability and Rehabilitation*, 14 (1), 23–26.

Aronow, H.U. (1987) Rehabilitation effectiveness with severe brain injury – translating research into policy. *Journal of Head Trauma Rehabilitation*, 2 (3), 24–36.

Association of Anaesthetists of Great Britain and Ireland (2009) *AAGBI safety guideline: Interhospital. Transfer* AAGBI, London.

Audit Commission (1999) *The place of efficient and effective critical are services within the acute hospital*. Audit Commission, London.

Audit Commission (2000) *The way to go home. Rehabilitation and remedial services for older people*. Audit Commission, London.

Avery, A. (1996) Eco-wellness nursing: getting serious about innovation and change. *Nursing Inquiry*, 3 (2), 67–73.

Bailey, K. (1987) *Human paleopsychology: Applications to aggression and pathological processes*. Lawrence Erlbaum Associates, Hillsdale, New Jersey.

Baker, M.J. (2011) Education requirements for nurses working with people with complex neurological conditions: Relatives' perceptions. *Nurse Education in Practice*, 11 (4), 268–272.

Baldo, V., Marcolongo, A., Floreani, A., et al. (2003) Epidemiological aspect of traumatic brain injury in Northeast Italy. *European Journal of Epidemiology*, 18 (11), 1059–1063.

Barker, D.J.P. (1982) *Practical epidemiology*, 3rd Edn. Churchill Livingstone, Edinburgh.

Barker-Collo, S. and Feigin, V. (2008) Memory deficit after traumatic brain injury: how big is the problem in New Zealand and what management strategies are available? *The New Zealand Medical Journal*, 121 (1268) [Online]. Available at: http://journal.nzma.org.nz/journal/121–1268/2903/ (24 September 2012).

Barnes, M.P. (1999a) Rehabilitation after traumatic brain injury. *British Medical Bulletin*, 55 (4), 927–943.

Barnes, M.P. (1999b) An overview of the clinical management of spasticity. In: Barnes, M.P. and Johnson, G.R. (eds) *Upper motor neurone syndrome and spasticity: Clinical management and neurophysiology*. Cambridge University Press, Cambridge, pp. 1–11.

Barnes, M.P. (2001) Spasticity: A rehabilitation challenge in the elderly. *Gerontology*, 47 (6), 295–299.

Barnes, M.P. and Radermacher, H. (2003) *Community rehabilitation in neurology*. Cambridge University Press, Cambridge.

Barquist, E., Amortequi, J., Hallal, A., et al. (2006) Tracheostomy in ventilator dependent trauma patients: A prospective, randomized intention-to-treat study. *Journal of Trauma*, 60 (1), 91–97.

Basso, A., Previgliano, I., Duarte, J.M. and Ferrari, N. (2001) Advances in management of neurosurgical trauma in different continents. *World Journal of Surgery*, 25 (9), 1174–1178.

Bauby, J-D. (1997) *The diving bell and the butterfly*. Knopf, New York.

Bay, E. and Donders, J. (2008) Risk factors for depressive symptoms after mild to moderate traumatic brain injury. *Brain Injury*, 22 (3), 233–241.

Beecham, J., Perkins, M., Snell, T. and Knapp, M. (2009) Treatment paths and costs for young adults with acquired brain injury in the United Kingdom. *Brain Injury*, 23 (1), 30–38.

Bell, M.D.D., Moss, E. and Murphy, P.G. (2004) Brain Death testing in UK, time for re–appraisal. *British Journal of Anaesthesia*, 92 (5), 632–640.

Bernardini, G.L. (2004) Diagnosis and management of brain abscess and subdural empyema. *Current Neurology and Neuroscience Reports*, 4 (6), 448–458.

Bloom, G.A., Horton, A.S., McCrory, P. and Johnston, K.M. (2004) Sport psychology and concussion: new impacts to explore. *British Journal of Sports Medicine*, 38 (5), 519–521.

BMJ Group and the Royal Pharmaceutical Society of Great Britain (2011) *British National Formulary*. BMJ Group/ Pharmaceutical Press, London.

Bobath, B. (1990) *Adult hemiplegia: Evaluation and treatment.* 3rd edn. Heinemann, Oxford.

Bobath, K. (1969) *The motor deficit in patients with cerebral palsy.* Spastics International Medical Publications in Association with William Heinemann Medical Books Ltd, Lavenham, Suffolk.

Boeree, C.G. (2009) *General psychology: The emotional nervous system* [Online]. Available at: http://webspace.ship.edu/cgboer/limbicsystem.html (accessed 24 September 2012).

Bogner, J.D., Corrigan, J.D., Mysiw, W.J., et al. (2001) A comparison of substance abuse and violence in the prediction of long–term rehabilitation outcomes after traumatic brain injury. *Archives of Physical Medicine and Rehabilitation.* 82 (5), 571–577.

*Bolam v Friern Hospital Management Committee* [1957] 1 WLR 582.

*Bolitho v City and Hackney Health Authority* [1998] AC 232.

Bornhofen, C. and McDonald, S. (2008) Emotion perception deficits following traumatic brain injury: a review of the evidence and rationale for intervention. *Journal International Neuropsychological Society,* 14 (4), 511–525.

Bos, S. (1997) Coma stimulation. *The Online Journal of Knowledge Synthesis for Nursing,* 4 (1), 1–6.

Bouderka, M., Fakhir, B., Bouaggad, A., et al. (2004) Early tracheostomy versus prolonged endotracheal intubation in severe head injury. *Journal of Trauma,* 57 (2), 251–254.

Boxall, K., Dowson, S. and Beresford, P. (2009) Selling individual budgets, consumer choice and control: Local and global influences on UK social care policy for people with learning disability. *Policy and Politics,* 37(4), 499–515.

Bradley, L.J., Kirker, G.B., Corteen, E., et al. (2006) Inappropriate acute neurosurgical bed occupancy and short falls in rehabilitation: Implications for the National Service Framework. *British Journal of Neurosurgery,* 20 (1), 36–39.

Brain Trauma Foundation (2000) Part 2: Early indicators of prognosis in severe traumatic brain injury. *Journal of Neurotrauma,* 17 (6–7), 555–627.

Brain Trauma Foundation (2008) Guidelines for prehospital management of traumatic brain injury, 2nd edn. *Prehospital Emergency Care,* 12 (Suppt 1), S1–52.

Breda, J., Shoenmaekers, D., Van Landeghem, et al. (2006) When informal care becomes a paid job: the case of Personal Assistance Budgets in Flanders. In C. Glendinning and P.A. Kemp (eds) *Cash and care: Policy challenges in the welfare state.* Policy Press, Bristol, pp. 155–170.

British Society of Rehabilitation Medicine (1998) *Rehabilitation after traumatic brain injury: A working party report of the British Society of Rehabilitation Medicine.* British Society of Rehabilitation Medicine.

British Society of Rehabilitation Medicine (2002) *Appendix 1: Standards for specialist in–patient and community rehabilitation services, 39–44* [Online]. British Society of Rehabilitation Medicine, London.

British Society of Rehabilitation Medicine (2008a) *Neurological Rehabilitation: A briefing paper for commissioners of clinical neurosciences, 1–8.* British Society of Rehabilitation Medicine, London.

British Society of Rehabilitation Medicine (2008b) *Measurement of outcome in rehabilitation. "Basket" of Measures.* British Society of Rehabilitation Medicine, London.

British Society of Rehabilitation Medicine (2009) *Standards for rehabilitation services, mapped on to the National service framework for long-term conditions.* British Society of Rehabilitation Medicine, London.

Brook, I. (2011) *Brain Abscess* [Online]. Available at: http://emedicine.medscape.com/article/212946-overview (accessed 24 September 2012).

Brown, A.W., Elovic, E.P., Kothari, S., et al. (2008) Congenital and acquired brain injury. 1. Epidemiology, pathophysiology, prognostication, innovative treatments, and prevention. *Archives of Physical Medicine and Rehabilitation,* 89 (3 Suppl 1), S3–S8.

Browne, G.J. and Lam, L.T. (2006) Concussive head injury in children and adolescents related to sports and other leisure physical activities. *British Journal of Sports Medicine,* 40 (2), 163–168.

Bruns, J.J. and Hauser, W.A. (2003) The epidemiology of traumatic brain injury: A Review. *Epilepsia,* 44 (Suppl. 10), 2–10.

Bryan, K. (2010) Policies for reducing delayed discharge from hospital. *British Medical Bulletin,* 95 (1), 33–46.

Bulger, E.M., Nathens, A.B., Rivara, F.P., et al. (2002) Management of severe head injury: Insititutional variations in care and effect on outcome. *Critical Care Medicine,* 30 (8), 1870–1876.

Bullock, M.R., Chesnut, R., Ghajar, J., et al. (2006) Surgical management of acute subdural hematomas. *Neurosurgery,* 58 (3), S16–24.

Bullock, R. and Teasdale, G. (1990) ABC of major trauma: Head injuries I. *British Medical Journal,* 300 (6738), 1515–1518.

Bulters, D. and Belli, A. (2009) A prospective study of the time to evacuate acute subdural and extradural haematomas. *Anaesthesia,* 64 (3), 277–281.

Campbell, M. (2000) *Rehabilitation for traumatic brain injury: Physical therapy in context,* Churchill Livingstone, Edinburgh.

Euro NCAP, (no date) *Car search results* [Online]. Available at: http://www.euroncap.com/carsearch.aspx (accessed 24 September 2012).

*Carers (Equal Opportunities) Act 2004: Elizabeth II.* Chapter 15 (2004) London: The Stationery Office.

Carr, J., Shepherd, R.B. and Ada, L. (1995) Spasticity: Research findings and implications for intervention. *Physiotherapy,* 81 (8), 421–429.

Carr, S. (2008) *SCIE Report 20: Personalisation: A rough guide.* SCIE, London.

Casarett, D., Kapo, J. and Caplan, A. (2005) Appropriate use of artificial nutrition and hydration– fundamental principles and recommendations. *The New England Journal of Medicine*, 353 (24), 2607–2612.

Cassidy, J.D., Carroll, L.J., Peloso, P.M., et al. (2004) Incidence, risk factors and prevention of mild traumatic brain injury: Results of the WHO Collaborating Centre Task Forces on Mild Traumatic Brain Injury. *Journal of Rehabilitation Medicine*, 43 (Suppl.), 28–60.

Cattelani, R., Roberti, R. and Lombardi, F. (2008) Adverse effects of apathy and neurobehavioural deficits on the community integration of traumatic brain injury subjects. *European Journal Physical Rehabilitation Medicine*, 44 (3), 245–251.

Chang, A.T., Boots, R.J., Hodges, P.W., et al. (2004) Standing with the assistance of a tilt table improves minute ventilation in chronic critically ill patients. *Archives of Physical Medicine and Rehabilitation*, 85 (12), 1972–1976.

Chartered Institute of Public Finance and Accountancy (CIPFA) (2007) *Direct Payments and Individual Budgets: Managing the Finances (CIPFA 2007).* Chartered Institute of Public Finance and Accounting in conjunction with 'In Control' supported by Department of Health. CIPFA, London.

Chatfield, D.A. and Menon, D.K. (2011) The Mental Capacity Act of 2005 and its impact in critical care. *Journal of the Intensive Care Society*, 12 (1), 47–51.

Chaudhry, M.A., Santarius, T., Wilson, L., et al. (2003) Head injuries: a prospective observational study evaluating the potential impact of the Galasko report on Accident and Emergency departments. *Injury*, 34 (11), 853–856.

Christensen, M.C., Nielsen, T.G., Ridley, S., et al. (2008) Outcomes and costs of penetrating trauma injury in England and Wales. *Injury*, 39 (9), 1013–1025.

Chua, K.S.G., Ng, Y-S., Yap, S.G.M. and Bok, C-W. (2007) A brief review of traumatic brain injury rehabilitation. *Annals of the Academy of Medicine, Singapore*, 36 (1), 31–42.

Chudley, S. (1994) The effect of nursing activities on intracranial pressure. *British Journal of Nursing*, 3 (9), 454–455.

Clayton, T.J., Nelson, R.J. and Manara, A.R. (2004) Reduction in mortality from severe head injury following introduction of a protocol for intensive care management. *British Journal of Anaethesia*, 93 (6), 761–767.

Clifton, G.L., Miller, E.R., Choi, S.C. and Levin, H.S. (2002) Fluid thresholds and outcome from severe head injury. *Critical Care Medicine*, 30 (4), 739–745.

Clini, E. and Ambrosini, N. (2005) Early physiotherapy in the respiratory intensive care unit. *Respiratory Medicine*, 99 (9), 1096–1104.

Coetzer, R. (2009) A clinical pathway including psychotherapy approaches for managing emotional difficulties after acquired brain injury. *CNS Spectrums*, 14 (11), 632–638.

Coles, J., Fryer, T., Coleman, M., et al. (2007) Hyperventilation following head injury: Effect on ischemic burden and cerebral oxidative metabolism. *Critical Care Medicine*, 35 (2), 568–78.

Cook, D.J., Fuller, H.D., Guyatt, G.H., et al. (1994) Risk factors for gastrointestinal bleeding in critically ill patients. *The New England Journal of Medicine*, 330 (6), 377–381.

Cooper, D.J., Rosenfeld, J., Murray, L., et al. (2011) Decompressive craniectomy in diffuse traumatic brain injury. *The New England Journal of Medicine*, 364 (16), 1493–1502.

Cope, D.N. and Hall, K. (1982) Head injury rehabilitation: Benefits of early intervention. *Archives of Physical Medicine and Rehabilitation*, 63 (9), 433–437.

Coronado, V.G., Thomas, K.E., Sattin, R.W. and Johnson, R.L. (2005) The CDC traumatic brain injury surveillance system: Characteristics of people aged 65 years and older hospitalized with a TBI. *Journal of Head Trauma Rehabilitation*, 20 (3), 215–228.

Cowen, T.D., Meythaler, J.M., DeVivo, M.J., et al. (1995) Influence of early variables in traumatic brain injury on functional independence measure scores and rehabilitation length of stay and charges. *Archives of Physical Medicine and Rehabilitation*, 76 (9), 797–803.

Crandall, J.R., Bhalla, K.S. and Madeley, N.J. (2002) Designing road vehicles for pedestrian protection. *British Medical Journal*, 324 (7346), 1145–1148.

Crimmins, D.W. and Palmer, J.D. (2000) Snapshot view of emergency neurosurgical head injury care in Great Britain and Ireland. *Journal of Neurology, Neurosurgery and Psychiatry*, 68 (1), 8–13.

Curley, G., Kavanagh, B. and Laffey, J. (2010) Hypocapnia and the injured brain: more harm than benefit. *Critical Care Medicine*, 38 (5), 1348–1359.

Daley, R.J., Rebuck, J.A., Welage, L.S. and Rogers, F.B. (2004) Prevention of stress ulceration: Current trends in critical care. *Critical Care Medicine*, 32 (10), 2008–2013.

Das-Gupta, R. and Turner-Stokes, L. (2002) Traumatic brain injury. *Disability and Rehabilitation*, 24 (13), 654–665.

*Data Protection Act 1998*: Elizabeth II (1998). The Stationery Office, London.

Davidson, J.A. (2005) Epidemiology and outcome of bicycle injuries presenting to an emergency department in the United Kingdom. *European Journal of Emergency Medicine*, 12 (1), 24–29.

Davies, P. (1994) *Starting again: Early rehabilitation after brain injury and other severe brain lesions.* Springer-Verlag, Berlin.

Dawodu, S.T. (2008) *Traumatic brain injury (TBI): Definition, epidemiology, pathophysiology* [Online]. Available at: http://www.emedicine.medscape.com/article/326510–overview (15 January 2012).

Dawodu, S.T. (2003) *Traumatic brain injury: Definition, epidemiology, pathophysiology* [Online]. Available at: http://www.emedicine.com/pmr/topic212.htm (accessed 24 September 2012).

Da Roit, B. and Le Bihan, B. (2008) *Cash–for–care schemes in Austria, Italy, France and the Netherlands: Effects on family support and care workers. Transforming elderly care at local, national and transnational levels*. International Conference at the Danish National Centre for Social Research, Copenhagen, 26–28 June 2008.

Deb, S. and Burns, J. (2007) Neuropsychiatric consequences of traumatic brain injury: A comparison between two age groups. *Brain Injury*, 21 (3), 301–307.

De Groot, Y.J., Jansen, N.E., Bakker, J., et al. (2010) Imminent brain death: Point of departure for potential heart–beating organ donor recognition. *Intensive Care Medicine*, 36 (9), 1488–1494.

Department of Health (1998) *Working together: Securing a quality workforce for the NHS*. HMSO, London.

Department of Health (1999) *Saving lives: Our healthier nation* [Online]. Available at: http://www.archive.official–documents.co.uk/document/cm43/4386/4386.htm (24 September 2012).

Department of Health (2000a) *Comprehensive critical care: A review of adult critical care services*. HMSO, London.

Department of Health (2000b) *The NHS plan: A plan for investment; a plan for reform*. HMSO, London.

Department of Health (2000c) *A health service for all talents: Developing the NHS workforce – consultation document on the review of workforce planning*. HMSO, London.

Department of Health (2000d) *No Secrets: Guidance on Developing and Implementing Multi–Agency Policies and procedures for the Protection of vulnerable Adults form Abuse*. TSO, London.

Department of Health (2001a) *National service framework for older people*. HMSO, London.

Department of Health (2001b) *Working together, learning together: A framework for lifelong learning for the NHS*. HMSO, London.

Department of Health (2003) *Discharge from hospital: Pathway, process and practice*. HMSO, London.

Department of Health (2004a) *Neuroscience critical care report: Progress in developing services*. HMSO, London.

Department of Health (2004b) *The NHS knowledge and skills framework (NHS KSF) and the development review process*. HMSO, London.

Department of Health (2005a) *The national service framework for long term conditions*. HMSO, London.

Department of Health (2005b) *Independence, wellbeing and choice*. TSO, London.

Department of Health (2005c) *Quality critical care. Beyond comprehensive critical care. Critical care stakeholder forum*. HMSO, London.

Department of Health (2006a) *Our health, our care, our say: A new direction for community services: A brief guide*. HMSO, London.

Department of Health (2006b) *Modernising nursing careers: Setting the direction*. HMSO, London.

Department of Health (2007a) *Best research for best health: A new national health research strategy*. HMSO, London.

Department of Health (2007b) Clinical governance standards for better health. HMSO, London.

Department of Health (2007c) *Our NHS, Our Future: NHS Next Stage Review: Professor Lord Darzi*. TSO, London.

Department of Health (2007d) *Putting people first –a shared vision and commitment to the transformation of adult social care*. TSO, London.

Department of Health (2007e) *Mental Capacity Act of 2007*. TSO, London.

Department of Health (2007f) *Towards a framework for post–registration nursing careers: Consultation response report*. HMSO, London.

Department of Health (2008a) *A high quality workforce: NHS next stage review*. HMSO, London.

Department of Health (2008b) *Evaluation of the individual budgets pilot programme: Final report*. HMSO, London.

Department of Health (2008c) *High quality care for all: NHS next stage review final report*, TSO, London.

Department of Health (2010a) *Essence of Care 2010* [Online]. Available at: http://www.dh.gov.uk/en/Publicationsandstatistics/Publications/PublicationsPolicyAndGuidance/DH_119969 (accessed 24 September 2012).

Department of Health (2010b) *A vision for adult social care: Capable communities and active citizens*. HMSO, London.

Department of Health (2010c) *Front line care: The nursing and midwifery in England. Report of the Prime Minister's commission on the future of nursing and midwifery in England* [Online]. Available at: http://www.dh.gov.uk/en/Publicationsandstatistics/Publications/PublicationsPolicyAndGuidance/DH_115295 (accessed 24 September 2012).

Department of Health (2011a) *Payment by results 2012–2013 road test package*. HMSO, London.

Department of Health (2011b) *Attendance at Accident and Emergency Departments* [Online]. Available at: http://www.dh.gov.uk/en/Publicationsandstatistics/Statistics/Performancedataandstatistics/AccidentandEmergency/DH_077485 (accessed 24 September 2012).

Department of Health (2011c) *Think local, act personal: Next steps for transforming adult social care*. HMSO, London.

Department of Health and Social Security (1990) *National Health Service and Community Care Act*. TSO, London.

Department of Transport (2007) *Think!* [Online]. Available at: http://think.direct.gov.uk/ (accessed 24 September 2012).

Department of Transport (2011) *Renewing your driving licence at 70 plus* [Online]. Available at: http://www.direct.gov.uk/en/Motoring/DriverLicensing/NeedANewOrUpdatedLicence/DG_4022086 (accessed 24 September 2012).

Dittrich, R. (2009) Personalisation and the future of adult social care: the views of Hampshire residents. *Research, Policy & Planning*, 27 (1), 3–16.

Dobkin, B.H. (2000) Functional rewiring of brain and spinal cord after injury: The three Rs of neural repair and neurological rehabilitation. *Current Opinions in Neurology*, 13 (6), 655–659.

Donabedian, A. (1996) *Evaluating the quality assurance and health promotion interventions in the EU-member States in 1996.* IUHPE/EURO, Saint–Denis Cedex, France.

Doty, P., Mahoney, K.J. and Simon-Rusinowitz, L. (2007) Designing the cash and counseling demonstration and evaluation. *Health Services Research*, 42 (1), 378–396.

Dowson, S. and Greig, R. (2009) The emergence of the independent support broker role, *Journal of Integrated Care*, 17 (4), 22–30.

Draper, K., Ponsford, J. and Schönberger, M. (2007) Psychosocial and emotional outcomes 10 years following traumatic brain injury. *Journal of Head Trauma Rehabilitation*, 22 (5), 278–87.

Drinkdriving.org (2011) *Worldwide BAC Limits – Worldwide Blood Alcohol Concentration (BAC) Limits* [Online]. Available at: http://www.drinkdriving.org/worldwide_drink_driving_limits.php (accessed 24 September 2012).

Drive and Stay Alive, Inc. (2011) *International Blood Alcohol Limits* [Online]. Available at: http://www.driveandstayalive.com/.

Drugs.com (2011) *Welcome to Drugs.com.* Available at: www.drugs.com (accessed 24 September 2012).

DuBois, J.M. (2011) Dead tired of repetitious debates about death criteria. *The American Journal of Bioethics*, 11 (8), 45–47.

Edwards, S. (ed.) (1996) *Neurological physiotherapy: A problem–solving approach*, Churchill Livingstone, Edinburgh.

Edwards, S. and Charlton, P. (2002) Splinting and the use of orthoses in the management of patients with neurosurgical disorders. In: Edwards, S. (ed.) *Neurological physiotherapy: A problem–solving approach*, 2nd edn. Churchill Livingstone, Edinburgh, pp. 219–254.

Elliott, H. (2011) *The Safest Cars Of 2011* [Online]. Available at: http://www.forbes.com/2011/01/15/safest–cars–2011–business–autos.html (8 September 2011).

Engberg, A.W. and Teasdale, T.W. (1998) Traumatic brain injury in children in Denmark: A national 15–year study. *European Journal of Epidemiology*, 14 (2), 165–173.

Engberg, A.W. and Teasdale, T.W. (2001) Traumatic brain injury in Denmark 1979–1996. A national study of incidence and mortality. *European Journal of Epidemiology*, 17 (5), 437–442.

Englander, J., Bushnik, T., Duong, T.T., Cifu, D.X., Zafonte, R., Wright, J., Hughes, R. and Bergman, W. (2003) Analyzing risk factors for late posttraumatic seizures: A prospec-

tive, multicenter investigation. *Archives of Physical Medicine and Rehabilitation*, 84 (3), 365–373.

*Equality Act 2010*: Elizabeth II (2010). The Stationery Office, London.

Espinosa-Aguilar, A., Reyes-Morales, H., Huerta-Posada, C., et al. (2008) Design and validation of a critical pathway for hospital management of patients with severe traumatic brain injury. *The Journal of Trauma Injury, Infection, and Critical Care*, 64 (5), 1327–1341.

European Campaign for Safe Road Design (2011) *Eurorap members leading call for safe road design in Europe* [Online]. Available at: http://saferoaddesign.eu/news.aspx (accessed 24 September 2012).

Evans, L. and Brewis, C. (2008) The efficacy of community–based rehabilitation programmes for adults with TBI. *International Journal of Therapy and Rehabilitation*, 15 (10), 446–458.

Farlam, J. (2011) *UK Speed Limits* [Online]. Available at: http://www.smartdriving.co.uk/Driving/DefensiveDriving/Speed/UK_Speed_limits.html (accessed 24 September 2012).

Faul, M., Xu, L., Wald, M.M. and Coronado, V.G. (2010) *Traumatic brain injury in the United States: Emergency department visits, hospitalizations and deaths 2002–2006.* Centers for Disease Control and Prevention, National Center for Injury Prevention and Control, Atlanta, GA.

Fortune, J.B., Feustel, P.J., Weigle, C.G. and Popp, A.J. (1994) Continuous measurement of jugular venous oxygen saturation in response to transient elevations of blood pressure in head-injured patients. *Journal of Neurosurgery*, 80 (3), 461–468.

Frank, J.S. and Earl, M. (1990) Coordination of posture and movement, *Physical Therapy*, 70 (12), 855–863.

*Freedom of Information Act 2000*: Elizabeth II (2000). The Stationery Office, London.

Giannoudis, P.V., Harwood, P.J., Court-Brown, C. and Pape, H.C. (2009) Severe and multiple trauma in older patients; incidence and mortality. *Injury*, 40 (4), 362–367.

Gilbert, T. and Powell, J.L. (2010) Power and Social Work in the United Kingdom. *Journal of Social Work*, 10 (1), 3–23.

Gill-Thwaites, H. (2006) Lotteries, loopholes and luck: Misdiagnosis in the vegetative state patient. *Brain Injury*, December, 20 (13–14), 1321–1328.

Glendinning, C., Challis, D., Fernandez, J., et al. (2008) *Evaluation of the Individual Budgets pilot programme: Final report.* Social Policy Research Unit, University of York, York.

Gordon, E., von Host, H. and Rudehill, A. (1995) Outcome of head injury in 2,298 patients treated in a single clinic during a 21-year period. *Journal of Neurosurgical Anesthesiology*, 7 (4), 235–247.

Granger, C.V., Hamilton, B.B. and Sherwin, F.S. (1986) *Guide for the use of the uniform data set for medical rehabilita-*

*tion*. New York: Uniform data system for medical rehabilitation project office. Buffalo General Hospital, NY.

Greaves, I., Porter, K. and Ryan, J. (2001) *Trauma Care Manual*. Arnold. London.

Green, E.M., Mulcahy, C.M. and Pountney, T.E. (1992) *Postural management theory and practice*. Active Design, Birmingham.

Greenwald, B.D., Burnett, D.M. and Miller, M.A. (2003) Congenital and acquired brain injury.1. Brain injury: Epidemiology and pathophysiology. *Archives of Physical Medicine and Rehabilitation*, 84 (3 Supp 1), S3–S7.

Greenwood, R. (2002) Head injury for Neurologists. *Journal of Neurology, Neurosurgery and Psychiatry*, 73 (Suppl 1), i8–i16.

Griffith, R. and Tengnah, C. (2008) *Law and professional issues in nursing*. Learning Matters Ltd, London.

Grossman, M.R., Sahrmann, S.A. and Rose, S.J. (1982) Review of length associated changes in muscle: Experimental evidence and clinical implications. *Physical Therapy*, 62 (12), 1799–1808.

Grubb, A. (1997) The persistent vegetative state: A duty (not) to treat and conscientious objection. *European Journal of Health Law*, 4, 39–60.

Guerrero, J.L., Thurman, D.J. and Sniezek, J.E. (2000) Emergency department visits associated with traumatic brain injury: United States, 1995–1996. *Brain Injury*, 14 (2), 181–186.

Halevy, A. and Brody, B. (1993) Brain death: Reconciling definitions, criteria, and tests. *Annals of Internal Medicine*, 119 (6), 519–525.

Hart, T., Millis, S., Novack, T., et al. (2003) The relationship between neuropsychologic function and level of caregiver supervision at 1 year after traumatic brain injury. *Archives of Physical Medicine and Rehabilitation*, 84 (2), 221–230.

Hatfield, A., Hunt, S. and Wade, D. (2003) The Northwick Park Dependency Score and its relationship to nursing hours in neurological rehabilitation. *Journal of Rehabilitation Medicine*, 35 (3), 116–120.

Hattie, H.A., Myers, J.E. and Sweeney, T.I. (2004) A factor structure of wellness: Theory, assessment, analysis, and practice. *Journal of Counseling & Development*, 82 (3), 354–364.

Headway: The Brain Injury Association (2011) *Welcome to Headway* [Online]. Available at: http://www.headway.org.uk (accessed 24 September 2012).

Hell, J.W. and Ehlers, M.D (eds.) (2008) *Structural and functional organization of the synapse*. Springer, New York.

Heskestad, B., Baardsen, R., Helseth, E., et al. (2009) Incidence of hospital referred injuries in Norway: A population based survey from the Stavanger region. *Scandinavian Journal of Trauma, Resuscitation and Emergency Medicine*, 17, 6.

Hessen, E., Nestvold, K. and Anderson, V. (2007) Neuropsychological functioning 23 years after mild brain injury: A comparison of outcome after paediatric and adult head injuries. *Brain Injury*, 21 (9), 963–979.

Hettler, B. (1980) Wellness promotion on a university campus. *Family & Community Health*, 3 (1), 77–95.

Hettler, B. (1984) Wellness: Encouraging a lifetime pursuit of excellence. *Health Values: Achieving High Level Wellness*, 8 (4),13–17.

Hoeman, S.P. (2008) *Rehabilitation Nursing: Prevention, interventions and outcomes*. 4th edn. Mosby Elsevier, USA.

Holsinger, T., Steffens, D.C., Phillips, C., et al. (2002) Head injury in early adulthood and the lifetime risk of depression. *Archives of General Psychiatry*, 59 (1), 17–22.

Honda, H. and Warren, D.K. (2009) Central nervous system infections: Meningitis and brain abscess. *Infectious Disease Clinics of North America*, 23 (3), 609–624.

Horak, F.B., Henry, S.M. and Shumway-Cook, A. (1997) Postural perturbations: New insights for treatment of balance disorder. *Physical Therapy*, 77 (5), 517–533.

Hudak, A.M., Trivedi, K., Harper, C.R., et al. (2004) Evaluation of seizure-like episodes in survivors of moderate and severe traumatic brain injury. *The Journal of Head Trauma Rehabilitation*, 19 (4), 290–295.

Hudson, C.M., Adams, D., DeRose, A. and Harro, C.C. (2008) Taking an interdisciplinary team approach to rehabilitation after a TBI. *Nursing*, 38 (Suppl Therapy), 7–11.

*Human Rights Act 1998: Elizabeth II* (1998). The Stationery Office, London.

*Human Tissue Act 2004: Elizabeth II* (2004). The Stationery Office, London.

Hunt, G.G. and Levine, C. (2006) *A Family Caregiver's Guide to Hospital Discharge Planning*. National Alliance for Caregiving, New York. Available at: www.caregiving.org (accessed 24 September 2012).

Hurvitz, E., Mandac, B.R., Davidoff, G., Johnson, J.H. and Nelson, V.S. (1992) Risk factors for heterotopic ossification in children and adolescents with severe traumatic brain injury. *Archives of Physical Medicine and Rehabilitation*, 73 (5), 459–462.

Jackson–Friedman, C., Lyden, P.D., Nunez, S., Jin, A. and Zweifler, R. (1997) High dose baclofen is neuroprotective but also causes intracerebral hemorrhage: A quantal bioassay study using the intraluminal suture occlusion method. *Experimental Neurology*, 147 (2), 346–352.

Jagger, J., Jane, J.A. and Rimel, R. (1983) The Glasgow coma scale: To sum or not to sum? *The Lancet*, 322 (8341), 97.

Jennett, B. (2005) Thirty years of the vegetative state: Clinical, ethical and legal problems. *Progress in Brain Research*, 150, 537–543.

Jennett B. (2002) Vegetative state: *Medical facts, ethical and legal dilemmas*. Cambridge University Press, Cambridge.

Jennett, B. (1996) Epidemiology of head injury. *Journal of Neurology, Neurosurgery & Psychiatry*, 60 (4), 362–369.

Jennett, B. and Bond, M. (1975) Assessment of outcome after severe brain damage: A Practical Scale. *The Lancet*, 305 (7905), 480–484.

Jennett, B. and Teasdale, G. (1977) Aspects of coma after severe head injury. *Lancet*, 1 (8071), 878–881.

Johansson, E., Rönnkvist, M. and Fugl-Meyer, A.R. (1991) Traumatic brain injury in northern Sweden, incidence and prevalence of long–standing impairments and disabilities. *Scandinavian Journal of Rehabilitation Medicine*, 23 (4), 179–185.

Johnson, K. and Davis, P.K. (1998) A supported relationship intervention to increase the social integration of persons with traumatic brain injuries. *Behavior Modifications*, 22 (4), 502–528.

Johnston, M.V. and Miklos, C.S. (2002) Activity related quality of life in rehabilitation and traumatic brain injury. *Archives of Physical Medicine and Rehabilitation*, 83 (12 Suppl 2), S26–38.

Johnstone, B., Vessell, R., Bounds, T., et al.(2003) Predictors of success for state vocational rehabilitation clients with traumatic brain injury. *Archives of Physical Medicine and Rehabilitation*, 84 (2), 161–167.

Joubert, J., Reid, C., Joubert, L., et al. (2006) Risk factor management and depression post–stroke: the value of an integrated model of care. *Journal of Clinical Neuroscience*, 13 (1), 84–90.

Joyce, T. (2009) Best interests. *Psychiatry*, 8 (12), 481–483.

Kandel, E.R., Schwartz, J.H. and Jessel, T.M. (1995) *Essentials of neural science and behavior*. McGraw-Hill, Maidenhead, Surrey.

Kannus, P., Niemi, S., Parkkari, J., et al. (2007) Alarming rise in fall–induced severe head injuries among elderly people. *Injury, International Journal of the Care of the Injured*, 38 (1), 81–83.

Kay, A. and Teasdale, G. (2001) Head injury in the United Kingdom. *World Journal of Surgery*, 25 (9), 1210–1220.

Kay, R.M., Rethlefsen, S.A., Fern-Buneo, A., et al. (2004) Botulinum toxin as an adjunct to serial casting treatment in children with cerebral palsy. *The Journal of Bone and Joint Surgery*, 86 (11), 2377–2385.

Kent and Medway Safety Camera Partnership (2011) *Home* [Online]. Available at: http://www.kmscp.org/ (accessed 24 September 2012).

Kiefer, R.A. (2008) An integrative review of the concept of well-being. *Holistic Nursing Practice*, 22 (5), 244–252.

Klauber, M.R., Marshall, L.F., Luerssen, T.G., et al. (1989) Determinants of head injury mortality: Importance of the low risk patient. *Neurosurgery*, 24 (1), 31–36.

Kleiven, S., Peloso, P.M. and von Holst, H. (2003) The epidemiology of head injuries in Sweden from 1987–2000. *Injury Control & Safety Promotion*, 10 (3), 173–180.

Klose, M., Juul, A., Poulsgaard, L., Kosteljanetz, M., et al. (2007a) Prevalence and predictive factors of post-traumatic hypopituitarism. *Clinical Endocrinology*, 67 (2), 193–201.

Klose, M., Juul, A., Struck, J., Morgenthaler, N.G., et al. (2007b) Acute and long–term pituitary insufficiency in traumatic brain injury: a prospective single-centre study. *Clinical Endocrinology*, 67 (4), 598–606.

Kotwica, Z. and Saracen, A. (2010). Severe head injuries in the elderly. *Hygeia Public Health*, 45 (2), 197–201.

Kraus, J.F. and McArthur, D.L. (1996). Epidemiologic aspects of brain injury. *Neurologic Clinics*, 14 (2), 435–450.

Kreimer, M. (2006) Developments in Austrian care arrangements: Women between free choice and informal care. In C. Glendinning and P.A. Kemp (eds) *Cash and Care: Policy challenges in the welfare state*. Policy Press, Bristol, pp. 141–153.

Kubler-Ross, E. and Kessler, D. (2005) *On grief and grieving: Finding the meaning of grief through the five stages of loss*. Scribner, New York.

Kurtoglu, M., Yanar, H., Bilsel, Y., et al. (2004) Venous thromboembolism prophylaxis after head and spine trauma: intermittent pneumatic compression devices versus low molecular weight heparin. *World Journal of Surgery*, 28 (8), 807–811.

Langlois, J.A., Rutland-Brown, W. and Thomas, K. (2004) *Traumatic brain injury in the United States: Emergency departmental visits, hospitalizations, and deaths*. Atlanta, GA, National Center for Injury Prevention and Control.

Langlois, J.A., Rutland-Brown, W. and Wald, M.M. (2006) The epidemiology and impact of traumatic brain injury: A brief overview. *The Journal of Head Trauma Rehabilitation*, 21 (5), 375–378.

Lannoo, E., Van Rietvelde, F., Colardyn, F., et al. (2000) Early predictors of mortality and morbidity after severe closed head injury. *Journal of Neurotrauma*, 17 (5), 403–414.

Leadbeater, C. (2004) *Personalisation through public participation*. Demos, London.

Leadbeater, C. (2008) This time it's personal, *The Guardian* (Society), 16 January [Online]. Available at: http://www.guardian.co.uk/society/2008/jan/16/care.budgets (accessed 24 September 2012).

Leatherman, M.E. and Goethe, K.E. (2009) Substituted decision making: Elder guardianship. *Journal of Psychiatric Practice*, 15 (6), 470–476.

Lecky, F., Bryden, D., Little, R., et al. (2008) *Emergency intubation for acutely ill and injured patients (Review)*. The Cochrane Collaboration, John Wiley and Sons Ltd, London.

Lenartova, L., Janciak, I., Wilbacher, I., et al. (2007) Severe traumatic brain injury in Austria III: Prehospital status and treatment. Wiener Klinische Wochenschrift. *The Middle European Journal of Medicine*, 119 (1–2), 35–45.

Leon-Carrion, J., Domingues-Morales, M.R. and Martin, J.M. (2005) Driving with cognitive deficits: Neurorehabilitation and legal measures are needed for driving again after severe traumatic brain injury. *Brain Injury*, 19 (3), 213–219.

Levy, A.S., Hawkes, A.P. and Rossi, G.V. (2007) Helmets for skiers and snowboarders: an injury prevention program. *Health Promotion Practice*, 8 (3), 257–265.

Lewine, J.D., Davis, J.T. Sloan, J.H., et al. (1999) Neuromagnetic assessment of pathophysiologic brain activity induced by minor head trauma. *American Journal of Neuroradiology*, 20 (5), 857–866.

Lippert-Grüner, M.L. and Terhaag, D. (2000) Multimodal early onset stimulation (MEOS) in rehabilitation after brain injury. *Brain Injury*, 14 (6), 585–594.

Lippert-Grüner, M., Wedekind, C., Ernestus, R.I. and Klug, N. (2002a) Early rehabilitative concepts in therapy of the comatose brain injured patients. *Acta Neurochirurgica Supplementum*, 79, 21–23.

Lippert-Grüner, M., Wedekind, C. and Klug, N. (2002b) Functional and psychosocial outcome one year after severe traumatic brain injury and early–onset rehabilitation therapy. *Journal of Rehabilitation Medicine*, 34 (5), 211–214.

Lippi, G. and Mattiuzzi, C. (2004) Mandatory wearing of helmets for elite cyclists: New perspectives in prevention of head injuries. *British Journal of Sports Medicine*, 38 (3), 364.

Liu, B.C., Ivers, R., Norton, R., Boufous, S., et al. (2009) *Helmets for preventing injury in motorcycle riders (Review)*. The Cochrane Collaboration. John Wiley & Sons, Ltd, London.

Lombardi, F., Tarrico, M., De Tanti, A., Telaro, E. and Liberati, A. (2002) Sensory stimulation of brain–injured individuals in coma or vegetative state. Results of a Cochrane systematic review. *Clinical Rehabilitation*, 16 (5), 464–472.

Lowenstein, D.H. (2009) Epilepsy after head injury: An overview. *Epilepsia*, 50 (Suppl 2), 4–9.

Lundsgaard, J. (2005) *Consumer direction and choice in long–term care for older persons including payments for informal care: How can it help improve care outcomes, employment and fiscal sustainability?* OECD, Paris.

Maas, A.I.R., Stocchetti, N. and Bullock, R. (2008) Moderate and severe traumatic brain injury in adults (Review). *The Lancet Neurology*, 7 (8), 728–741.

Macan, J., Bundalo-Vrbanac, D. and Romić, G. (2006) Effects of the new karate rules on the incidence and distribution of injuries. *British Journal of Sports Medicine*, 40 (4), 326–330.

Mahoney, F.I. and Barthel, D.W. (1965) Functional evaluation: The Barthel index. *Maryland State Medical Journal*, 14, 61–65.

Malec, J.F. and Basford, J.S. (1996) Postacute brain injury rehabilitation. *Archives of Physical Medicine and Rehabilitation*, 77 (2), 198–207.

Mallonee, S., Shariat, S., Stennies, G., et al. (1996) Physical injuries and fatalities resulting from the Oklahoma City bombing. *The Journal of the American Medical Association*, 276 (5), 382–387.

Manthorpe, J., Stevens, M., Rapaport, J., et al. (2009) Safeguarding and system change: Early perceptions of the implications for adult protection services of the English individual budgets pilots – A quantitative study. *British Journal of Social Work*, 39 (8), 1465–1480.

Maslow, A.H. (1968) *Toward a psychology of being*, 2nd edn. Van Nostrand Reinhold, New York.

Mathias, J.L. and Wheaton, P. (2007) Changes in attention and information processing speed following severe traumatic brain injury: A meta-analytic review. *Neuropsychology*, 21 (2), 212–223.

Mathiowetz, V. and Haugen J.B. (1994) Motor behavior research: Implications for therapeutic approaches to central nervous system dysfunction. *American Journal of Occupational Therapy*, 48 (8), 733–745.

Mauritz, W., Wilbacher, I., Majdan, M., et al. (2008) Epidemiology, treatment and outcome of patients after severe traumatic brain injury in European regions with different economic status. *The European Journal of Public Health*, 18 (6), 575–580.

Mayoclinic.com (2012) *Answers* [Online]. Available at: www.mayoclinic.com (accessed 24 September 2012).

Mayrose, J. (2008) The effects of a mandatory motorcycle helmet law on helmet use and injury patterns among motorcyclist fatalities. *Journal of Safety Research*, 39 (4), 429–432.

McAllister, T.W., Sparling, M.B., Flashman, L.A., et al. (2001) Differential working memory load effects after mild traumatic brain injury. *Neuroimage*, 14 (5), 1004–1012.

McBeth, P.B., Ball, C.G., Mulloy, R.H. and Kirkpatrick, A.W. (2009) Alpine ski and snowboarding traumatic injuries: incidence, injury patterns, and risk factors for 10 years. *The American Journal of Surgery*, 197 (5), 560–564.

McCabe, P., Lippert, C., Weiser, M., et al. (2007) Community reintegration following acquired brain injury. Brain *Injury*, 21 (2), 231–257.

McCrory, P. (2002a) The role of helmets in skiing and snowboarding. *British Journal of Sports Medicine*, 36 (5), 314.

McCrory, P. (2002b) Boxing and the brain. *British Journal of Sports Medicine*, 36 (1), 2.

McIntosh, A.S., McCrory, P., Finch, C.F., et al. (2009) Does padded headgear prevent head injury in rugby union football? *Medicine & Science in Sports & Exercise*, 41 (2), 306–313.

Medical Research Council (1981) *Aids to the examination of the peripheral nervous system, Memorandum no. 45.* The Stationery Office, London,

Medicinenet.com (2012) *Home* [Online]. Available at: www.medicinenet.com (accessed 24 September 2012).

*Mental Capacity Act 2005: Elizabeth II.* (2005) TSO, London.

Meyer, M.J., Megyesi, J., Meythaler, J., et al. (2010) Acute management of acquired brain injury part I: An evidence–based review of non–pharmacological interventions. *Brain Injury*, 24 (5), 694–705.

Miller, F.G. and Truog, R.D. (2009) The incoherence of determining death by neurological criteria: A commentary on controversies in the determination of death, a white paper by the President's Council on Bioethics. *Kennedy Institute of Ethics Journal*, 19 (2), 185–193.

Misra, U., Kalita, J., Pandey, S. and Mandal, S.K. (2003) Predictors of gastrointestinal bleeding in acute intracerebral haemorrhage. *Journal of the Neurological Sciences*, 208 (1–2), 25–29.

Mitchell, W. and Glendinning, C. (2008) Risk and adult social care: What does UK research evidence tell us? *Health, Risk and Society*, 10 (3), 279–315.

Mitchell, A.J., Kemp, S., Benito-León, J. and Reuber, M. (2010) The influence of cognitive impairment on health–related quality of life in neurological disease. Review article. *Acta Neuropsychiatrica*, 22 (1), 2–13.

Mitchell, S., Bradley, V.A., Welch, J.L. and Britton, P.G. (1990) Coma arousal procedure: A therapeutic intervention in the treatment of head injury. *Brain Injury*, 4 (3), 273–279.

Mittenberg, W. and Strauman, S. (2000) Diagnosis of mild head injury and the postconcussion syndrome. *Journal of Head Trauma Rehabilitation*, 15 (2), 783–791.

Mohr, J.D. (1990) Management of the trunk in adult hemiplegia: The Bobath concept. In: *Topics in neurology: Lesson 1*, American Physical Therapy Association in Touch Series, pp. 1–12.

Moppet, I.K. (2007) Traumatic brain injury: Assessment, resuscitation and early management. *British Journal of Anaesthesia*, 99 (1), 18–31.

Moran, N. (2006) *Early experiences of implementing individual budgets*. Social Policy Research Unit, University of York, York.

Morrell, R.F., Merbitz, C.T., Jain, S. and Jain, S. (1998) Traumatic Brain Injury in Prisoners. *Journal of Offender Rehabilitation*, 27 (3–4), 1–8.

Mortenson, P.A. and Eng, J.J. (2003) The use of casts in the management of joint mobility and hypertonia following brain injury in adults: A systematic review. *Physical Therapy*, 83 (7), 648–658.

Mountain, D. and Shah, P. (2008) Recovery and the medical model. *Advances in Psychiatric Treatment*, 14, 241–244.

MRC CRASH trial collaborators (2008) Predicting outcome after traumatic brain injury: Practical prognostic models based on large cohort of international patients. *British Medical Journal*, 336 (7641), 425–429.

Müller-Staub, M., Needham, I., Odenbreit, M., et al. (2008) Implementing nursing diagnostics effectively: cluster randomized trial. *Journal of Advanced Nursing* 63 (3), 291–301.

Müller-Staub, M., Needham, I., Odenbreit, M., et al. (2007) Improved Quality of Nursing Documentation: Results of a Nursing Diagnoses, Interventions, and Outcomes Implementation Study. *International Journal of Nursing Terminologies and Classifications*, 18 (1), 5–17.

Murray, G.D., Butcher, I., McHugh, G.S., et al. (2007) Multivariable prognostic analysis in traumatic brain injury: Results from the IMPACT study. *Journal of Neurotrauma*, 24 (2), 329–337.

Muzumdar, D., Jhawar, S. and Goel, A. (2010) *Brain abscess: An overview. International Journal of Surgery*, 9 (2), 136–144.

Myers, J.E. and Sweeney, T.J. (2004) The indivisible self: An Evidence-based model of wellness. *Journal of Individual Psychology*, 60 (3), 234–245.

Myers, J.E. and Sweeney, T.J. (2008) Wellness Counseling: The evidence base for practice. *Journal of Counseling and Development*, 86, 482–493.

Myers, J.E., Sweeney, T.J. and Witmer, M. (2000) Counseling for wellness: A holistic model for treatment planning. *Journal of Counseling and Development*. 78 (3), 251–266.

Nair, M. and Peate, I. (eds) (2009) *Fundamentals of applied pathophysiology: An essential guide for nursing students*. John Wiley and Sons, Chichester, West Sussex.

Nakamura, N., Yamaura, A., Shigemori, J.O., et al. (2002) Epidemiology, prevention and countermeasures against severe traumatic brain injury in Japan and abroad. *Neurological Research*, 24 (1), 45–53.

NANDA-I (2012) *Nursing Diagnoses: Definitions and Classification 2012–2014*. Wiley-Blackwell, Des Moines, IA.

National Health Service Institute of Innovation and Improvement (2011a) *QIPP standards* [Online]. Available at: http://www.improvement.nhs.uk/qipp/ (accessed 24 September 2012).

National Health Service Institute of Innovation and Improvement (2011b) *High Impact Actions* [Online]. Available at: http://www.institute.nhs.uk/building_capability/general/aims/ (accessed 24 September 2012).

National Leadership and Innovation Agency for Healthcare (NLIAH) (2008) *Passing the baton: A practical guide to effective discharge planning* [Online]. Available at: http://www.wales.nhs.uk/sitesplus/829/page/36467 (accessed 24 September 2012)

Neil-Dwyer, G. and Lang, D.A. (1997) 'Brain attack' – Aneurysmal subarachnoid haemorrhage: Death due to delayed diagnosis. *Journal of the Royal College of Physicians of London*, 31 (1), 49–52.

Nell, V. and Brown, D.S.O. (1991) Epidemiology of traumatic brain injury in Johannesburg-- II. Morbidity, mortality and etiology. *Social Science & Medicine*, 33 (3), 289–296.

*NHS and Community Care Act 1990: Elizabeth II*. Chapter 19 (1990) London: The Stationery Office.

References 327

NHS Choices (2010) *Brain abscess* [Online]. Available at: http://www.nhs.uk/Conditions/Brain–abscess/Pages/Introduction.aspx (25 March 2012).

NICE (2003) *Head injury: Triage, assessment, investigation and early management of head injury in infants, children and adults. NICE Clinical Guideline 4*. NICE, London.

NICE (2007) *Head injury: Triage, assessment, investigation and early management of head injury in infants, children and adults. NICE Clinical Guideline 56* [Online]. Available at: http://www.nice.org.uk/guidance/CG56/NICEGuidance (accessed 24 September 2012).

Nicholson, T.R.J., Cutter, W. and Hotopf, M. (2008) Assessing mental capacity: The Mental Capacity Act. *British Medical Journal*, 336 (7639), 322–325.

Nickson, C. (2010) *Safe driving in Europe. Worldwide BAC limits* [Online]. Available at: http://www.safetravel.co.uk/europedrinkdrivinglimits.html (accessed 24 September 2012).

NMC (2006) *Standards of proficiency for nurse and midwife prescribers*. NMC, London.

Norton, D., McLaren, R. and Exton–Smith, A.N. (2002) An investigation of geriatric nursing problems. In: Rafferty, A.M. and Traynor, M. (eds) *Exemplary research for nursing and midwifery*. Routledge, London, pp. 69–99.

Norwood, S., Berne, J., Rowe, S., et al. (2008) Early venous thromboembolism prophylaxis with enoxaparin in patients with blunt traumatic brain injury. *Journal of Trauma*, 65 (5), 1021–1027.

Novack, T.A., Bush, B.A., Meythaler, J.M. and Canupp, K. (2001) Outcome after traumatic brain injury: Pathway analysis of contributions from premorbid, injury severity, and recovery variables. *Archives of Physical Medicine and Rehabilitation*, 82 (3), 300–305.

Nursing and Midwifery Council (2008) *The NMC code of professional conduct: Standards for conduct, performance and ethics* [Online]. Available at: http://www.nmc–uk.org/ (20 November 2011).

Nyein, K., Turner-Stokes, L. and Robinson, I. (1999) The Northwick Park Care Needs Assessment (NPCNA): A measure of community care needs: Sensitivity to change during rehabilitation. *Clinical Rehabilitation*, 13 (6), 482–491.

O'Brien, L. (2007) Achieving a successful and sustainable return to the workforce after ABI: A client–centred approach. *Brain Injury*, 21 (5), 465–478.

Oddo, M., Levine, J., Frangos, S., et al. (2009) Effect of mannitol and hypertonic saline on cerebral oxygenation in patients with severe traumatic brain injury and refractory intracranial hypertension. *Journal of Neurology, Neurosurgery and Psychiatry*, 80 (8), 916–920.

Office of the Surgeon General (US) and Office on Disability (US) (2005) *The Surgeon General's call to action to improve the health and wellness of persons with disabilities*. Office of the Surgeon General, Rockville, Maryland.

Orem, D.E. (1983) *The self-care deficit theory of nursing: A general theory*. In: Clements, I.W. and Roberts, F.B. (eds) *Family health: A theoretical approach to nursing care*. John Wiley & Sons, New York, pp. 205–217.

Ouellet, M.C., Savard, J. and Morin, C.M. (2004) Insomnia following traumatic brain injury: A review. *Neurorehabilitation Neural Repair*, 18 (4), 187–98.

Pagulayan, K.F., Hoffman, J.M., Temkin, N.R., et al. (2008) Functional limitations and depression after traumatic brain injury: examination of the temporal relationship. *Archives of Physical Medicine and Rehabilitation*, 89 (10), 1887–1892.

Palmer, J.D. (1998) The epidemiology of head injuries. *Current Medical Literature: Neurology and Neurosurgery*, 14 (2), 31–36.

Patel, H.C., Menon, D.K., Tebbs, S., et al. (2002) Specialist neurocritical care and outcome from head injury. *Intensive Care Medicine*, 28 (5), 547–553.

Peek-Asa, C., McArthur, D., Hovda, D. and Kraus, J. (2001) Early predictors of mortality in penetrating compared with closed brain injury. *Brain Injury*, 15 (9), 801–810.

Perel, P., Roberts, I., Bouamra, O., Woodford, M., et al. (2009) Intracranial bleeding in patients with traumatic brain injury: A prognostic study. *BMC Emergency Medicine*, 3 (9), 15–22.

Perna, R.B. and Geller, S.E. (2000) Understanding postconcussion syndrome. *Journal of Cognitive Rehabilitation*, 18 (1), 12–15.

Pickard, J., Seeley, H.M., Kirker, S., et al. (2004) Mapping rehabilitation resources for head injury. *Journal of the Royal Society of Medicine*, 97, 384–389.

Plant, R. (1998) Theoretical basis of treatment concepts. In: Stokes, M. (ed.) *Neurological physiotherapy*. Mosby International Limited, London, pp. 271–286.

Pohl, M., Mehrholz, J. and Rückriem, S. (2003) The influence of illness duration and level of consciousness on the treatment effect and complication rate of serial casting in patients with severe cerebral spasticity. *Clinical Rehabilitation*, 17 (4), 373–379.

Pope John Paul II (2004) *Life sustaining treatments and vegetative state: Scientific advances and ethical dilemmas* [Address of John Paul II to the participants in the international congress]. 20 March. Available at: http://www.vatican.va/holy_father/john_paul_ii/speeches/2004/march/documents/hf_jp–ii_spe_20040320_congress–fiamc_en.html (accessed 24 September 2012).

Pope, P.M. (2002) Posture management and special seating. In: Edwards, S. (ed.) *Neurological physiotherapy. A problem–solving approach*, 2nd edn. Churchill Livingstone, London, pp. 135–160.

Post, M., Visser-Meily, J. and Gispen, L. (2002) Measuring nursing needs of stroke patients in clinical rehabilitation: A comparison of validity and sensitivity to change between the Northwich Park dependency score and the Barthel Index. *Clinical Rehabilitation*, 16 (2), 182–189.

Powell, J.L. (2005) Aging and family policy in the UK. *Journal of Sociology and Social Welfare*, 32 (2), 63–75.

Powell, J.L. (2009) From 'Trust Society' to the 'Risk Society'? The case of aging and welfare in Europe'. *Hallym International Journal of Aging*, 11 (1), 65–76.

Powell, J.L. and Gilbert, T. (2011) Personalisation and sustainable care. *Journal of Care Services Management*, 5 (2), 79–86.

Prime Minister's Strategy Unit (2005) *Improving the life chances of disabled people*. Prime Minister's Strategy Unit, London.

Pryor, J. (2002) Rehabilitation nursing: A core nursing function across all settings. *Collegian*, 9 (2), 11–15.

Rabiee, P. and Moran, N. (2006) *Interviews with early individual budget holders*. Social Policy Research Unit, York.

Rassovsky, Y., Satz, P., Alfano, M.S., et al. (2006) Functional outcome in TBI II: verbal memory and information processing speed mediators. *Journal Clinical Experimental Neuropsychology*, 28 (4), 581–591.

Reid-Arndt, S.A., Nehl, C. and Hinkebein, J. (2007) The Frontal Systems Behaviour Scale (FrSBe) as a predictor of community integration following a traumatic brain injury. *Brain Injury*, 21 (13–14), 1361–9.

Reiff, D., Haricharan, R., Bullington, N., et al. (2009) Traumatic brain injury is associated with the development of deep vein thrombosis independent of pharmacological prophylaxis. *Journal of Trauma*, 66 (5), 1436–1440.

Reynolds, F.D., Dietz, P.A., Higgins, D. and Whitaker, T.S. (2003) Time to deterioration of the elderly, anticoagulated, minor head injury patient who presents without evidence of neurologic abnormality. *The Journal of Trauma*, 54 (3), 492–496.

Rice-Oxley, M. and Turner-Stokes, L. (1999) Effectiveness of brain injury rehabilitation. *Clinical Rehabilitation*, 13 (Suppl. 1), 7–24.

Richardson, D.L. (1991) The use of the tilt table to effect passive tendo–achilles stretch in a patient with head injury. *Physiotherapy Theory and Practice*, 7, 45–50.

Richmond, R., Aldaghlas, T.A., Burke, C., et al. (2011) Age: Is it all in the head? Factors influencing mortality in elderly patients with head injuries. *The Journal of Trauma*, 71 (1), E8–E11.

Rivara, F.P. (2008) Evaluating the effect of an injury prevention intervention in a population. *American Journal of Preventative Medicine*, 34 (4), S148–152.

Rivara, F.P. and Sattin, R.W. (2011) Preventing bicycle-related injuries: next step. *Injury Prevention*, 17 (3), 215.

Road Safety Act 2006: *Elizabeth II. Chapter 49* (2006) London: The Stationery Office.

Road Safety Partnership for Gloucestershire County Council (2011) *Partnership's temporary advice signs move on* [Online]. Available at: http://roadsafety–gloucestershire.org.uk/partnerships-temporary-advice-signs-move-on (15 December 2011).

Rodriguez-Arias, D., Smith, M.J. and Lazar, N.M. (2011) Donation after circulatory death: Burying the dead donor rule. *The American Journal of Bioethics*, 11 (8), 36–43.

Roper N., Logan, W. and Tierney, A. (2000) *The Roper Logan and Tierney Model of Nursing*. Churchill Livingstone, Edinburgh.

Rosenbaum, P. and Stewart, D. (2004) The World Health Organization international classification of functioning, disability and health: A model to guide clinical thinking, practice and research in the field of cerebral palsy. *Seminars in Pediatric Neurology*, 11 (1), 5–10.

Rosso, A., Brazinova, A., Janciak, I., et al. (2007) Severe traumatic brain injuries in Austria II: Epidemiology of hospital admissions. Wiener Klinische Wochenschrift. *The Middle European Journal of Medicine*, 11 (1–2), 29–34.

Roy, C.W., Thornhill, S. and Teasdale, G.M. (2002) Identification of rehabilitation problems after head injury. *Brain Injury*, 16 (12), 1057–1063.

Royal College of Nursing (2004) *Discharge Planning. Sheet 4*. RCN, London. Available at: http://www.institute.nhs.uk/quality_and_service_improvement_tools (accessed 24 September 2012).

Royal College of Nursing (2007a) *Role of the rehabilitation nurse*. Royal College of Nursing, London.

Royal College of Nursing (2007b) *Maximising independence. The role of the nurse in supporting the rehabilitation of older people*. Royal College of Nursing, London.

Royal College of Physicians (2010) *Medical rehabilitation in 2011 and beyond. Report of a working party*. RCP, London.

Royal College of Physicians (1995) Criteria for the diagnosis of brain stem death. *Journal of the Royal College of Physicians of London*, 29, 381–382.

Royal College of Physicians and British Society of Rehabilitation Medicine (2003) *Rehabilitation following acquired brain injury. National guidelines*. Turner–Stokes, L. (ed.). Royal College of Physicians and British Society of Rehabilitation Medicine, London.

Royal College of Physicians, National Council for Palliative Care and British Society of Rehabilitation Medicine (2008) *Long-term neurological conditions: Management at the interface between neurology, rehabilitation and palliative care. Concise Guidance to Good Practice series, No 10*. Royal College of Physicians, London.

Royal College of Surgeons of England (1999) *Report of the working party on the management of patients with head injuries*. Royal College of Surgeons of England, London.

Royal College of Surgeons of England (2005) The Royal College of Surgeons of England: A position paper on the acute management of patients with head injury. *Annals of the Royal College of Surgeons of England*, 87 (5), 323–325.

Royal College of Surgeons of England (2007) *Improving your elective patient's journey*. Patient Liaison Group, Royal College of Surgeons of England, London.

Ruedl, G., Kopp, M. and Burtscher, M. (2011) The protective effects of helmets in skiers and snowboarders. *British Medical Journal*, 342 (Editorial), 394–395.

SafetyNet (2009) *Vehicle safety [Online]*. Available at: http://ec.europa.eu/transport/road_safety/specialist/knowledge/vehicle/index.htm (accessed 24 September 2012).

Salvarani, C.P., Colli, B.O and Carlotti Junior, C.G. (2009) Impact of a program for the prevention of traffic accidents in a Southern Brazilian city: A model for implementation in a developing country. *Surgical Neurology*, 72 (1), 6–14.

Samuel, M. (2008) Social care experiencing 'Its Most Important Year'. *Community Care*, 31 July 2008.

Sander, A.M., Sherer, M., Malec, J.F., et al. (2003) Preinjury emotional and family functioning in caregivers of persons with traumatic brain injury. *Rehabilitation*, 84 (2), 197–203.

Satz, P., Alfano, M.S., Light, R., et al. (1999) Persistent post-concussive syndrome: A proposed methodology and literature review to determine the effects, if any, of mild head and other bodily injury. *Journal of Clinical and Experimental Neuropsychology*, 21 (5), 620–628.

Schmit, B.D., Dewald, J.P. and Rymer, W.Z. (2000) Stretch reflex adaptation in elbow flexors with repeated passive movements in unilateral brain–injured patients. *Archives of Physical Medicine and Rehabilitation*, 81 (3), 269–278.

Schulz, M.R., Marshall, S.W., Mueller, F.O., et al. (2004) Incidence and risk factors for concussion in high school athletes, North Carolina, 1996–1999. *American Journal of Epidemiology*, 160 (10), 937–944.

Scottish Intercollegiate Guidelines Network (SIGN) (2009) *Early management of patients with a head injury* [Online]. Available at: www.sign.ac.uk (accessed 24 September 2012).

Scribd.com (2011) *Neuroglial Cells* [Online]. Available at: http://www.scribd.com/doc/187365/Neuroglial–Cells (accessed 24 September 2012).

Seeley, H.M. (2007) Developing services for head injury: obtaining data. *Health Informatics Journal*, 13 (2), 135–153.

Seeley, H.M., Maimaris, C., Hutchinson, P.J., et al. (2006) Standards for head injury management in acute hospitals: evidence from the six million population of the Eastern region. *Emergency Medicine Journal*, 23 (2), 128–132.

Seelig, J.M., Becker, D.P., Miller, J.D., et al. (1981) Traumatic acute subdural haematoma: major mortality reduction in comatose patients treated within four hours. *The New England Journal of Medicine*, 304, 1511–1518.

Semelyn, J.K., Summers, S.J. and Barnes, M.P. (1998) Aspects of caregiver distress after severe head injury. *Journal of Neurologic Rehabilitation*, 12 (2), 53–60.

Servadei, F., Verlicchi, A., Soldano, F., et al. (2002) Descriptive epidemiology of head injury in Romagna and Trentino. *Neuroepidemiology*, 21 (6), 297–304.

Sesperez, J., Wilson, S., Jalaludin, B., et al. (2001) Trauma case management and clinical pathways: Prospective evaluation of their effect on selected patient outcomes in five key trauma conditions. *The Journal of Trauma Injury, Infection, and Critical Care*, 50 (4), 643–649.

Sharpf, F.W. (2002) The European Social Model. *Journal of Common Market Studies*, 40 (4), 645–670.

Shepperd, S., McClaren, J., Phillips, C.O., et al. (2010) *Discharge planning from hospital to home (Review)*. The Cochrane Collaboration. John Wiley & Sons Ltd, London.

Simon-Rusinowitz, L.S., Bochniak, A.M., Mohoney, K.J., et al. (2000) Implementation issues for consumer–directed programs: A survey of policy experts. *Generations*, 24 (1), 34–40.

Simon-Rusinowitz, L.S., Marks, L.N., Loughlin, S.M., et al. (2002) Implementation issues for consumer–directed programs: Comparing views of policy experts, consumers and representatives. *Journal of Aging and Social Policy*, 14 (3/4), 95–118.

Singer, B.J., Jegasothy, G.M., Singer, K.P. and Allison, G.T. (2003) Evaluation of serial casting to correct equinovarus deformity of the ankle after acquired brain injury in adults. *Archives of Physical Medicine and Rehabilitation*, 84 (4), 483–491.

Singh, R., Venkateshwara, G., Kirkland, J., et al. (2012) Clinical pathways in head injury: Improving the quality of care with early rehabilitation. *Disability and Rehabilitation*, 34 (5), 439–442.

Skills for Health (2011) *Skills for health: Developing a better skilled, more productive workforce*. Available at: www.skillsforhealth.org.uk (accessed 24 September 2012).

Skole, K., Deshpande, N. and Licht, H. (2007) *Gastrointestinal bleeding in a woman with head trauma* [Online]. Available at: http://www.hcplive.com/publications/Resident-and-Staff/2007/2007-10/2007-10_03 (25 January 2012).

Slaughter, B., Fann, J.R. and Ehde, D. (2003) Traumatic brain injury in a county jail population: Prevalence, neuropsychological functioning and psychiatric disorders. *Brain Injury*, 17 (9), 731–741.

Smith, D., Meaney, D. and Shull, W. (2003) Diffuse axonal injury in head trauma. *Journal of Head Trauma Rehabilitation*, 18 (4), 307–316.

Social Care Institute for Excellence/Putting People First (SCIE) (2011) *Think Personal Act Local: A sector wide commitment to moving forward with personalisation and community based support*. SCIE, London.

Spotlight (2010) Palliative care beyond cancer. *British Medical Journal*, 341, 643–662.

Stanley, D., Gilbert, A. and Penhale, B. (2011) *Phase III: Financial abuse of older adults in England: A policy analysis perspective. Detecting and preventing financial abuse of older adults*. NDA project, Uxbridge.

Steudel, W.I., Cortbus, F. and Schwerdtfeger, K. (2005) Epidemiology and prevention of fatal head injuries in Germany – trends and the impact of the reunification. *Acta Neurochirurgica*, 147 (3), 231–242.

Strucken, M.A., Clark, A.N., Sander, A.M., et al. (2008) Relation of executive function and social communication measures to functional outcomes following traumatic brain injury. *NeuroRehabilitation*, 23 (2), 185–198.

Stucki, G., Stier–Jarmer, M., Grill, E. and Melvin, J. (2005) Rationale and principles of early rehabilitation care after an acute injury or illness. *Disability and Rehabilitation*, 27 (7–8), 353–359.

Sulheim, S., Holme, I., Ekeland, A. and Bahr, R. (2006) Helmet use and risk of head injuries in alpine skiers and snowboarders. *The Journal of the American Medical Association*, 295 (8), 919–924.

Susman, M., Di Russo, S.M., Sullivan, T., et al. (2002) Traumatic Brain Injury in the elderly: increased mortality and worse functional outcome at discharge despite lower injury severity. *The Journal of Trauma*, 53 (2), 219–224.

Swenson, R. (2006) *Limbic System* [Online]. Available at: http://www.dartmouth.edu/~rswenson/Neurosci/chapter_9.html (accessed 24 September 2012).

Tagliaferri, F., Compagnone, C., Korsic, M., et al. (2006) A systematic review of brain injury epidemiology in Europe. *Acta Neurochirurgica (Wien)*, 148 (3), 255–268.

Tanriverdi, F., Senyurek, H., Unluhizarci, K., et al. (2006) High risk of hypopituitarism after traumatic brain injury: A prospective investigation of anterior pituitary function in the acute phase and 12 months after trauma. *Journal of Clinical Endocrinology & Metabolism*, 91 (6), 2105–2111.

Teasdale, G. and Jennett, B. (1974) Assessment of coma and impaired consciousness. A practical scale. *Lancet*, 2 (7872), 81–84.

Tennant, A. (2005) Admission to hospital following head injury in England: Incidence and socio–economic associations. *BMC Public Health*, 5, 21.

The Neurological Alliance. (2003) *Neuro numbers: A brief review of the numbers of people in the UK with a neurological condition*. Neurological Alliance.

The SAFE study investigators. (2007) Saline or albumin for fluid resuscitation in patients with traumatic brain injury. *The New England Journal of Medicine*, 357, 874–884.

Thompson, H.J. and Mauk, K. (2011) *Care of the patient with mild traumatic brain injury*. American Association of Neuroscience Nurses and American Association of Rehabilitation Nurses, USA.

Thorn, S. (2000) Neurological rehabilitation nursing: A review of the research. *Journal of Advanced Nursing*, 31 (5), 1029–1038.

Thornhill, S., Teasdale, G.M., Murray, G.D., et al. (2000) Disability in young people and adults one year after head injury: Prospective cohort study. *British Medical Journal*, 320 (7250), 1631–1635.

Thurman, D.J. and Guerrero, J. (1999) Trends in Hospitalization Associated With Traumatic Brain Injury. *The Journal of the American Medical Association*, 282 (10), 954–957.

Thurman, D.J., Branche, C.M., Sniezek, J.E. (1998) The epidemiology of sports–related traumatic brain injuries in the United States: Recent developments. *Journal of Head Trauma Rehabilitation*, 13 (2), 1–8.

Tortora, G.J. and Derrickson, B.H. (2011b) *Principle of anatomy and physiology. Maintenance and continuity of the human body. Volume 2*. 13th edn. John Wiley and Sons Inc., Asia.

TraumaticBrainInjury.Com (2011) *Traumatic Brain Injury* [Online]. Available at: http://traumaticbraininjury.com/ (accessed 24 September 2012).

Travis, J.W. (2011) *Wellness Education: A new model for health* [Online]. Available at: http://www.thewellspring.com/flex/the-wellness-paradigm/1951/wellness-education-a-new-model-for-health.cfm (accessed 24 September 2012).

Travis, J.W. and Ryan, R.S. (2004) *Wellness workbook: How to achieve enduring health and vitality* (3rd edn.). Celestial Arts, Berkeley, CA.

Treacy, P.J., Reilly, P. and Brophy, B. (2005) Emergency neurosurgery by general surgeons at a remote major hospital. *ANZ Journal of Surgery*, 75 (10), 852–857.

Trivedi, M. and Coles, J.P. (2009) Blood pressure management in acute head injury. *Journal of Intensive Care Medicine*, 24 (2), 96–107.

Tsang, K.K. and Whitfield, P.C. (2011) Traumatic brain injury: review of current management strategies. *British Journal of Oral and Maxillofacial Surgery*, 50 (4), 298–308.

Tseng, J.H. and Tseng, M.Y. (2006) Brain abscess in 142 patients: Factors influencing outcome and mortality. *Surgical Neurology*, 65 (6), 557–562.

Turner-Stokes, L. (2007) Developing casemix classifications for rehabilitation in the UK. *BMC Health Services Research*, 7 (1), A4.

Turner-Stokes, L. (2004) The evidence for the cost–effectiveness of rehabilitation following acquired brain injury. *Clinical Medicine*, 4 (1), 10–12.

Turner-Stokes, L., Hassan, N., Pierce, K. and Clegg, F. (2002) Managing depression in brain injury rehabilitation: the use of an integrated care pathway and preliminary report of response to sertraline. *Clinical Rehabilitation*, 16 (3), 261–268.

Turner-Stokes, L., Nyein, K. and Haliwell, D. (1999a) The Northwick Park Care Needs Assessment (NPCNA): A directly costable outcome measure in rehabilitation. *Clinical Rehabilitation*, 13, 253–267.

Turner-Stokes, L., Nyein, K., Turner-Stokes, T. and Gatehouse, C. (1999b) The UKFIM+FAM: Development and evaluation. Functional Assessment Measure. *Clinical Rehabilitation*, 13 (4), 277–287.

Turner-Stokes, L., Paul, S. and Williams, H. (2006) Efficiency of specialist rehabilitation in reducing dependency and costs of continuing care for adults with complex acquired brain injuries. *Journal of Neurology, Neurosurgery and Psychiatry*, 77, 634–639.

Turner-Stokes, L., Sykes, N. and Silber, E. (2008) Long-term neurological conditions: Management at the interface between neurology, rehabilitation and palliative care. *Clinical Medicine*, 8 (2), 186–191.

Turner-Stokes, L., Tonge, P., Nyein, K., et al. (1998) The Northwick Park Dependency Score (NPDS): A measure of nursing dependency in rehabilitation. *Clinical Rehabilitation*, 12, 304–318.

Turner-Stokes, L., Williams, H. and Siegert, R.J. (2010) The rehabilitation complexity scale version 2: A clinimetric evaluation in patients with severe complex neurodisability. *Journal of Neurology, Neurosurgery and Psychiatry*, 81, 146–153.

UKTransplant (No Date) *Become a donor* [Online]. Available at: https://www.organdonation.nhs.uk/ukt/how_to_become_a_donor/questions/answers/answers_3.asp#q7 (accessed 24 September 2012).

United Kingdom Acquired Brain Injury Forum (UKABIF) (2004) *Mapping survey of social service provision for adults aged 16 years and over with acquired brain injury and their carers in England.* UKABIF, London.

Ungerson, C. and Yeandle, S. (eds) (2006) *Cash for care in developed welfare states.* Palgrave Macmillan, Basingstoke.

United States of America. Department of Health and Human Services (1998) *National Institutes of Health. Office of the Director.* Rehabilitation of persons with Traumatic Brain Injury: NIH Consensus Statement. October 26–28. Bethesda, Md: National Institutes of Health, 16 (1), 1–41.

Urban, R.J., Harris, P. and Masel, B. (2005) Anterior hypopituitarism following traumatic brain injury. *Brain Injury*, 19 (5), 349–358.

Urbenjaphol, P., Jitpanya, C. and Khaoropthum, S. (2009) Effects of the sensory stimulation program on recovery in unconscious patients with traumatic brain injury. *Journal of Neuroscience Nursing*, 41 (3), E10–E16.

Vakil, E. (2005) The effects of moderate to severe traumatic brain injury (TBI) on different aspects of memory: A selective review. *Journal of Clinical and Experimental Neuropsychology*, 27 (8), 977–1021.

Valadka, A.B., Gopinath, A.P. and Robertson, C.S. (2000) Midline shift after severe head injury: Pathophysiologic implications. *Journal of Trauma*, 49 (1), 1–10.

Vanier, M., Lamoureux, J., Dutil, E. and Houde, S. (2002) Clinical Efficacy of stimulation programs aimed at reversing coma or vegetative state (VS) following traumatic brain injury. Review. *Acta Neurochirurgica Supplementum*, 79, 53–57.

Vazuka, F.A. (1962) *Essentials of the neurological examination.* Smith Kline and French Laboratories, Philadelphia.

Verplanke, D., Snape, S., Salisbury, C.F., et al. (2005) A randomised controlled trial of botulinum toxin on lower limb spascitiy following acute acquired severe brain injury. *Clinical Rehabilitation*, 19 (2), 117–125.

Vetruba, K.L., Rapport, L.J., Vangel, S.R. Jr., et al. (2008) Impulsivity and traumatic brain injury: The relations among behavioral observation, performance measures and rating scales. *Journal of Head Trauma Rehabilitation*, 23 (2), 65–73.

Vitaz, T.W., McIlvoy, L., Raque, G.H., et al. (2001) Development and implementation of a clinical pathway for severe brain injury. *The Journal of Trauma Injury, Infection, and Critical Care*, 51, 369–375.

Wade, D. (2011) Complexity, case-mix and rehabilitation: The importance of the holistic model of illness. *Clinical Rehabilitation*, 25 (5), 387–395.

Wade, D.T. (2005) Describing rehabilitation interventions. *Clinical Rehabilitation*, 19 (8), 811–818.

Wade, D.T. and Collin, C. (1988) The Barthel ADL index: A standard measure of physical disability? *International Disability Studies*, 10 (2), 64–67.

Wade, D.T. and De Jong, D.A. (2000) Recent advances in rehabilitation. *British Medical Journal*, 320 (7246), 1385–1388.

Wade, D.T., King, N.S., Wenden, F.J., et al. (1998) Routine follow up after head injury: A second randomised controlled trial. *Journal of Neurology, Neurosurgery and Psychiatry*, 65 (2), 177–183.

Waters, K.R. and Luker, K.A. (1996) Staff perspectives on the role of the nurse in rehabilitation wards for elderly people. *Journal of Clinical Nursing*, 5 (2), 105–114

Webb, A.C. and Samuels, O.B. (2011) Reversible brain death after cardiopulmonary arrest and induced hypothermia. *Critical Care Medicine*, 39 (6), 1538–1542.

Weinstein, C.S., Seidman, L.J., Ahern, G. and McClure, K. (1994) Integration of neuropsychological and behavioral neurological assessment in psychiatry: A case example involving brain injury and polypharmacy. *Psychiatry: Interpersonal and Biological Processes*, 57 (1), 62–76.

Wenden, F.J., Crawford, S., Wade, D.T., et al. (1998) Assault, post–traumatic amnesia and other variables related to outcome following head injury. *Clinical Rehabilitation*, 12 (1), 53–63.

Westerberg, H. and Klingberg, T. (2007) Changes in cortical activity after training of working memory: A single-subject analysis. *Physiology and Behaviour*, 92 (1–2), 186–192.

Whyte, J., Cifu, D., Dikmen, S. and Temkin, N. (2001) Prediction of functional outcomes after traumatic brain injury: A comparison of 2 measures of duration of unconsciousness. *Archives of Physical Medicine and Rehabilitation*, 82 (10), 1355–1359.

Wiener, J., Tilly, J. and Cuellar, A.E. (2003) *Consumer-directed home care in the Netherlands, England and Germany.* AARP Public Policy Institute, Washington DC.

Wilberger, J.E., Harris, M. and Diamond, D.L. (1991) Acute subdural haematoma: morbidity, mortality and operative timing. *Journal of Neurosurgery*, 74 (2), 212–218.

Wilde, E.A., McCauley, S.R., Kelly, et al. (2010) Feasibility of the neurological outcome scale for traumatic brain injury (NOS-TBI) in adults. *Journal of Neurotrauma*, 27 (6), 975–981.

Wijdicks, E.F.M., Varelas, P.N., Gronseth, G.S. and Greer, D.M. (2010) Evidence-based guideline update: Determining brain death in adults. Report of the quality standards subcommittee of the American Academy of Neurology. *Neurology*, 74 (23), 1911–1918.

Williams, H., Harris, R. and Turner-Stokes, L. (2007) Can the Northwick Park Care Needs Assessment be used to estimate nursing staff requirements in an in-patient setting? *Clinical Rehabilitation*, 21 (6), 535–544.

Williams, P.E. (1990) Use of intermittent stretch in the prevention of serial sarcomere loss in immobilised muscles. *Annals of the Rheumatic Diseases*, 49 (5), 316–317.

Williams, W.H., Mewse, A.J., Tonks, J., et al. (2010) Traumatic brain injury in a prison population: Prevalence and risk for re-offending. *Brain Injury*, 24 (10), 1184–1188.

Wilson, B. (2008) Neuropsychological rehabilitation. *Annual Review of Clinical Psychology*, 4, 141–162.

Wilson, B.A., Gracey, F., Evans, J.J. and Bateman, A. (2009) *Neuropsychological rehabilitation: Theory, models, therapy and outcome*. Cambridge University Press, UK.

Witmer, J.M., Sweeney, T.J. and Myers, J.E. (1998) *The wheel of wellness*. Authors, Greensboro, N.C.

Woertgen, C., Rothoerl, R.D., Schebesch, K.M. and Albert, R. (2006) Comparison of craniotomy and craniectomy in patients with acute subdural haematoma. *Journal of Clinical Neuroscience*, 13 (7), 718–721.

Wood, L.I. and Yurdakul, L.K. (1997) Change in relationship status following traumatic brain injury. *Brain Injury*, 11 (7), 491–501.

Wood, R.L. (1991) Critical analysis of the concept of sensory stimulation for patients in vegetative states. *Brain Injury*, 5 (4), 401–409.

World Health Organization (1958) Constitution of the World Health Organization, Annex. WHO, Geneva, Switzerland.

World Health Organization (2001) *International Classification of Functioning, Disability and Health (ICF)* [Online]. Available at: http://www.who.int/classifications/icf/e?n/ (21 September 2011).

Yates, P.J., Williams, W.H., Harris, A., et al. (2006) An epidemiological study of head injuries in a UK population attending an emergency department. *Journal of Neurology, Neurosurgery and Psychiatry*, 77 (5), 699–701.

Zampolini, M., Zaccaria, B., Tolli, V., et al. (2012) Rehabilitation after traumatic brain injury in Italy: A multi-centred study. *Brain Injury*, 26 (1), 27–35.

Zeman, A. (2001) Consciousness. *Brain*, 124 (1), 1263–1289.

Zhao, Q-J., Zhang, X.G. and Wang, L.X. (2011) Mild hypothermia therapy reduces blood glucose and lactate and improves neurologic outcomes in patients with severe traumatic brain injury. *Journal of Critical Care*, 26 (3), 311–315.

Zink, B.J. (2001) Traumatic brain injury outcome: Concepts for emergency care. *Annals of Emergency Medicine*, 37 (3), 318–332.

# Index

Note: page numbers in *italic* refer to figures. Page numbers in **bold** refer to tables.

*Neurotrauma: Managing Patients with Head Injuries*, First Edition. Edited by Nadine Abelson-Mitchell.
© 2013 Blackwell Publishing Ltd. Published 2013 by Blackwell Publishing Ltd.